# Stuttering

# Stuttering

Joseph Kalinowski, Ph.D.
Tim Saltuklaroglu, Ph.D.

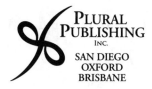

PLURAL
PUBLISHING
INC.

SAN DIEGO
OXFORD
BRISBANE

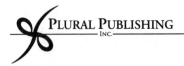

PLURAL PUBLISHING
INC.

5521 Ruffin Road
San Diego, CA 92123

e-mail: info@pluralpublishing.com
Web site: http://www.pluralpublishing.com

49 Bath Street
Abington, Oxfordshire OX14 1EA
United Kingdom

Typeset in 11/13 Palatino by Flanagan's Publishing Services, Inc.
Printed in the United States of America by McNaughton and
Gunn

ISBN-13: 978-1-59756-011-5
ISBN-10: 1-59756-011-1
**Library of Congress Control Number:** 2005908768

# Contents

# Preface

The opportunity to write a book about stuttering is a dream come true for us. We are people who stutter and having this disorder has guided our vocational paths with the ultimate goal of better serving those who stutter and contributing to the body of knowledge surrounding this enigmatic disorder or, at least, raising some worthwhile questions for debate. Writing this book has not only allowed us to share the scientific ideas arising from our body of research, but also our heartfelt feelings and experiences with stuttering, which we believe most other people who stutter will relate to, especially those who have undergone countless hours of therapy with its inherent ups and downs. Although we believe that this text is a step toward this goal, judgment of its success or failure is not for us to decide. Instead it will be judged in the natural history and progression of science, as well as by people who stutter, their families, and the clinicians who treat them.

Joseph Kalinowski, Ph.D.
Timothy Saltuklaroglu, Ph.D.

# Acknowledgments

This book is the result of a very circuitous path and would not have reached fruition without the help of numerous individuals and institutions. First and foremost, we thank Andy Stuart, an audiologist and experimental psychologist. We thank him for his tireless effort, dedication, inspired research abilities, and friendship. Back in the early 1990s Andy and the author (JK) made numerous treks to SUNY Geneseo from Dalhousie University in Halifax, Nova Scotia. While at Geneseo, they spent endless days collecting data and debating notions about speech perception. These treks led to the summer residential stuttering program at Geneseo and some fundamental ideas about stuttering that have allowed our research to flourish ever since. Although speech pathologists and audiologists usually share the same academic department, they rarely seem to collaborate. However, when they do the meshing of ideas can be highly productive and make all the difference in the world.

We would like to thank the people at Haskins Laboratories for revealing to us the power of Motor Theory (i.e., notions about speech perception). As well as being groundbreaking in the areas of speech perception and production, these ideas are critical to our notions of stuttering and we believe they can be functionally applied to make the lives of those who stutter much easier. We would especially like to thank Bruno Repp for his comments and advice over the last decade or so on a number of projects. We would be remiss not to thank others from Haskins who have helped and advised us over the years, especially when the first author (JK) was studying there. These include Michael D'Angelo, Arthur Abramson, Phil Rubin, Vince Gracco, Robin Story, and Joy Armson (also of Dalhousie University). That laboratory and its scholars shaped much of our current way of thinking and our approach to research. Whenever we called for help on a project, they always provide advice and suggestions.

The author's (JK) working relationships with Andy Stuart and Joy Armson at Dalhousie University in Halifax, Nova Scotia from 1991 to 1995 began in earnest with the first work examining the effects of altered feedback and speech rate on stuttering frequency. This working relationship was meaningful, thought-provoking, and wonderful. In 1995, the author (JK) moved to East Carolina University where Mike Rastatter was the new departmental Chair and was beginning a new doctoral research program from the ground level. Mike had already published a number of papers on stuttering and hired the author, and later Andy Stuart to come and collaborate with him at ECU. While working with Andy and Mike at ECU, the research efforts continued to expand. As well as publishing extensively together, this team created a patent for the SpeechEasy™, the first all-in-the-ear device that produces altered feedback for the purpose of helping those who stutter speak more fluently. The University supported the research and the doctoral program, bringing in students from all over the Unites States as well as Canada, Turkey, China, and India. This is how the second author (TS) came aboard in 2000. All these students have taught us wonderful things about their culture and how they view communication disorders, as well as contributing to our ideas and helping us collect data. Nothing is more exciting than unbridled youthful enthusiasm for scholarship. The students who have helped along the way include Vijaya Guntupalli, Chayadevie Nanjundeswaran; Jianliang Zhang; Kerry Lynch; Helen Glover, M.S.; Lee Thorne, M.S; Vikram Dayalu, Ph.D. at Seton Hall; Greg Snyder, Ph.D.; and Saravanan Elangovan, Ph.D.

We must also thank various other individuals who have supported our work. These include Greg Givens, Ph.D., Chair, Communication Sciences and Disorders at East Carolina University; Ms. Marti Van Scott, Technology Transfer Office at East Carolina University; Tao Jiang, Ph.D., of Micro-DSP; Darwin Richards, President, and Alan Newton, Vice President, of Janus Development Group; and Ms. Julie Richardson of Myers & Bigel.

In addition, we are grateful to the many speech pathologists who have provided us with hundreds of data points, referred patients to us, and provided feedback regarding our methods and ideas. We must also thank Allison Motluk of New Scientist magazine for mentioning mirror neurons to us. It took us a year to follow up (and a conference at Harvard on that topic), but we finally believe we have made some sense of the way in which mirror neurons may be involved in the inhibition of stuttering.

We must extend our sincere gratitude to the multitude of stuttering individuals who have allowed us to work with them, treat them and use the manifestations of their pathology to advance our research. In the last few years, since the inception of portable altered feedback devices, we have had the opportunity to treat hundreds of patients. We have learned more about the nature of stuttering, altered feedback, motoric behaviors, and synergistic stuttering inhibition from them than from any stuttering course or journal article. They were masters at telling us what worked and what did not and this book is dedicated to them.

To my wife, Barbara, and daughters, Alissa, and Amy who allow me to take them to the movies more than they want. And to my mother, Mary, and my late father Tony, whose support and selflessness to that troubled stuttering child will never be forgotton. We went through a lot!

JK

To my parents, who patiently waited for me to do things "my way" and never gave up on me.

TS

# 1

# Introduction

> *"The universe is full of magical things, patiently waiting for our wits to grow sharper."*
> —*Eden Phillpotts*

## A Changing Field

"Stuttering"—The word elicits images of a struggle to speak, anxiety, frustration, and a host of other negative behaviors and emotions associated with a breakdown in communication. Yet, how many of us can provide an accurate description of this debilitating communicative disorder, let alone know how to react to it or effectively treat it? Welcome to the study of the fascinating, complex, and often misunderstood disorder of stuttering. While many students in the field of communication disorders may know a person who stutters, may have a friend or family member who stutters, or may even stutter themselves, we suspect that, for most, this is the first time the disorder is being tackled academically. Let us begin by stating that the academic views and clinical treatment approaches to stuttering appear to be changing (Dayalu & Kalinowski, 2002). Subscribing to the contents of this book may represent a departure from some commonly held beliefs about stuttering and may contradict some notions found elsewhere. For this reason we do not wish to

1

begin in the standard manner, providing a standard definition of stuttering and then progressing to discussing some of the "facts" regarding the nature and treatment of stuttering. While a few accepted notions about stuttering do continue to survive, most of what has been previously theorized regarding its nature and treatment will be questioned and held up to scientific scrutiny. For this reason, we choose to re-examine the field of stuttering from a perspective that is most probably different from that held by the majority of other academics in this field. We will re-evaluate previously held beliefs and highlight what we consider to be novel changes in the way that stuttering is both understood and treated. We intend to provide new, alternative, logical, and compelling explanations for the behavioral, cognitive, and neurophysiologic phenomena associated with this enigmatic disorder based primarily on what we consider to be scientific and empirical research.

Why do we choose this approach to this textbook? Simply because our scientific, clinical, and personal experiences have indicated it is time for a change in the way stuttering is viewed and treated. Both authors are "stutterers" (we do not mind using this word as we are members of this group or "club," though others prefer to be referred to as "persons who stutter"). We have grown up with the disorder, we have been treated for the disorder, and we entered this field to learn more about the disorder and help others suffering from it. Though we have both been relatively successful in managing our stuttering (Kalinowski, 2003), it has not been without a price. We have endured most of the hardships that those who stutter are subjected to while growing up (which are substantial and discussed in the next chapter). We have repeatedly failed to conquer the disorder using traditional therapeutic means and have often failed to provide a remedy to others seeking help. Stated bluntly, we have been the "cheaters and the cheated" (Saltuklaroglu & Kalinowski, 2002). However, we have learned much from our research, our mistakes, and from the research and mistakes of others. We now consider ourselves lucky enough to be in the position of having garnered a better understanding than most of this strange and complex pathology. In this text, we intend to share what we have learned and we hope to provide students entering the field not only with a complete "toolbox" for treating stuttering, but also the knowledge of how best to use each tool in that box.

Typical graduate-level stuttering courses espouse the teachings of researchers who have viewed stuttering in a similar manner for the last 40 years or so. By the same token, these theoretical frameworks have taught clinicians to treat stuttering using a variety of similar methods, many of which have been somewhat effective for relieving stuttering in the short-term, yet require substantial effort and compromises to speech naturalness, but still often fail to provide long-term relief (Andrews, 1984; Boberg, 1981; Craig & Calver, 1991; Dayalu & Kalinowski, 2002; Kalinowski, Noble, Armson, & Stuart, 1994). One reason for the lack of progress in treatment is that stuttering still has no known cause and without a known cause, a cure cannot be on the immediate horizon. We are optimistic that both cause and cure for stuttering will eventually be found. Advancements in neuroimaging (brain mapping), genetic research, and neurophysiology may hold the key to uncovering the source of stuttering. These technologies may advance to the point where we will be able to understand the manner in which neurons in the brain communicate with each other, transmitting their chemical messages for the purposes of encoding and decoding speech and other complex cortical activities. As such, the underlying etiology of stuttering as well as a host of other centrally originating disorders may become readily apparent. When we are able to identify the true source of stuttering, the proverbial "pink pill" that attacks its origin is more likely to follow. However, knowledge of causation does not always imply that a cure is forthcoming. For example, the HIV virus has long been known to be the cause of AIDS, and though considerable advances have been made toward managing and controlling the effects of the virus, a cure for this tragic disease has yet to be uncovered. Thus, though we remain optimistic and are driven by our ongoing desire to help those who stutter, realistically we do not expect the miracle cure to present itself at least until we have a much better understanding of the basic neurophysiologic processes that underlie speech production and perception.

Without losing track of searching for the cure, our immediate task consists of "managing" stuttering. This means that we attempt to reduce its impact on communication to the greatest extent possible. Communication is fundamental to nearly all aspects of life. Humans are arguably the most proficient communicators on the planet, and for most people speech is a primary modality for effective and efficient communication. In this context, by stating that speech is effective for this purpose, we mean that speech adequately serves the purposes of fluent and natural-sounding communication. By stating that speech is efficient for this purpose, we mean that effective communication is accomplished as quickly as possibly with the least amount of effort expended. Needless to say, speech may be considered a "gift" that many people (especially those outside the field) take for granted. Seen from this perspective, it becomes evident how stuttering can have an impact on nearly every aspect of life. A continuous compromise to our primary mode of communication can permeate all social and vocational interactions (Hayhow, Cray & Enderby, 2002; Klein & Hood, 2004; Peters & Starkweather, 1989;), reducing the efficiency and effectiveness in the communicative process. Successful management of stuttering, then, means that the symptoms of stuttering should be suppressed sufficiently to eliminate as much as possible their negative impact on life and, hence, increase communicative efficiency and effectiveness. Considering that in today's world of advanced medicine and technology, stuttering continues to have an impact on communication and is a source of anxiety and distress to those afflicted (Kraaimaat, Vanryckeghem, & Dam-Baggen, 2002; Messenger, Onslow, Packman, & Menzies, 2004), it appears that there is still room for improvement in its treatment. Perhaps treatment has often failed because of our inability to emulate nature's own recovery mechanisms (e.g., repetitions and prolongations) as treatment modalities when the critical recovery window has passed. However, the relative lack of progress in stuttering management and the inability to produce better treatments over a long time course, as that we and others have observed, suggests some fundamental flaws in the way people view stuttering. Therefore, we suggest that it is time to adopt an alternative point of view to the nature and treatment of stuttering. Our view is that successful management of stuttering reduces its impact on communication, to the greatest extent possible by using nature's own recovery mechanisms or derivatives thereof. Exploring these natural recovery mechanisms is the focus of this book. Simply put: the goal for successful stuttering remediation becomes optimizing the effects of naturally occurring fluency-enhancing mechanisms.

Over the last 12 years or so, we have accumulated a body of research that has not only allowed, but required us to view the disorder differently from others. This alternative viewpoint appears to explain more phenomena associated with stuttering than any previously held views, and has led to new avenues for viable and effective treatment of stuttering. Namely, we view repetitions and prolongations that commonly characterize stuttering are the answer rather than the problem to the stuttering syndrome (Kalinowski et al., 2000; Kalinowski et al., 2004). Stuttering is somewhat analogous to a fever. At first, it seems intuitive that to heal, one should reduce a fever. However, science has shown that fever serves a biological purpose, allowing the body to fight infections more efficiently, and by reducing fever via medication one may prolong the diseased state. In the same vein, uncomfortable though they may be, the aberrant speech behaviors we observe when someone is stuttering may actually be natural compensations to release a block occurring in the brain and may be a necessary part of stuttering management. Thus, in sharing this information we hope to lead students down a path of science and logic to the point where they have a clear understanding of the disorder and feel comfortable providing treatment. Ultimately, we hope they are able to use the contents herein to provide the best therapeutic course for anyone afflicted with this debilitating disorder. The fact that the ideas presented here may be somewhat controversial and may dispute previously held notions should be comforting rather than intimidating as the field of stuttering can withstand some re-examination of its fundamental tenets.

## Paradigm Shifts

Let us be clear about one thing. When we state that the field is changing, we mean the way in which the disorder is being viewed in some scientific and clinical arenas is changing, such that the very definition of stuttering may vary significantly from those found in other texts. This is not the first time that the field is changing, nor will it be the last. This does not mean that the pathology itself is changing. Stuttering probably manifests and develops in the same way today as it has since the time of Demosthenes (the great Greek orator was known to stutter).

The change in orientation in the field of stuttering simply marks one step in the progression of science, through what Thomas Kuhn called a series of "Paradigm Shifts" in his seminal text *The Structure of Scientific Revolutions* (Kuhn, 1996). Scientific paradigms are viewpoints from which research is conducted and explained. When scientists believe they are in possession of a viable theoretical framework to explain a certain set of phenomena within their chosen field, they have a paradigm in which the majority of their data can be safely interpreted. Most scientists are generally content to work within their chosen paradigm and interpret their data through the accepted theories that form the foundation of that paradigm. It is not until "anomalous" data points begin to arise or strange phenomena are observed that cannot be explained within the context of a given paradigm, that the paradigm is questioned (Kuhn, 1996, p. 6). Others, who are often younger members of the scientific community and are not heavily "invested" in that particular way of thinking, generally bring about this questioning of the paradigm. Psychologic or paradigmatic investment is similar to a financial investment in that time, effort, or money are not easily compromised once there is enough on the line. Therefore, older members of a field, who have adopted a way of thinking and spent their careers propagating a particular paradigm are less likely than younger members to consider and accept alternative viewpoints.

It takes a series of anomalous events to shake a paradigm to a critical point that may likely cause a "shift." A paradigm shift begins to occur with the change in thinking that is required to explain the previously unexplainable observations (Kuhn, 1996, p. 65). Therefore, it makes sense that new paradigms generally have better "explanatory power" than the ones they supplant. However, it should be noted that paradigms do not shift quickly nor easily. Remember that many of those espousing an old paradigm are heavily invested in their beliefs. Though they may see evidence that contradicts their viewpoints, they often do not give up without a fight. In fact, it is thought by some, that for one paradigm to completely give way to another, those propagating the losing paradigm must literally die out (Kuhn, 1996, p. 151). For an example, we may look to the field of psychology, a field which has undergone numerous paradigmatic shifts. Freud's psychoanalysis was supplanted by Skinner's behaviorism, Perl's gestalt therapy, Beck's cognitive therapy, and today's psychopharmacologic cornucopia. However, even today there are practitioners who continue to treat a variety of problems by psychoanalytically attempting to uncover and resolve internal conflicts through cathartic release.

An extreme yet very well-known example of how consequential paradigm shifting can be found is in our current notions regarding the role of the earth in the solar system. Until Nicholas Copernicus' work became accepted, the earth was considered the center of the solar system and the sun revolved around the earth in a circular orbit (Kuhn, 1996, p. 67–69). The church had propagated these geocentric notions for hundreds of years, since the time of Ptolemy, the ancient Greek astronomer. Copernicus' calculations provided strong evidence that the earth was not the center of the universe. However, at the time the church was arguably the most powerful entity in Europe and its teachings were simply not questioned, let alone challenged. In the eyes of the church, Copernicus' science was reprehensible and the penalties for his interpretations were extreme. Luckily for Copernicus, he published his best work, *De Revolutionibus*, on his deathbed. Simply put, challenging a paradigm requires good science, as well as conviction, persistence, and guts. Copernicus proved convincingly that the sun was indeed the center of the solar system and all the planets revolved around the sun, advancing the paradigm of a "heliocentric" solar system to replace the previous "geocentric" paradigm. Once this paradigm had shifted and Copernicus' views became widely accepted, scientific advancement in the field of astronomy was required based on Copernicus's findings, to show evidence of a true shift in thinking. Furthermore, it was not until Kepler re-examined the work of Brahe that previously unexplained planetary behaviors began to make sense. Kepler discovered that planetary orbits are elliptical rather than circular, further advancing our understanding of planetary motion and creating another scientific leap forward in the field of astronomy.

Another example of a new paradigm may be found in the birth of quantum mechanics. It was found that the behavior of subatomic particles had different physical properties and behaved differently under various forces than larger entities (Kuhn, 1996). These differences could not be explained by conventional Newtonian physics. Consequently, this paradigm shift opened the door to a new age of physics, one that continues to push the boundaries of science and allows for the creation of ever more impressive technologic feats.

At each stage of scientific advancement (i.e., each paradigm shift), new theories supplant old ones, similar to the way that one government replaces another in a political revolution. Old political systems overstay their welcome and are replaced by what the people expect to be new systems (Kuhn, 1996, p. 92). The three most famous political revolutions are the American Revolution, the French Revolution, and the Russian Revolution, which brought Communism and created the Soviet Union. The new governments came into power, wrote new laws, developed fundamentally different economic systems, and made irrevocable changes in the conception of government, the rights of man and society, and the social contract. New paradigms come to fruition, gain power, replace old ones, and are eventually supplanted in a similar fashion. That is what happened when Lenin replaced Czar Nicholas II in the Russian revolution and what will usually happen in this "construct-destruct" phenomenon. There is no permanence in science—only shifting sands of science. When paradigms shifts occur in science, new textbooks are written and students learn according to the new paradigm (Kuhn, 1996, p. 26), often unaware of the history of scientific turmoil that was necessary to achieve the current understanding in a given field. Oftentimes, during a paradigm shift, students are subjected to more than one set of ideas and have to "pick a side." As such, the written word or rhetoric becomes important. Paradigm shifts not only depend on the strength of the science supporting them, but on the strength of the rhetoric propagating them. For a paradigm to flourish, it must be presented in a manner that is attractive enough to encourage others to want to explore it and propagate the ideas it espouses. Powerful rhetoric permeates our history books. One excellent example is Lincoln's "Gettysburg Address." This 282-word presentation at the dedication of the National Cemetery at Gettysburg resounds today with a fervor that has seldom been achieved by any other political rhetoric and gave purpose to a great calamity that befell the United States. Readers can look to Garry Wills for a brilliant analysis of "the Address" (Wills, 1992).

How does the discussion of scientific progression relate to this textbook and the field of stuttering? In its relatively short history, the field of stuttering has undergone a few paradigmatic shifts. Our definition of a paradigm is loose, in that we suggest it is the prevailing notion held my most scientists, clinicians, parents, and so forth. We note that Kuhn's (1996) explanation was restricted to the hard sciences (e.g., astronomy and physics). However, the exclusivity of paradigms to hard sciences appears to be somewhat rigid and perhaps not wholly accurate. We consider the notion of paradigms somewhat more loosely, extending it to the behavioral sciences and clinical practices emanating from these sciences. Thus, we believe that the evidence presented here is cause for a paradigmatic shift in the field of stuttering. While this text is not intended to be a history lesson in stuttering, we believe that it is important for students to have an understanding of the way in which scientists, clinicians, and persons who stutter have seen the disorder through various paradigms and how the shortcomings of past paradigms have begged for alternative avenues of research and thus helped shape our current understanding of the disorder. We believe the paradigmatic approach to the disorder to be of utmost importance. The way we see the disorder has a direct impact on the manner in which it is treated. The inadequacies of previous paradigmatic approaches are directly reflected in the apparent lack of progress in the treatment of stuttering. However, rather than be immediately discarded, past approaches should be embraced and viewed as stepping stones toward the eventual eradication of the disorder. Until a cure is found, the field of stuttering cannot rest on its laurels. Paradigm shifts founded in empirical data that push the understanding of the pathology to higher levels should always be welcomed. Thus, the rich history of research and treatment in stuttering can be put to best use by reinterpreting previous data in light of current ideas that we believe provide the best possible explanation for the bulk of research conducted in this field. Needless to say, though the ideas presented herein may reflect a changing of the guard and the most current under-standing of the disorder, the natural progression of science should ensure that these ideas may be similarly supplanted, or at least amended, to explain an ever growing corpus of knowledge.

When a paradigm changes, the phenomena that is being observed does not change, but the perspective and the ideas adopted by those studying the phenomena change. Or, as Kuhn (1996) states, "scientists see rabbits where once they saw ducks" (Kuhn, 1996. p 114), making reference to the famous duck-rabbit optical illusion. What follows is a brief history of a few theoreti-cal approaches to stuttering that have predominated over the years, followed by our attempts to clearly differentiate the rab-bits from the ducks in the field of stuttering.

## Lee Edward Travis

The work of Samuel Orton and, to a greater extent, his student Lee Edward Travis at the University of Iowa, provided one of the earliest and, arguably, one of the most influential theories of stut-tering, known as the cerebral dominance or handedness theory (Travis, 1931). Based on early findings by pioneers in neurolin-guistics such as Paul Broca and Hughlings Jackson, it was gener-ally accepted that the left cerebral hemisphere was dominant for speech and language in right-handed individuals. That is, the left cerebral hemisphere should be dominant for timing the nerve impulses associated with speech and language in those who are right-handed. However, numerous reports at the time seemed to indicate that many people with defective speech, including many who stuttered, were left-handed. This suggested that being left-handed or ambidextrous may reflect abnormal or incomplete cerebral dominance for speech and language pro-duction and may be a red flag for a communicative disorder. It may be of interest that the word "sinister," which is generally used to denote evil or threatening may also mean left-handed (from the Latin for "left").

Under these auspices, Travis explored the possibility of pre-venting stuttering by binding a limb (often by using a cast) in an effort to counteract any incomplete cerebral dominance responsible for stuttering. In fact, reports exist of Wendell Johnson and Charles Van Riper (discussed next) being part of a group of 30 or so people who stutter doing outdoor activities (e.g., playing badminton) on the Iowa campus with one hand bound in a cast (Moeller, 1975). It should also be noted that, at this time, children who displayed left-handed tendencies were often forced to switch to their right hand, possibly to prevent the onset of speech disorders such as stuttering. However, Wingate (1997) provides accounts of children beginning to stutter after switching to a non-dominant right hand and later becoming more fluent when allowed to return to using their preferred left hand. It is quite possible that the handedness exercises did not play any role in the presence or absence of stuttering. It may simply be that many of the children for whom these reports exist were simply following nature's recovery schedule, in which about 70 to 80% of children who begin to stutter naturally and spontaneously recover (Kalinowski et al., 2002; Yairi & Ambrose, 1992, 1999). Regardless, these data do not support the concept of cerebral dominance as a viable theory for the source of stuttering. Not surprisingly, though Travis' work generated a great deal of interest, it was also controversial. It could not adequately predict those who would stutter from those who would not, nor did it yield any satisfactory reduction in stuttering. Peripheral limitation of the limbs does not appear to affect dominance. Johnson and Van Riper stuttered for the rest of their lives and went on to develop their own theories and therapeutic courses as the ideas behind cerebral dominance began to wane in popularity. As for Travis himself, he left Iowa in 1938, took up numerous other positions, and his views of stuttering later became influenced by the psychodynamic approach that was beginning to gain popularity. However, since the espousal of this theory, the question of laterality and cerebral dominance has never been completely answered and has continued to provide a source of interest and speculation for researchers in the field of stuttering (e.g., Webster, 1986), especially considering technologic advances that now allow for scientists to map patterns of cerebral activation and note differences in cerebral anatomy (Foundas, Bolich, Corey, Hurley, & Heilman, 2001) and physiology (Fox et al., 1996; Fox et al., 2000; Ingham, 2001) associated with stuttering when compared to nonstuttering populations.

# Psychoanalysis

Views of stuttering have been heavily influenced by dominant psychologic paradigms. There appears to be something attractive about attempting to control an inherently involuntary disorder. The pursuit may be character-building or spiritual in nature, not unlike a 12-step meeting for managing substance abuse. Freudian psychoanalysis gained popularity in the early part of the previous century and it provided a plausible explanation for stuttering. Under this paradigm, stuttering was thought to emanate from a need to satisfy either oral or anal erotic needs, covertly express hostility, or unconsciously suppress speech (Bloodstein, 1995; Fenichel, 1945). For example, Fenichel stated that stuttering was "a pregenital conversion neurosis where an inner conflict is converted to the external." The supposed conflicts espoused by these repressed need theories were generally thought to originate in childhood and be overtly displayed in the form of stuttering. However, many of the psychoanalysts (e.g., Barbara, 1954; Coriat, 1928) held different opinions with respect to the onset time and the site of the neurosis associated with stuttering. Clearly, psychoanalysis was not founded in science, but rather a somewhat radical belief system of emotional needs and conflicts based on the teachings of Freud. In fact, reading excerpts from textbooks written from a psychoanalyst's perspective has often evoked startling bewilderment from students in our classes. These excerpts have been described "amusing," "sick," and even "pornographic." Consequently, consistent with this theoretical approach psychoanalytical therapy under this paradigm often consisted of numerous hours spent revealing traumatic childhood experiences to a trained therapist. An emotional catharsis was reached that was thought to resolve the deep-rooted conflict believed to be causal to the stuttering behaviors.

Like other approaches that preceded it, and many that would follow, psychoanalysis essentially failed in yielding an effective treatment for stuttering. In fact, Abraham Brill, a prominent psychoanalyst in the 1920s, reported only being able to help 4 of 69 patients that he had treated (Brill, 1923). Not surprisingly, the popularity of psychoanalysis began to wane in a similar fashion to the school of cerebral dominance when the prescribed therapy failed to adequately reduce the symptoms. However, the passing of the torch from one failing paradigm to another serves to illustrate a salient point: no matter how complex or simple a theoretical perspective may be, a desperate client who just wants to see results does not care about the orientation and will try the prescribed therapy. This is common across many chronic pathologies whereby management is characterized by intermittent recoveries and relapses such as obesity, depression, and alcoholism. The failure of psychotherapy eventually gave way to learning theory, but not without a substantial degree of overlap between schools of thought.

## Johnsonian Theory

Wendell Johnson, an Iowa protégé of Travis, provided another theory of stuttering that was among the first to address the development of stuttering in children. His approach heavily influenced treatment, especially in children until the 1980s. Even today, and casts a shadow of guilt on some parents of children who stutter. Although his viewpoint was not without psychoanalytical underpinnings (e.g., the strong parental influences and lasting disability), Johnson propagated a more "semantic" view of the disorder. Indeed, the difference between his view and those of the psychoanalysts may only exist on a semantic level. In stark contrast to Orton and Travis' ideas of cerebral dominance, Johnson's diagnosogenic or semantogenic theory (Johnson, 1955b) assumed no organic etiology to the disorder. In other words, Johnson did not believe there was anything inherently different about the brain or speech-motor system of the person who stutters. Rather, Johnson espoused the idea that stuttering was defined by those listening to it. That is, normally developing children who exhibited nonfluent behaviors during the early periods of speech and language development (e.g., tension-free whole word repetitions, interjections, or revisions), could be converted into children who stutter by parents placing "unrealistic" (Bloodstein, 1995, p. 77) demands on their speech. With the blame for stuttering falling squarely on the shoulders of parents and caregivers, the therapeutic course targeted parents and caregivers. They were taught to avoid labeling the child as a stutterer. To do this, mothers were taught to ignore all speech aberrations in their children and refrain from drawing any negative attention to their speech. By applying the stuttering label to a child Johnson believed that disruptive speech behaviors could be permanently ingrained into the psyche or neuronal firing patterns of a young child. It appears that Johnson may have seen countries go to war over made-up problems (e.g., World War I), that millions had died for surreal causes, and that perhaps many of the problems people had were simply brought about by their own perceptions. To Johnson, stuttering was just such a problem, created by the listener's overly perfectionistic expectations of speech. It seemed, to Johnson anyway, that stuttering would subside when the expectations were relaxed—at least in about 72% of cases (Johnson, 1955b). The ensuing "pseudoscientific" (untestable—"circular argument") assumption was that children who recovered from stuttering had parents who did not draw attention to their disrupted speech, and children in whom stuttering persisted had parents that continued to stigmatize their children. Johnson's approach to working with stuttering children and their caregivers remained seminal and the "gold standard" for decades. In other words, when working with children, a "hands-off" (or indirect) approach was required. The key was to work with the parents and teach them to avoid uttering the word "stutterer," "stuttering," or any derivation thereof. Caregivers and therapists alike feigned ignorance of stuttering behaviors, simply pretending that the disorder did not exist in young children. A powerful semantic bugaboo pertaining to stuttering appeared to exist and the fear of the label appeared to make it real and palpable in parents, clinicians, and family members. How did Johnson get away with this argument? For starters, his treatment methods targeting parents (not the stuttering children) probably yielded about an 80% success rate, which is not bad by anyone's standards—if he had been achieving these results without any help. From a paradigmatic point of view, the 20% or so who did not recover did not seem to represent enough of an anomaly to question the paradigm until much later. When we look at the development of stuttering in children, we will again examine Johnson's recovery rates in light of those achieved by others and what naturally occurs in stuttering children.

For the 20% or more of children who continued to stutter, Johnson began to advocate direct therapy, but only in their school-aged years. To him, it was apparent that their mothers or caretakers had failed in their attempts to refrain from drawing negative attention to their children and adversely labeling them. This may have occurred via either verbal or nonverbal (e.g., facial strain when stuttering) forms of punishment, thus creating the pathologic condition within the child. As such, the time had come for direct stuttering intervention. In some sense it was to point out that the "emperor had no clothes," or that it was time for the denial to end and for everyone to acknowledge the presence of a true pathologic condition. Johnson came to refer to stuttering as an "anticipatory, apprehensive, hypertonic, avoidance reaction" (Bloodstein, 1995, p. 65). This meant that the moment of stuttering is an anticipatory reaction to an emotional fear of stuttering. Or paradoxically stated, stuttering is what a person does to avoid stuttering—again an untestable statement. This was even paradoxic to Johnson because to him the problem began innocuously in the ear of the mother or caregiver, yet had been somehow transferred to the psyche of the child and now required the use of behavioral speech machinations and self-analysis to purge it. Johnson's consistent view that stuttering was an emotional disorder rather than a symptom of physiologic or organic pathology led to a therapeutic approach that consisted primarily of dealing with fear associated with stuttering (Johnson, 1959). With this in mind, he taught methods of easy stuttering such as the "bouncing" technique which was essentially easy, tension-free, voluntary stuttering consisting of the production of syllabic repetitions (e.g., buh, buh, buh, balloon). Bouncing was used with the intention of providing those who stutter with a means of overcoming their fears and tendencies to avoid stuttering (Johnson, 1959). This method would also later influence Van Riper's approach, and interestingly Johnson's technique had "inhibitory" powers over stuttering but probably not primarily due to fear reduction as he theorized (Saltuklaroglu et al., 2004). That is, as we will later describe, artificial or voluntary stuttering may actually impact the brain at some level to suppress true stuttering. Johnson also began to use slowed-speech models and reinforced the notions of a loving, caring environment, aspects of therapy that continue to be appropriate today. However, unlike the criteria for intervention today, Johnson refrained from administering direct therapy to stuttering children until they were, by all standards, confirmed stutterers with little probability of recovery.

While for years Johnson was revered as a premier authority in the field of stuttering, his name has recently been maligned. It appears that in 1939 Johnson did find a way to test his own theory. Recall that, according to Johnsonian theory, normally fluent children could be morphed into stuttering children by negative parental reactions. Accordingly, Johnson took a group of 22 fluent children from an orphanage in Iowa and divided them into two groups of 11. For five months, one group received positively reinforcing speech therapy while the children in the other group were continually subjected to chastisement and harassment based on their speech. They were told stuttering and needed to stop speaking unless they could do it without stuttering. If stuttering was truly to be found in the ear of the listener, this type of treatment should have turned normally fluent children into children who stutter. However, it did not. None of the children who were subjected to these extreme conditions began to stutter and this study was not made public until recently.

The fact that the experiment failed and essentially disproved Johnsonian theory was probably the primary reason that this experiment was not made public for so long. The other reason may have been the ethical considerations. While this type of research may not have been subjected to strong ethical considerations when it was conducted in 1939, by today's standards, however, it is considered highly unethical.

## Joseph Sheehan

Joseph Sheehan (1953; 1958) was another pioneer in stuttering research and treatment. His theories drew from research done on rats that examined approach-avoidance conflicts with respect to reaching a desired target. He viewed stuttering as a conflict between drives to speak and refrain from speaking. The untestable argument that he presented was that when the drive to speak outweighed the drive to remain silent, fluent speech was produced, and when the drive to refrain from speaking was stronger, the person remained silent. However, when the two drives were approximately equal, speech was stuttered. At the time this theory became popular it drew from both psychoanalysis and Johnsonian approaches (i.e., unresolved conflicts and anticipatory fear). In addition, Sheehan developed a famous analogy, which is still apropos for describing stuttering as a "syndrome." He compared stuttering to an iceberg, with only a small portion visible, and the rest of the mass, invisible, yet looming tempestuously beneath the surface (Sheehan, 1970). As such, Sheehan advocated overt confrontation, openness, and acceptance of stuttering. He believed that only by exposing the hidden portion of the pathology could stuttering be adequately treated (Sheehan, 1958). The need to refrain from speaking was supposedly caused by an inner shame and hatred associated with stuttering. This was considered a deep psychologic conflict that was required to be overcome with willpower and resolve. Sheehan and his followers would conduct group therapy sessions to try to instill such traits in their patients. At the initial stages of treatment, the focus was on acceptance of stuttering within the self and putting aside expectations of immediate fluency. Rather, it focused on coping with stuttering. It was not until later in the treatment course when some of the fears had been overcome (i.e., conflicts underlying stuttering had been resolved) that fluency was considered more of a realistic goal and could be incorporated into treatment protocols. Sheehan's theories achieved some popularity and his therapies are still currently available.

## Behaviorism

Around the 1960s, thanks primarily to the influence of B. F. Skinner, behaviorism gained popularity in the field of psychology. This paradigm assumed that all human behaviors were under voluntary control and desirable behaviors could be taught or shaped using the appropriate schedules of reinforcement. Under the assumptions of this simple learning theory, it was thought that undesirable behaviors could be extinguished or eliminated and replaced with their desirable counterparts by systematic reinforcement and punishment (Andrews & Ingham, 1972). Speech was not to be excluded from this line of thinking. In fact, just about all forms of speech therapy that are practiced today have strong behavioral components. If you are a student in the field, you will probably have started to work with patients in the clinic. Examine how your therapy goals are written for children with articulation difficulties or language disorders, as well as any adult clients that you may be treating. Most goals are written such that a long-term objective is determined, which is divided into smaller incremental goals. Advancement through the smaller goals is generally based on a client's behavioral progress toward a goal, which is thought to be shaped by the stimulus, level of cueing, and the forms of reinforcement provided (Ryan, 1974; Webster, 1974). The very nature of therapy is such that it warrants the shaping of desirable communicative behaviors.

The treatment of stuttering also fits nicely into this line of thinking. Behaviorists noted the ease with which stuttering could be reduced when certain modifications were made to the manner of speaking. For example, many noticed that simply by reducing speech rates, stuttering behaviors could be significantly reduced. It should not be surprising that rate reduction has formed the cornerstone for most behavioral speech therapies since the 1960s. Furthermore, the observed decreases in stuttering may possibly have taken some of the onus off finding the origin of stuttering. Learning theory assumed that stuttering was due to "poor speaking habits" but did not provide any explanation for the sources of those poor habits (i.e., the etiology of the pathology) (Webster, 1974). However, for therapeutic purposes it did not matter. The important observation was the fact that stuttering could be reduced if speech was properly "shaped." Again it should be noted that people seeking remission from painful pathologies care little about theories—just results. Learning theorists assumed that their behavioral modifications were simply correcting poorly learned speaking habits.

Later in the 1980s technologic advances allowed scientists to uncover kinematic and acoustic differences between stuttered speech and fluent speech and even between the fluent speech of those who stutter and those who are normally fluent. A new theoretical paradigm was born that propagated the notion that stuttering occurred due to a discoordination between the dynamics of the speech subsystems (i.e., respiratory, laryngeal, and articulatory) (Caruso, Abbs, & Gracco, 1988). It was assumed that those who stutter suffered from a temporal motor deficit that did not allow for adequate muscular coordination during speech production. The theoretical shift in thinking was significant. Once again, stuttering was thought to possess an organic component. People who stutter were thought to possess a compromised speech motor system that was in need of "repair." Stuttering appeared to manifest at the level of the speech articulators, larynx, and lungs, and therefore, appeared to be a surface level disorder of the motor speech periphery. It seemed logical that by appropriately shaping one's manner of speech production, normal or fluent speech patterns could replace patterns of stuttering resulting from the "broken" speech system.

However, this new theoretical orientation did not produce any new treatment methods. Behaviorism continued to dominate. The only thing that was different was that those providing treatment began to assume that their methods were somehow "repairing" or "correcting" the assumed temporal motor deficit (Packman & Onslow, 2002). This approach was supported by the simple observation of stuttering behaviors and their suppression upon the imposition of some simple behaviorally based "speech techniques." Rate reduction continued to form the foundation of therapies. It was assumed that correcting the temporal motor deficits and instilling fluent speech was most easily accomplished by beginning at slow speech rates. In other words, the rationale for using behavioral techniques was further validated with the inception of the speech motor dynamics paradigm. Rather than just believing that operant conditioning was replacing bad speaking habits with good ones, it could now be assumed that the operant schedules of speech retraining were actually correcting an organically based disorder of speech production.

Two major approaches to treating stuttering were spawned from this line of thinking. Both therapies provided the option of intensive or extended treatment schedules. Intensive therapies often consisted of 100 or more therapy hours condensed into a one-month period. In contrast, extended schedules allowed for therapies to be conducted once, twice, or three times a week, for months or years, as long as the client and clinician saw the need to continue. Having just described these therapy schedules, is there something unsettling about these approaches? What is "special" about speech that it may not be amenable to behavioral shaping (i.e., disorders such as stuttering), and why is behavioral therapy for stuttering often continued for months, years, or even over the course of a lifetime?

## Charles Van Riper's Therapy

Charles Van Riper, whose clinical contributions to the field of stuttering are arguably unmatched, viewed stuttering as a neuromotor disorder that could be brought under "voluntary" control using his therapy His approach was in effect "stuttering modification" or to " stutter fluently." Van Riper was a very severe stutterer himself who had also come through Iowa and practiced the methods he espoused. Even today, the Stuttering Foundation of America offers sets of videotapes showing Van Riperian therapy in action, providing an example of a master clinician. He developed a four-stage program of identification, desensitization, modification, and stabilization (Van Riper, 1973). Essentially, those participating in his program were first taught to identify their most miniscule moments of stuttering, as well as negative emotions and avoidance behaviors associated with stuttering (which may sound like an easy task, but can be difficult and emotionally draining for many who stutter). Pseudo- or artificial stuttering was an integral portion of therapy and often made people uncannily free of most of their stuttering behavior. Purposefully stuttering in an intense manner created long periods of fluency where clients could now work on modifying their stuttering when it occurred. Van Riper suggested that pseudo- or artificial stuttering was desensitizing clients to their own stuttering (however, we will discuss later the powerful inhibitory action these methods can have on the central nervous systems of those who stutter). Unlike Johnson's bouncing techniques, which were exclusively repetitive in nature, Van Riper's pseudostuttering was a combination of repetitions and prolongations implemented with the notion that controlling the number of repetitions and the duration of the prolongations would bring the involuntary pathology under some form of voluntary control. It was thought that by overcoming the fear of stuttering and achieving some control over the pathology, methods for modifying the actual moment of stuttering could be more successfully implemented. It should be pointed out that Van Riper also may have been unaware of the true value of pseudostuttering as a method for reducing true stuttering events. Participants were then taught to modify or behaviorally shape their stuttering behaviors into milder or more controlled forms of stuttering that could be easily produced without greatly impeding communication. Finally, upon mastering the first three stages, the stabilization stage was designed to promote carryover of the learned skills into the outside world, improve speech naturalness and functionality, and generally allow therapy participants to generalize the therapeutic process. These methods were effective for some in reducing the frequency and severity of speech disruptions as well as teaching coping strategies. However, their appeal was limited. Stuttering modification involved a truly artful and introspective confrontation with the disorder, requiring those who stutter to dissect their stuttering behaviors, one at a time, and understand the sources of fears that may been present for years. It required participants to try to overcome both the overt stuttering behaviors and associated fears by replacing them with the more desirable, behaviorally shaped alternatives.

Van Riper attracted a dedicated core group of followers who were taught to use his methods and style. However, his approach was not standardized and was only practiced by those who spent long hours being specifically schooled to administer the specialized techniques. As such, though his approach was effective for some, its appeal was somewhat limited by the strong emotional content of therapies, the long hours of training required to become skilled in these methods, and the use of non-standardized methods that may not have appealed to the majority of practicing clinicians. Thus, what the field drew from Van Riper was a need for standardized therapeutic protocols that most clinicians could follow without specialized training. These protocols needed to be data driven, empirical in nature, and not quite so intuitive, so that they could be implemented by the masses who did not have the experience of icons such as the Van Ripers, Johnsons, Sheehans, and their loyal followers. In other words, the field was in need of an effective approach that could be implemented more efficiently, without years of training at the master's feet. Such an approach would also allow for easier access to treatment as it would not be restricted to a few specialized university clinics under the supervision of these specialists.

## Fluency-Shaping Therapies

A slew of behaviorists in the 1960s and early 1970s set up protocols that used learning theory to change stuttering. They really did not care what caused stuttering because they were so excited about their results in amelioration of stuttering. As stated, overt stuttering behaviors (i.e., repetitions and prolongations of speech sounds) can be amenable to immediate suppression. So, these behaviorists had reason to be excited—at least at first. We do not want to mislead readers as to the importance of one protocol over another. Bruce Ryan (1974) developed the gradual increase in length and complexity of utterances program (GILCU), which is an excellent example of a behavioral speech protocol progressing hierarchically from very simple to complex extended productions. Perkins (1973a, 1973b) used delayed auditory feedback (DAF) to establish appropriate speaking rates. The effects of DAF and its history will be discussed in much more detail as data from DAF studies provide some of the foundations for our theoretical perspectives. Cooper (1976) had his fluency initiating gestures (FIGS), which were a set of speaking techniques designed to induce fluency (e.g., slow, deep, loud, and smooth speech) that were first taught individually and then in combination. Behavioral psychologist Ronald Webster (1974; 1975) at Hollins College in Roanoke, Virginia had a powerful impact on stuttering therapy by not only standardizing therapy, but also intensifying therapy to 8 hours a day for 19 days and offering year-round therapy at his center and later at other satellite centers. At his therapy center, clients could retrain speech using computers or voice monitors that provided biofeedback. They could train and monitor themselves to accurately produce speech targets that were thought to be compatible with fluent speech production. Behaviors were monitored and counted and the goal was to retrain the speech system, "shocking" it back to normalcy. The use of these systems did not require the presence of a speech pathologist as the computers provided reinforcement for accurate "target" productions. Typically clients would practice for about 20 minutes at a time on the biofeedback devices and then come out for a 10-minute transfer with another speaker. Sessions adhered to strict behavioral regimes of 8 to 10 hours a day. These strict regimens and criteria for speech targets were much different from the easygoing cigar-smoking manner of the Van Riperian school, even though some clinicians training under Van Riper might have called him a "martinet."

Thus, in contrast to stuttering modification methods, fluency-shaping offered standardized protocols that were considerably easier to learn and administer, making them more attractive to the general community of speech therapists. Rather than the hours of training and specific understanding of the disorder that Van Riperian therapy advocated, fluency-shaping techniques were essentially standardized recipes for fluent speech that could be administered by almost any therapist who was familiar with the general underpinnings of behavioral therapies and simple learning theory. In addition, the therapeutic focus shifted from confronting stuttering to ingraining fluent speech patterns, making it appealing to vast numbers of potential clients as well as therapists who may not have firsthand experience in dealing with this complex syndrome. It became the next popular step in the sequence of stuttering treatments. As the speech motor paradigm dictated, it was believed that with practice of correct speaking techniques, speech could be "reprogrammed" in those who stutter, allowing fluent speech patterns to supplant stuttering behaviors (Boberg & Kully, 1994; Onslow, Costa, Andrews, Harrison, & Packman, 1996; Webster, 1980). The therapies under this paradigm propagated the notion that speech could be taught in a manner similar to other motor skills requiring muscular coordination (e.g., skating or riding a bicycle). Intensive speech retraining can last for hundreds of hours, during which speech rates can be reduced to as low as two seconds per syllable uttered, and a client's speech output may be limited to a syllable or a single word until, if we adhere to the assumptions of speech motor dynamics, proper coordination of speech subsystems is established via mastery of the endorsed "techniques."

Although numerous data sets have suggested that these therapies produced short-term remission of stuttering, they should be interpreted with caution as these protocols may not be effective for many over the long term. Relapse to stuttering following these therapies has been found to be at least 70% (Craig & Calver, 1991; Craig & Hancock, 1995; Dayalu & Kalinowski, 2002). It may be even higher, depending on how we define "relapse." Among the problems with these therapies that may contribute to the high relapse rates are unstable speech patterns (i.e., the techniques are difficult to generalize and may fail to reduce stuttering when needed most), unnatural sounding speech (stuttered speech may be less conspicuous than post-therapeutic speech), and difficulties in implementation (i.e., the techniques espoused may feel unnatural and may not be easily reproducible at all times). All these qualities are examined in detail as we continue to examine the nature of fluent speech relative to stuttering and examine what constitutes viable, efficient, and effective stuttering management. However, these complaints are clearly suggestive of some fundamental problems within this paradigm. First of all, how many types of motoric skills require continued training after the skill is learned? Once a person learns to skate or ride a bike, they do not relapse to a state where the fundamentals must be relearned again and again (Saltuklaroglu et al., 2003). Children do not actively learn to talk. Speech and language develop naturally in most children if they are in reasonably conducive environments (i.e., relatively normal interactions with caregivers). Thus, as we discuss speech production and stuttering, it should be evident that speech is a specialized and relatively automatic process for human beings. In addition, stuttering is considered to be an involuntary pathology. Therefore, it seems unlikely that behavioral speech retraining alone is the long-term answer to solving stuttering and ingraining speech patterns that may override stuttering. Lastly, the notion of a temporal motor deficit that forms the foundation for these therapies may not be accurate. A recurring theme in this text is the separation between cause and effect (Armson & Kalinowski, 1994). In other words, when interpreting any research, we must continue to ask ourselves if the effects seen are causal to stuttering, or simply reflect some effect of stuttering. If the speech motor paradigm is scrutinized in this manner, how do we know that the observed differences in phonation, breathing patterns, jaw and lip movements, and articulatory trajectories found even in the fluent speech of those who stutter, are not simply effects of a deeper-rooted pathology, rather than being causal to the pathology?

## The Next Step

We have very briefly described five theoretical orientations that have helped shape the field of stuttering over the last century. However, the intent of this section was not to provide a complete view of each, nor to examine the data (or lack thereof) gathered to support each perspective. Bloodstein's *Handbook on Stuttering* (1995) provides a much more comprehensive description of the various schools of thought and makes an invaluable reference for anyone digging into the history of stuttering. Instead, these basic overviews provide reference points for describing key theories and clinical findings that will be reinterpreted as we unveil our paradigmatic approach to the nature and treatment of stuttering.

## References

Andrews, G. (1984). Evaluation of the benefits of treatment. In W. H. Perkins (Ed.), *Stuttering disorders*. New York: Thieme-Stratton.

Andrews, G., & Ingham, R. J. (1972). An approach to the evaluation of stuttering therapy. *Journal of Speech and Hearing Research, 15*, 296–302.

Armson, J., & Kalinowski, J. (1994). Interpreting results of the fluent speech paradigm in stuttering research: Difficulties in separating cause from effect. *Journal of Speech and Hearing Research, 37*, 69–82.

Barbara, D. A. (1954). *Stuttering: A psychodynamic approach to its understanding and treatment*. New York: Julian Press.

Bloodstein, O. (1995). *A handbook on stuttering* (5th ed.). San Diego, CA: Singular Publishing Group.

Boberg, E. (1981). Maintenance of fluency: An experimental program. In E. Boberg (Ed.), *Maintenance of fluency: Proceedings of the Banff Conference*. New York: Elsevier.

Boberg, E., & Kully, D. (1994). Long-term results of an intensive treatment program for adults and adolescents who stutter. *Journal of Speech and Hearing Research, 37,* 1050–1059.

Brill, A. A. (1923). Speech disturbances in nervous and mental diseases. *Quarterly Journal of Speech Education, 9,* 129–135.

Caruso, A. J., Abbs, J. H., & Gracco, V. L. (1988) Kinematic analysis of multiple movement coordination during speech in stutterers. *Brain, 111,* 439–456.

Cooper, E. B. (1976). *Personalized fluency control therapy: An integrated behavior and relationship therapy for stutterers.* Austin, TX: Learning Concepts.

Coriat, I. H. (1928). Stammering: A psychoanalytic interpretation. *Nervous and Mental Diseases, 47,* 1–68.

Craig, A. R., & Calver, P. (1991). Following up on treated stutterers: Studies of perceptions of fluency and job status. *Journal of Speech and Hearing Research, 34,* 279–284.

Craig, A. R., & Hancock, K. (1995). Self-reported factors related to relapse following treatment for stuttering. *Australian Journal of Human Communication Disorders, 23,* 48–60.

Dayalu, V. N., & Kalinowski, J. (2002). Pseudofluency in adults who stutter: The illusory outcome of therapy. *Perceptual and Motor Skills, 94,* 87–96.

Fenichel, O. (1945). *The psychoanalytic theory of neurosis.* New York: W. W. Norton.

Fox, P. T., Ingham, R. J., Ingham, J. C., Hirsch, T. B., Downs, J. H., Martin, C., Jerabek, P., Glass, T., & Lancaster, J. L. (1996). A PET study of the neural systems of stuttering. *Nature, 382,* 158–161.

Fox, P. T., Ingham, R. J., Ingham, J. C., Zamarripa, F., Xiong, J. H., & Lancaster, J. L. (2000). Brain correlates of stuttering and syllable production. A PET performance-correlation analysis. *Brain, 123,* 1985–2004.

Foundas, A. L., Bollich, A. M., Corey, D. M., Hurley, M., & Heilman, K. M. (2001). Anomalous anatomy of speech-language areas in adults with persistent developmental stuttering. *Neurology, 57,* 207–215.

Hayhow, R., Cray, A. M., & Enderby, P. (2002). Stammering and therapy views of people who stammer. *Journal of Fluency Disorders, 27,* 1–17.

Ingham, R. J. (2001). Brain imaging studies of developmental stuttering. *Journal of Communication Disorders, 34,* 493–516.

Johnson, W. (1955a). The time, the place, and the problem. In W. Johnson & R. R. Leutenegger (Eds.), *Stuttering in children and adults.* Minneapolis: University of Minnesota Press.

Johnson, W. (1955b). A study of the onset and development of stuttering. In W. Johnson & R. R. Leutenegger (Eds.), *Stuttering in children and adults.* Minneapolis: University of Minnesota Press.

Johnson, W. (1959). *The onset of stuttering: Research, findings and implications.* Minneapolis: University of Minnesota Press.

Kalinowski, J. (2003). Self-reported efficacy of an all in-the-ear-canal prosthetic device to inhibit stuttering during one hundred hours of university teaching: An autobiographical clinical commentary. *Disability and Rehabilitation, 25*, 107–111.

Kalinowski, J., Dayalu, V. N., & Saltuklaroglu, T. (2002). Cautionary notes on interpreting the efficacy of treatment programs for children who stutter. *International Journal of Language and Communication Disorders, 37*, 359–361.

Kalinowski, J., Dayalu, V. N., Stuart, A., Rastatter, M. P., & Rami, M. K. (2000). Stutter-free and stutter-filled speech signals and their role in stuttering amelioration for English-speaking adults. *Neuroscience Letters, 293*, 115–118.

Kalinowski, J., Noble, S., Armson, J., & Stuart, A. (1994). Naturalness ratings of the pretreatment and post-treatment speech of adults with mild and severe stuttering. *American Journal of Speech Language Pathology, 3*, 61–66.

Kalinowski, J., Saltuklaroglu, T., Guntupalli, V. K., & Stuart, A. (2004). Gestural recovery and the role of forward and reversed syllabic repetitions as stuttering inhibitors in adults. *Neuroscience Letters, 363*, 144–149.

Klein, J. F., & Hood, S. B. (2004). The impact of stuttering on employment opportunities and job performance. *Journal of Fluency Disorders, 29*, 255–273.

Kraaimaat, F. W., Vanryckeghem, M., & Dam-Baggen, R. V. (2002). Stuttering and social anxiety. *Journal of Fluency Disorders, 27*, 319–331.

Kuhn, T. S. (1996). *The structure of scientific revolutions* (3rd ed.). Chicago: The University of Chicago Press.

Messenger, M., Onslow, M., Packman, A., & Menzies, R. (2004). Social anxiety in stuttering: Measuring negative social expectancies. *Journal of Fluency Disorders, 29*, 201–212.

Moeller, D. (1975). *Speech pathology and audiology: Iowa origins of a discipline.* Iowa City: University of Iowa Press.

Onslow, M., Costa, L., Andrews, C., Harrison, E., Packman, A. (1996). Speech outcomes of a prolonged-speech treatment for stuttering. *Journal of Speech and Hearing Research, 4*, 734–749.

Packman, A., & Onslow, M. (2002). Searching for the cause of stuttering. *Lancet, 360*, 655–656.

Perkins, W. (1973a). Replacement of stuttering with normal speech. I. Rationale. *Journal of Speech and Hearing Disorders, 38*, 283–294.

Perkins, W. (1973b). Replacement of stuttering with normal speech. II. Clinical procedures. *Journal of Speech and Hearing Disorders, 38*, 295–303.

Peters, H. F. M., & Starkweather, W. C. (1989). Development of stuttering throughout life. *Journal of Fluency Disorders, 14,* 303–321.

Ryan, B. (1974). *Programmed therapy for stuttering in children and adults.* Springfield, IL: Charles C Thomas.

Saltuklaroglu, T., & Kalinowski, J. (2002). The end-product of behavioural stuttering therapy: Three decades of denaturing the disorder. *Disability and Rehabilitation, 24,* 786–789.

Saltuklaroglu, T., Kalinowski, J., Dayalu, V., Guntupalli, V. K., Stuart, A., & Rastatter, M. (2003). A temporal window for the central inhibition of stuttering via exogenous speech signals in adults. *Neuroscience Letters, 349,* 120–124.

Saltuklaroglu, T., Kalinowski, J., Dayalu, V. N., Stuart, A., & Rastatter, M. P. (2004). Voluntary stuttering suppresses true stuttering: A window on the speech perception-production link. *Perception and Psychophysics, 66,* 249–254.

Sheehan, J. G. (1953). Theory and treatment of stuttering as an approach-avoidance conflict. *Journal of Psychology, 36,* 27–49.

Sheehan, J. G. (1958). Conflict theory of stuttering. In J. Eisenson (Ed.), *Stuttering: A symposium.* New York: Harper & Row.

Sheehan, J. G. (1970). *Stuttering: Research and therapy.* New York: Harper & Row.

Travis, L. E. (1931). *Speech pathology.* New York: D. Appleton-Century.

Van Riper, C. (1973). *The nature of stuttering.* Englewood Cliffs, NJ: Prentice-Hall.

Webster, R. L. (1974). A behavioral analysis of stuttering: treatment and theory. In K. Calhoun et al. (Eds.), *Innovative treatment methods in psychopathology.* New York: John Wiley & Sons.

Webster, R. L. (1975). *The precision fluency shaping program: Speech reconstruction for stutterers.* Roanoke, VA: Communication Development Corporation.

Webster, R. L. (1980). Evolution of a target-based behavioral therapy for stuttering. *Journal of Fluency Disorders, 5,* 303–320.

Webster, W. G. (1986). Neuropsychological models of stuttering–II. Interhemispheric interference. *Neuropsychologia, 24,* 737–741.

Wills, G., (1992). *Lincoln at Gettysburg.* New York: Touchstone.

Wingate, M. (1997). *Stuttering: A short history of a curious disorder.* Westport, CT: Bergin & Garvey.

Yairi, E., & Ambrose, N. G. (1992). A longitudinal study of stuttering in children: A preliminary report. *Journal of Speech and Hearing Research, 35,* 755–760.

Yairi, E., & Ambrose, N. G. (1999). Early childhood stuttering I: Persistency and recovery rates. *Journal of Speech, Language and Hearing Research, 42,* 1097–1112.

# 2

# Stuttering and the Person Who Stutters

> *"It is impossible for a man to learn what he thinks he already knows."*
>
> —*Epictetus*

In this chapter, we start to build our definition and model of stuttering, beginning with the generally accepted notion that stuttering originates as a neural block "somewhere in the brain" (Fox et al., 1996; Saltuklaroglu et al., 2004; Sommer et al., 2002). However, for our definition to make sense to those relatively new to the field, it is important that we describe the disorder and differentiate it from other forms of "nonfluency" found in people who do not stutter. The descriptions that follow may be somewhat similar to those found in other texts. After all, we have been observing the same pathology with the same epidemiology, symptomatology, and phenomenology for years. The manifestations of the disorder have not changed. It is our interpretations of these observations that separate our view of stuttering from that of others.

## Incidence, Prevalence, and Genetics

Stuttering is found in every race, culture, and language. Though it was once speculated that cultures that more highly valued good verbal communication displayed higher incidences of stuttering, that does not appear to be the case. Interestingly, the word "stuttering" has an onomatopoeic quality in most languages. Its only significant basis for discrimination seems to be gender. Males seem to be afflicted with stuttering more often than females by a ratio of 3 to 1 (Bloodstein, 1995, p. 117). We are often perplexed by the ratio. However, there is one hypothesis that links a number of other brain disorders such as dyslexia, autism, Tourette's syndrome, and dyslexia with prenatal testosterone levels, and this seems provocative (e.g., Lutchmaya, Baron-Cohen, Raggatt, Knickmeyer, & Manning, 2004).

There also seems to be some genetic predisposition to stuttering that may play a role in determining the gender ratio. This genetic predisposition is evident in familial or hereditary patterns of stuttering. People who stutter often have immediate relatives who stutter. Andrews et al. (1983) found that people who stutter were three times more likely than those who do not to have a first-degree relative who also stuttered. However, many people who stutter are the only ones in the family displaying the pathology, suggesting that for a child to begin to display stuttering behaviors, any genetic predisposition may need to be compounded by other factors. In fact, evidence exists against the possibility of a simple sex-linked or autosomal dominant (only one parent must have the gene in order to inherit the disorder), or recessive genetic linkage (both parents must have the genes in order to inherit the disorder). Instead, it seems more likely that adopting a more complex polygenic model (two or more genes) may better explain the inherited predisposition to stuttering (Andrews & Harris, 1964; Kidd, Kidd, & Records, 1978; Meyer, 1945). In turn, actual surfacing of the symptoms may occur as a result of the genetic predisposition plus environmental influences (Bloodstein, 1995, p.131; Kidd, 1977; Kidd, Heimbuch, & Records, 1981). In addition, twin studies have indicated that there is not 100% concordance for identical twins, although the persistence of stuttering in identical twins is much higher than for fraternal twins who would have genetic material similar, but not identical, to that of their sibling. All this suggests that genetics plays a role in stuttering but does not apparently have a clear-cut link to the manifestations found in other disorders (e.g., Duchenne's muscular dystrophy, hemophilia, cystic fibrosis, Huntington's disease).

Stuttering can be found to exist in isolation or concomitantly with other disorders. Reports of high incidences of stuttering among children with Down syndrome, Tourrette's syndrome, attention deficit disorder, phonological disorders, and other neurological pathologies are common. However, the association in all these disorders is not clear, although these observations again suggest a genetic predisposition for stuttering and have been the target of investigations seeking a common gene for the different disorders (Comings et al., 1996). One population in which stuttering seems to be lower is those who are congenitally hearing impaired. However, evidence exists of an individual with severe hearing impairment who stuttered in sign language suggesting that stuttering can permeate "gestural" (see chapter 5) communication in both oral and manual mediums (Montgomery & Fitch, 1988).

## Stuttering Versus Normal Nonfluency

The early years of language acquisition and development are characterized by growth spurts in vocabulary, phonology, syntax, and morphology. At this time, children learn new words every day, and learn to combine sounds in different ways. They combine words in appropriate forms to construct an ever growing number of utterances, add appropriate endings to words, and basically learn to use speech and language to interact effectively in a variety of environments. Considering this exponential growth rate, it is not surprising that a few mistakes are made along the way. These naturally occurring mistakes are what we refer to as normal nonfluency and though there is some overlap between the characteristics of normal nonfluencies and those of incipient stuttering, there are aspects that can help distinguish between the two.

Stuttering is often associated with "repetitions." As described below, part-word or syllabic repetitions are one of the defining elements of stuttering. However, normal nonfluency may be characterized by "whole word repetitions" or "phrase repetitions." "Revisions" are another type of normal nonfluency, whereby the child realizes that he or she has made an error in producing speech and chooses to self-correct or revise the utterance. "Interjections" such as inserting "um," "er," and so forth between words are also characteristic of normal nonfluency and may be just another example of the child requiring time to synthesize novel linguistic forms. It should be noted that children who stutter may also display these normally disfluent behaviors, but, in addition, will also show the diagnostic characteristics of stuttering outlined below. Differential diagnosis between the two forms of disfluency (normal versus stuttering) may be easy or difficult, depending on the relative amounts of each. Of course, stuttering is more easily diagnosed when the speech behaviors become more tense, increase in duration, and are accompanied by other struggle behaviors. The point we make is that the observable behaviors that characterize normal nonfluency and stuttering need not fall into dichotomous or categoric distinctions, rather they can often represent ends of a continuous scale. That is, the diagnosis is more like determining hair color, which can fall anywhere on a wide-ranging scale, than gender, in which people fall distinctly into a particular category. It will become clear, however, that the observable behaviors may not represent what is going on "below the surface." At the level of the brain, there appears to be something different going on in those who stutter.

Others in this field have determined guidelines for differentiating between normal nonfluency and stuttering. For example, it has been suggested that incipient stuttering has 10 or more disfluencies per 100 words, any less than that would be considered normal disfluency (Adams 1977; Peters & Guitar, 1991). Another suggestion is that repetitions should consist of one unit, as in whole words (Yairi, 1981). However, these criteria should be considered guidelines and not rules. Exceptions can always be found. For example, both Yairi and Ambrose (1992) and Johnson et al. (1959) found normally nonfluent children with 25 or more disfluencies per 100 words, some of which exhibited either one or two repetition units. As we begin to examine the "gestural" nature of speech as well as stuttering, it will become clear that these behavioral criteria are really "made up," and it may often be impossible to determine what is normal nonfluency and what is incipient stuttering.

It should also be noted that normal nonfluencies can occur after the initial stages of language development. In fact, almost no one is completely fluent all the time. Just watch a news reporter on television or your lecturers. Even though their speech is clearly not stuttered, if one listens carefully it is common to note the occasional word or phrase repetition, inter-jection, or revision. Many normally fluent speakers report non-fluency during times of anxiety, fatigue, or stress. It may not come as a surprise that even for those who do not stutter, public speaking is a task that evokes high levels of fear and anxiety. Some have even claimed to stutter at these times. However, in most cases the disfluencies are fleeting, unexpected, not word or sound specific, and are not accompanied with the tension and loss of control that are the characteristics of true stuttering. Simply put, these normal nonfluencies are not true stuttering behaviors.

## Overt (Observable) Behaviors

Wingate (1964) provided a descriptive definition of stuttering based on two salient and observable behaviors—repetitions and prolongations of speech sounds. Van Riper (1982) also described repetitions and prolongations as the "core" stuttering behaviors. These discrete signature behaviors are indicative of a struggle to speak and are often necessary to obtain a diagnosis of stuttering from a speech-language pathologist. The repetitions produced by most people who stutter take the form of repeated syllables and have also been called "part-word" repetitions, as in "ba-ba-ba-balloon." Syllabic repetitions are not typical of speech in people who do not stutter; when people who do not stutter are anxious or have linguistic formulation or retrieval problems they may simply repeat simple whole words or phrases. Syllabic repetitions and prolongations are not an overt strategy used by those who do not stutter. They are produced almost exclusively by those who do stutter. Thus, syllabic repetitions are a clear diagnostic marker of stuttered behavior and generally differentiate stuttering from normal nonfluencies.

Repetitions of sounds occur for all sounds, regardless of the manner and place of their articulation. They are typically the first strategy observed in the onset and development of stuttering. Prolongations occur on continuant sounds such as /s, r, w, l, m, n/, and all vowels. For example, the prolongation of the word "milk" may sound like "mmmmmmmilk." The manner of articulation during the production of stops such as /b, p, d, t, g, k/ does not allow for them to be prolonged. At this point we will be describing these behaviors, but we urge readers to keep the structure of these speech disruptions in mind (they turn out to be important in recovery from the disorder and in techniques that temporarily alleviate its symptoms). In our controlled experiments, we add a third category of overt stuttering behaviors which we call "silent postural fixations." These behaviors often characterize more advanced forms of the disorder. During a silent postural fixation the flow of speech is completely impeded and no sound is produced. It appears to be an indication that the speech system is frozen or "locked up." The postural fixation is often produced as the person struggling to speak places the articulators (e.g., jaw, lips, tongue) in the position to produce the desired sound. As you may imagine, postural fixations can often be the most difficult to treat, as some type of endogenous (self-produced) sound production is needed to facilitate ongoing speech and release the stuttering block.

Having described these three types of overt stuttering events, we caution that true overt stuttering behaviors are rarely neatly assigned to a particular category; stuttered behaviors really lie on a continuum. Many stuttering events possess characteristics of repetitions and prolongations, prolongations and postural fixations, repetitions and postural fixations, or even all three types of behaviors combined. When we attempt to classify stuttering events we simply choose the behavior that is most salient. However, it becomes apparent that although we categorically distinguish overt stuttering into only three types, a stuttered speech disruption can take on an almost infinite variety of acoustic forms as repetitions, prolongations, and postural fixations are combined. Perhaps what is most interesting about overt stuttering behaviors, is that though they represent the oscillatory struggle associated with the disorder, they are most likely produced with a purpose, namely to release the speech system from the block or struggle (Dayalu et al., 2001, Kalinowski et al., 2000). This may seem counterintuitive at first, as most people see oscillatory struggle behaviors as the "core" stuttering problem, we continue to argue that overt stuttering behaviors are actually nature's solution to the stuttering block.

It should not be surprising that we have never met two people who stutter in the same way. Stated otherwise, everyone who stutters exhibits an individual pattern of stuttering. In fact, it would not be unreasonable to liken stuttering patterns to fingerprints. Individual stuttering patterns are shaped as the disorder develops in a person and may even change in any given person over the course of a lifetime. It is fair to say that stuttering is a truly heterogeneous disorder, both among and within individuals. Stated simply, no two people stutter in the same way and stuttering patterns are variable within individuals. Aside from the variability in the types of core behaviors observed, numerous other variables help differentiate among those who have the pathology. These variables include:

1. *Stuttering severity:* The severity of stuttering is often, but not always, related to both the frequency and duration of overt stuttering behaviors. Frequency and duration of overt stuttering events provide a large source of heterogeneity in the disorder and can help define individual stuttering patterns. Typical assessment tools attempt to determine how many stuttered words or syllable per minute are observed during reading, monologue, and conversation. The mean duration and range of durations in the stuttered events can also be measured, providing information on the severity of observable behaviors for a particular speaking task in a particular setting.

2. *Difficult words or sounds:* As stuttering progresses, some sounds or words are stuttered more frequently than others. As a result, a fear and anticipation of stuttering begins to develop for these particular sounds or words. This anticipation of stuttering is self-fulfilling, and a repertoire of difficult

sounds or words develops. Typically, when a particular sound proves to be difficult, the difficulty will generalize to other similar sounds. For example, many people who have difficulty with words starting with "p" also have difficulty with those starting with "t" and "k"—that is, other voiceless plosives. Feared sounds or words are signature events for each person who stutters, unique to their own personal battle with the disorder. They are much more prone to stutter on these feared sounds or words than others, and will typically try to avoid them. It should be noted that most people who stutter have difficulty saying their own name. One reason for this is because it is a word that cannot be substituted by an other word (though we have reports of people who try to occasionally call themselves by names that they feel are easier to say and less likely to induce stuttering).

3. *Extraneous speech productions:* Sometimes, while stuttering, speech sounds are produced that are unrelated to the sound or word on which the struggle is actually occurring. These sounds can often seem to have no acoustic form, but they are typically vocalic and oscillatory in nature. However, these behaviors and their acoustic manifestations develop as aids to initiate difficult sound or words and can soon become ingrained into stereotypical motor responses to anticipated speech failures. They were initially thought to be distracters but we now suspect they serve a more fundamental purpose similar to those of the core behaviors—to release the involuntary block. These stereotypical responses become ingrained and habituated over time, becoming additional unwanted symptoms of the stuttering syndrome.

4. *Ancillary behaviors:* As core stuttering behaviors develop, "ancillary" struggle behaviors may develop concomitantly. These are overt behaviors that are not directly related to speech production but are indicative of the tension and difficulty that a person is experiencing while attempting to produce speech. They include, but are not limited to: head jerking, arm jerking, leg movement, eye blinking, nostril flaring, lip biting, tongue protrusion, and almost any other form of bodily contortion. In the past, these behaviors may have been thought to be helpful in "distracting" a person

from stuttering, a condition once suspected as being helpful for inducing fluency. However, the problem with this hypothesis is that an increase in distracting stimuli (e.g., increases in extraneous body movements), did not create proportional decreases in stuttering, as would be expected under such a hypothesis. In later chapters we present a more plausible biological purpose for ancillary behaviors, especially those associated with oscillatory struggle.

5. *Covert behaviors:* Until now, we have been describing "the visible portion of the iceberg," according to Joseph Sheehan's analogy of stuttering. Covert stuttering behaviors are the bulk of the pathology. They are the portion of the iceberg that lies invisible, beneath the surface of the disorder. They clearly affect not only patterns of overt stuttering, but can also become cemented in the psyche of an individual and help shape entire lives. As such, we will describe in detail covert stuttering behaviors.

## Linguistic Aspects of Stuttering

Although stuttering can occur at any place or time during speech production, the locus of overt stuttering events in connected speech has been a topic of strong interest over the years, and certain linguistic trends have been found that can exist independently of the anticipated stuttering on certain sounds. In both children and adults who stutter, stuttering has been found to occur more frequently in the first few words of a sentence (Brown, 1945; Wingate, 1982). Furthermore, in both age groups, stuttering occurs more frequently in longer words (Brown, 1945; Williams et al., 1969). However, this latter phenomenon has also been observed related to normal nonfluencies and is, therefore, not a true characteristic of stuttering.

It has been found that stuttering is most likely to occur on the initial syllable of a word. The reason for this has yet to be adequately explained, though the combination of increased frequency at the beginning of an utterance with increased frequency on the initial phoneme has for years led researchers to believe that stuttering is associated with an inherent difficulty in initiating speech. This theory has influenced therapeutic orientations and, hence, it is a theory that cannot be dismissed lightly. In the 1970s, Adams and colleagues suggested that voicing and voice initiation was a primary factor in stuttering manifestations. As a result, the speech motor control paradigm in stuttering exploded as a research avenue and a therapy rationale, with an emphasis on retraining the laryngeal anatomy for "better" voice initiation. Acoustic laryngeal reaction time (ALRT), lip perturbations (McClean et al., 1991), electromyography (EMG) (Hulstijn et al., 1991), and photoglottography (PGG) were all used to examine the temporal motor and spatial capacities of those who stutter against those who did not, with an eye toward speech initiation and speech motor dynamics. Differences were found between the two populations across various parameters of speech, and these differences were interpreted as evidence of difficulty in initiating speech and exerting motor control over the speech musculature. Linguists had alternative orientation. They saw this initiation problem differently and explained it to be related to the initial timing and access problems. As we begin to examine the breadth and depth of this pathology, and see how stuttering can even have an influence over speech that otherwise appears perceptually fluent, we discuss a phenomenon known as "subperceptual stuttering" that will explain these differences and call for a theoretical orientation with more explanatory power. For now it is sufficient to say that stuttering probably occurs most on initiation because the brain has yet to receive an appropriate signal to help suppress the neural stuttering block.

Another topic regarding the loci of stuttering events that has been the subject of much debate is the distribution of stuttering across "content" words such as nouns, adjectives, verbs, and adverbs; and function words such as pronouns, prepositions, or conjunctions. Though children have been observed stuttering more on function words, the trend seems to shift in adults, who seem to stutter more on content words (Howell et al., 1999). It was thought that this occurs because content words carry higher levels of "propositionally" or weight with regard to their meaning in an utterance. However, this concept has also been recently revisited. In a study that examined stuttering frequency on 63 content and 63 function words matched for initial sound and number of syllables, Dayalu et al. (2002) concluded that the best predictor of stuttering on any given word was its inverse frequency of use in the English language. That is, words that were more commonly used were found to be stuttered less than those used less frequently. As such, stuttering frequency was not thought to be directly related to content or function categories per se. The authors explained this phenomenon by a generalized adaptation effect (i.e., stuttering less frequently upon repeated productions) to the small list of 100 to 200 function words that are repeatedly used in the English language. This view may also find some support in the finding that stuttering occurs more on words that are less familiar to those producing them (Hubbard & Prins, 1994). Therefore, it appears that, generally speaking, the more times a word is used, the less chance there is of stuttering on it.

## Adaptation and Consistency Effects

Two phenomenon associated with stuttering frequency and loci have been observed over the years. The first is called the adaptation effect. This simply refers to the fact that if a person who stutters were to read the same passage repeatedly, the frequency of stuttering would start to diminish on the second reading and keep decreasing upon further readings. This observation has been found repeatedly in both children and adults who stutter (Johnson & Knott, 1937; Neeley & Timmons, 1967; Shulman, 1955; Williams, Silverman, & Kools, 1968). Many explanations for this phenomenon have been proposed, including the extinction of a learned response (Wischner, 1950), reduction in anxiety related to anticipation of stuttering (Johnson & Knott, 1937), reduction of fear due to stuttering in the first reading (Sheehan, 1958), and mental rehearsal of the reading material (Eisenson, 1958). We believe it is simply a case of some engagement of the neural mechanism for fluency that tends to respond favorably to repeated productions. It should be noted that the adaptation effect degrades when the reading material differs. Even when passages using the same words are punctuated differently, to produce different meanings, the adaptation effect can diminish (Wingate, 1966). Thus, when conducting experiments testing conditions that reduce stuttering, different passages should always be used for each condition and a sufficient time interval introduced between conditions to negate any potential adaptation effects that may confound results. In other words, if the same passages are used for each condition, it may be impossible to tell whether the experimental condition being tested is responsible for the reductions in stuttering or whether it is simply due to an adaptation effect rom consecutive readings.

The second effect, the consistency effect, is somewhat analogous. It refers to the observation that upon repeated productions of the same material, stuttering tends to occur in the same places. Therefore, even though some adaptation may occur and the frequency of stuttering may be reduced upon consecutive readings, the stuttering that remains will probably occur on the same words or sounds. This may be related to the fact that those who stutter acquire their own patterns and may begin to anticipate stuttering on particular sounds or words.

## Involuntary Nature

One characteristic of stuttering that we continue to stress throughout this textbook is that stuttering is an "involuntary disorder." The speech disruptions (e.g., repetitions and prolongations) that characterize stuttering are overt intermittent manifestations of uncontrolled oscillatory or fixated behavior. This defining involuntary characteristic is integrated in many descriptive definitions of stuttering.

The World Health Organization (WHO, 1977) defined stuttering disorders as

> Disorders in the rhythm of speech, in which the individual knows precisely what he wishes to say, but at the same time is unable to say it because of an involuntary, repetitive prolongation or cessation of a sound (p. 202).

According to The Stuttering Foundation of America (1997),

> Stuttering is a communication disorder characterized by excessive involuntary disruptions in the smooth and rhythmic flow of speech, particularly when such disruptions consist of repetitions or prolongations of a sound or syllable, and when they are accompanied by emotions such as fear and anxiety, and behaviors such as avoidance and struggle (p. 56).

Perkins (1984) said,

> Stuttering is a "temporary overt or covert loss of control of the ability to move forward fluently in the execution of linguistically formulated speech (p. 431).

Simply put, the essential character of stuttering is its involuntary nature (not subject to the control of the will). Highlighting the involuntary nature of the disorder carries important theoretical and therapeutic implications. Hence, therapeutic techniques taught to reduce stuttering frequency (e.g., rate control, breath control) may be effective in stuttering inhibition for periods of time but when these techniques fail to work, they cannot be faulted, because of the inherent and essential involuntary nature of the stuttering. When stuttering occurs despite use of such techniques, it is most likely that the technique in question was not sufficiently powerful to override or release the stuttering block for that specific moment in time and place. Stuttering, in other words, is difficult to treat because assessment results can change across situations and the potency of any therapeutic strategy can change according to time and place. These are the problems associated with generalization (moving stuttering therapy outside the clinic room) and relapse (difficulty in maintaining gains over long periods of time).

With the inherent involuntary nature of stuttering in mind and knowing that stuttering can be inhibited or reduced for periods of time via conscious behaviors, albeit not completely removed, the onus of responsibility for inhibiting an involuntary pathology cannot lie on the shoulders of a person who stutters simply because they were "taught" a set of inhibition techniques "believed" to reduce stuttering. By the same token, the therapists cannot be blamed for failing to provide the correct inhibition techniques. They may not be well enough equipped to deal with all manifestations of the stuttering in situational context. Thus, though speech can be temporarily brought under some degree of voluntary control, it is a relatively automatic and specialized process. In turn, stuttering persists as an involuntary and heterogeneous pathology that may continue to keep resurfacing like "the heads of the hydra" (Saltuklaroglu & Kalinowski, in press).

## Covert Behaviors

By viewing overt repetitions and prolongations as core markers of the disorder, we essentially limit ourselves to measuring and treating observable behaviors (what we hear or see). A limited definition of stuttering such as the one offered by Wingate (1964) does not encompass all that constitutes the pathology. Overt stuttering behaviors are just the tip of the iceberg but the behaviors beneath (e.g., avoidance and expectancy behaviors) are often as insidious and restraining as those overt behaviors. Beneath the surface lies a whole "syndrome" of compensations that is experiential in nature and cannot be seen by outsiders. These compensation strategies are only experienced and felt by the stuttering individual and others suffering from the same disorder. Simply put, this is what the person who stutters does to avoid stuttering. It is the hidden pathology that hides much of the overt stuttering that would occur but does not because of avoidance of people, places, and speaking situations. Conversations may be cut short so that opportunities to hear stuttering are not available, or they are not started at all. (Why talk when the world may crash in on you and everybody, especially an unsuspecting stranger, will know that you are different from others?) Why would one subject oneself to the bewildered looks and discomfort of those listening and watching? Before going into detail, we should point out that covert strategies are self-rewarding because while in silence a person who stutters remains the same as others. Speaking, on the other hand, may carry a façade of normalcy for short periods, but only until it is time to stutter.

Imagine what sort of tensions, anxieties, frustrations, and other negative reactions may arise if every time you began to speak, you ran the risk of not being able to complete your sentences. How would you begin to feel? What would you do to cope? Imagine the anticipatory fears of knowing you will be put under pressure to communicate and not be able to do so effectively. When approaching any speaking situation, people who stutter have a few choices. In the beginning the compensatory behaviors can be very relatively unobtrusive but as the disorder progresses (repetitions and prolongations), the covert strategies also progress and can become more of an impediment to communication. Avoidance of certain sounds evolves into avoiding words or phrases, then avoidance of talking to authority figures, and finally failure to speak to one's own parents. (Kalinowski et al., 1998). Simply put, the safest way to avoid the social penalty of overt stuttering is "escape" or to avoid those situations where the person who stutters knows that failure and perceived social punishment are inevitable. Nobody can identify a person who stutters until they open their mouth and begin to speak, so the avoidance of situations is a commonly used strategy and is self-rewarding. By avoiding a situation, a person who stutters avoids any negative repercussions that would likely follow should they choose to expose their disorder. You may consider people who stutter to be anxious, shy, or introverted. Maybe this is just another symptom of stuttering. A vivid memory shared by many people who stutter is of being a child in a classroom. On the first day of a new school year, the teacher often systematically asks each member of the class to say their names. Imagine the lump in the throat of the child that stutters on that first day of class as each student effortlessly introduces themselves and the countdown begins . . . five more students until it's my turn, four more, three more. The tension builds, the anticipation of stuttering and the fear associated with it becomes more and more salient until finally the inevitable—a blockage of speech and the bewildered attention of the entire classroom, including the teacher who may also find him- or herself at a loss for words. It is truly a feeling of terror and cannot be taken lightly. The stuttering child immediately stands out from the rest of the class, and will probably become the butt of jokes, teasing, and ostracizing from the other members of the class. Many children who stutter may simply feign illness that day so as not to participate and suffer the humiliation and instant "labeling." Furthermore, many teachers may refrain from drawing attention to the student thereafter, resulting in the student feeling segregated and inferior throughout the remainder of the year. This is a victory and a loss all in one. It is a short-term victory for the child who does not have to feel the repeated anxiety of anticipation, and the inevitable failure. Yet with that victory comes lost opportunities, separation, the feeling of looking in from the outside, and the reinforcement of covert escape behaviors. Other commonly used strategies are the use of substitutions and circumlocutions, which may also be considered forms of avoidance (as hard sounds or words are still being avoided). As stated, people who stutter are often adept at anticipating their stuttering and may choose words that they consider easier to say. This is what we call "substitution." As a result, people who stutter often prepare in advance what they want to say or recite it over and over to help ensure that they will be able to produce the desired sentence without any overt stuttering.

People who stutter may use "circumlocutions." Describing an object or a person is a symptom often seen in an aphasic or brain-injured person when he or she has difficulty retrieving a word. The use of substitutions and circumlocutions can be both awkward and tiring. It often makes the person who stutters appear to be less intelligent than he or she is, as shifting words may not always be appropriate for communicating an intended message. The constant search for alternative and easier words is a constant strain and a game that is never won, as word substitution simply continues to increase anxiety and just seems to prolong the eventual overt stuttering. However, there may be a small bright side. As the person who stutters develops some resiliency to the pathology, these compensation strategies may allow the person to develop a vocabulary and be able to choose from a wide variety of synonyms for a particular word—a skill that may be useful in one's education and vocation. The brain can be truly wondrous for blocking certain words, but at the same time, opening up a neuronal "thesaurus" that works its magic around difficult sounds and words.

The effectiveness of these strategies varies, reducing overt stuttering sometimes yet not others. However, this type of intermittent reinforcement schedule is among the most powerful known to man—just ask any compulsive gambler in Atlantic City or Las Vegas. A covert strategy to reduce stuttering is analogous to playing a slot machine. Sometimes the compensations (e.g., avoidances, substitutions, circumlocutions, lip biting, etc.) pay off and sometimes they do not, and that is the rub. When they work the payoff is big and one sounds normal and gets away with it. The person who stutters has a rush of adrenaline and a feeling of being "normal for just this minute." That may not seem much of a "rush" for those who do not stutter, but for those who do, it is quite a powerful feeling to make it through a conversation successfully without being labeled or marked as different. We are all social beings and social acceptance is an innate drive that we carry to survive. Those who stutter use covert strategies for social acceptance and to increase their gambler's stock. However, like all gamblers they "bust" sometimes, usually on the next few rolls of the dice or the next few hands. In stuttering, the disorder never runs out, so the gambling on speech output becomes a way of life. Even after therapy the game continues, playing the odds to sound as normal as possible and using substitutions and circumlocutions to improve the odds. Thus, the goal of people who stutter is to use everything in their arsenal to hide the disorder. Covert strategies allows this to be possible, even if only on an intermittent basis. We might call it poker, blackjack, craps, or roulette.

Every time a person who stutters begins to speak, it is as if they are required to traverse a minefield and sustain the least amount of injury (i.e., stuttering). One could travel straight ahead in this minefield and throw caution to the wind, but in the short term, an increase in stuttering behaviors would likely occur. The cascade of stuttering would most likely begin with the anticipation of the first difficult word. The anticipatory fears associated with entering this minefield, the strategies used to carefully maneuver through it without being hurt, and the scarring from being repeatedly injured are real and have been described as constituting up to 80% of the stuttering syndrome. These invisible components of stuttering are the "covert" characteristics of the disorder. Traversing a minefield does not come without a cost, even if you miss all the metaphoric stuttering mines. The amount of energy spent engineering an avoidance strategy, engaging that strategy, and constantly evaluating that strategy are costly endeavors. The avoidance of stuttering comes at a price too. The important point to be made here is that one may have spoken to a person who stutters who was "not stuttering" per se but was engaged in a set of circumlocutions, substitutions, and avoidances that masked the disorder. On the surface they may have appeared to be communicating effectively, even relatively fluently. However, below the surface, the battle for just getting through the next sentence rages on—whether to stutter overtly, avoid, substitute, or circumlocute. This suggests that even when a person who stutters appears to be fluent, the disorder is not at bay, but is simply manifesting outside the realm of observability, due to the diligent use of circumlocutions; substitutions and avoidances, which are his or her covert behaviors.

We are suggesting that observable behaviors such as repetitions and prolongations of speech sounds do not capture the true essence of stuttering. While seeing these behaviors along with other overt struggle behaviors may tell us that a person is stuttering, there may be plenty of other occasions when a person appears to be speaking "normally" but is simply engaged in the covert battle. They may even be feeling the tension associated with stuttering, and experiencing speech blocks that are not perceived by the listener but are salient and real to the person who stutters (Armson & Kalinowski, 1994). As such, the covert behaviors also may be considered true symptoms of the pathology and not just byproducts of overt behaviors. In fact, in our model of stuttering, covert behaviors represent what may be just an example of stuttering symptoms that occur in the brain. The point is this: if we just aim to remove the core behaviors are we really treating stuttering? We suggest the answer is "no" and in order to provide effective and efficient treatment, conditions need to be created in which a person who stutters is "invulnerable" to stuttering so that all characteristics of the disorder are removed. Thus, any adequate and comprehensive definition of stuttering should consider the broad range of covert behaviors that inevitably develop soon after a child begins to stutter overtly.

# Impact

Another relatively undisputed notion is that stuttering is often a debilitating pathology. Stuttering, one must remember, is a disorder unlike many others. Its essence is chronic and hidden, unobtrusive until the inevitable. Once oral communication is initiated anything is possible, from a ½-second fleeting stuttering moment to an endless 3-minute block, with all the associated ancillary behaviors; this may occur even when covert compensations are being simultaneously used. These stuttering moments can be the most conspicuous, salient, and visceral behaviors in the communicative interaction. They evoke powerful visceral responses that are analogous to those evoked by viewing surgery (Guntupalli, Kalinowski, Nanjundeswaran, Saltuklaroglu, & Everhart, under review). Stuttering can shape the lives of people who stutter in ways that can be detrimental to their hopes and aspirations. It can impact academics, vocations, social lives, marriage, and every other aspect of life in which communication is required (Klein & Hood, 2005). If you do not stutter, try to imagine what it would be like if every time you began to speak the possibility arose that you would not be able to say what you wanted to say . . . and for no visible or apparent reason. The feeling one needs to grasp is the inevitable failure to communicate. In other words, before the person who stutters communicates he or she knows that there will be failure followed by a repeated re-enactment of embarrassment and shame; however, communication is necessary for survival in this world so repeated attempts are made with the necessary compensations. Think of the stares that would be forthcoming, how other people would react, and how you would feel.

A typical experience for a mild-to-moderate person who stutters would entail going into a restaurant, like McDonalds, and ordering a meal. The first thing that happens when volitional control fails is a typical audible struggle on the first word. It is most likely that the cashier takes about a tenth of a second to look up from the cash register to focus on the face of the person speaking to identify the source of the communication breakdown and then reacts reflexively, with an uncomfortable giggle.

The giggle or smirk is reflexive in nature and not intended to be mean-spirited (at least not for most adults). It is something that occurs merely because a very unusual behavior has been witnessed, one that is seemingly out of the normal communicative context. The cashier may have taken orders from 300 customers that day and, most likely, none of the others had exhibited this particularly strange behavior. In other words, the cashier was caught "off guard." We have found that stuttering elicits changes in autonomic responses in those witnessing it. A recent study reports changes in galvanic skin responses (e.g., differences in skin conduction) and heart rate when normally fluent individuals were asked to watch videotapes of the speech of both stuttering and normally fluent individuals. While observing the stuttering population, the participants showed an increase in galvanic skin response and a decrease in heart rate relative to observing the fluent group. These autonomic (involuntary) responses are evidence of discomfort and uneasiness associated with witnessing stuttering (and remember that in the Guntupalli et al. [under review] experiment the participants were not required to interact with anyone who stutters).

Under conscious control, the reflexive giggle becomes one of uneasiness and confusion. The cashier may remember the event for the rest of the day and perhaps later tell friends or coworkers about it. For the time being, in order to fulfill the food order, the cashier places a "cognitive governor" on the unease and waits patiently for the order. Such an experience will happen repeatedly through the life of a person who stutters, from childhood onward. For the person who stutters it is another event to "handle," in a never-ending chain of similar events. However, he or she must move on and learn to cope with such situations.

There are a number of ways that people who stutter may learn to cope with situations such as the encounter described above. Some may be able to laugh at themselves. Laughter can be a powerful medicine and it may allow the person who stutters to feel some degree of acceptance if one can laugh at one's pathology in the same way that others do. However, the comedy that the person who stutters is required to engage in countless times may often mask and even compound the true pain and suffering beneath the surface. To be able to truly laugh at oneself and see this debilitating pathology as just a way of being different from others can most often take years of introspective reflection, along with a strong sense of security and self-esteem that usually develops later in life, perhaps after having achieved success in other facets of life. Perhaps it is for this reason that reports exist of stuttering becoming less severe or easier to manage later in life (Silverman, 2004).

Another means of coping with reactions to stuttering is withdrawal. As previously stated, nobody can identify people who stutter until they open their mouth and begin to talk (not even by taking pictures of their brain, which we will discuss). Thus, the simplest means of evading the immediate repercussions of stuttering is found in the art of avoidance. Though this may begin as a simple avoidance of certain sounds, it can soon escalate to include the avoidance of words, phrases, particular speaking situations, even places and people. For example, many teenagers and adults who stutter are terrified of using the telephone. Why does the telephone evoke so much fear? Without other cues that send communicative intent (e.g., facial cues, hand gestures, body orientation), the whole communicative load is placed upon speech and the auditory channel for receiving it. Therefore, any breakdown, pause, hesitation, in speech is highlighted. Many people who stutter report having people hang up on them or be excessively rude or impatient when they stutter on the telephone. Similar events were reported by a group of nonstuttering graduate students when they made phone calls pretending to stutter (pseudostuttering) as a required course assignment (Rami et al., 2003). Hence, it is not surprising that the telephone may very quickly become a source of fear and a common avoidance. It may also not be surprising that many teenagers who stutter are often described as withdrawn, shy, quiet, having few friends, and so forth. Their personal battles with stuttering may have reached the point where they are no longer worth fighting in public. They choose to stutter overtly only in the presence of those around whom they feel most comfortable, or sometimes not at all. Not surprisingly, we have consulted with many teenagers who stutter and their parents regarding the possibility of psychological counseling to help cope with the day-to-day trials of stuttering, though we have heard relatively few instances of psychological intervention helping to ease the pain.

It becomes clear that stuttering can be a source of pain, embarrassment, and insecurity throughout the formative years of childhood and adolescence. It will come as no surprise that stuttering continues to be a source of anguish in adulthood. Like others, people who stutter as they enter their late teens or early adulthood are required to choose a vocation. Imagine how limited your choice of job opportunities would be if your ability to communicate was impeded. Though literature on stuttering is filled with examples of stutterers who have "overcome" their stuttering to become successful actors, singers, politicians, and sports stars, it is fair to say that for the stuttering masses, the decision to choose a particular vocation is not one that is taken lightly. The reality is that sports stars are judged not by how they talk, but how they perform on the field of play; singers who stutter are always fluent when they sing (more on that later too). Most of the other famous stutterers who have succeeded were perhaps mild-to-moderate overt stutterers, able to hide their disability to a certain extent in many speaking situations. Celebrities such as James Earl Jones, Marilyn Monroe, Winston Churchill, and Bruce Willis claim stuttering in their past, without it having a gross impact on their careers. It may even continue to impact their day to day lives to some extent, though that is doubtful. However, the knowledge that they once stuttered comes as a revelation, or "shock" to the world. It seems more likely that these icons had either recovered to some extent or mastered strategies to hide their stuttering for it not to impede their successes. For most of us who stutter moderately to severely, the revelation of our stuttering to the world is not a shock. It is analogous to the sun rising in the morning. Many of us who stutter moderately to severely often choose a vocation, at least initially in our lives, that will entail as little speaking as possible—especially if we stutter moderately to severely. For those seeking jobs requiring postsecondary education, common choices include accounting, computers, or finance. There is something comforting about working with numbers and keyboards all day. They do not require a person to talk to them, nor do they talk back. For others not lucky enough to have the option of postsecondary education, vocational options may only consist of different forms of labor. In fact, before entering academia, the first author (JK) was a security guard on the third (late night) shift—a job that would only require him to monitor a building and keep the coffee pot full. This allowed him to hide until people started calling on the telephone and walkie-talkie. Then he found he could not hide from speaking tasks, even when situated in the remotest of places and at the oddest of times. The second author (TS) would have been happy to make a career of "tree-planting," a lonely piecework job in unpopulated regions of Canada.

To highlight the impact of stuttering, a powerful exercise in our classes is the pseudo- (fake) stuttering assignment. Students in our graduate level stuttering class are required to make ten phone calls to businesses, asking three or four questions per phone call, while pretending to stutter by using fake or pseudostuttering. They are asked to stutter as well as they can, with the notion that there is no right or wrong way to do it. We usually have to teach them by example because they want to do as little stuttering as possible. We stutter a lot in class to make them comfortable with overt stuttering manifestations before the assignment. Students are reminded that for the person who stutters, this is a chronic pathology and they are only walking in that person shoes (i.e, pseudostuttering) for a short period of time in order to attempt to empathize with the feelings of stuttering. It should be noted, however, that nonstuttering students are never able to fully empathize with the involuntary nature of the disorder, as they are able to decide when, where, and how long they will stutter, unlike those who truly have the disorder. Upon hearing about this course requirement, many students develop an intense fear of the assignment. Some have reported not sleeping the night before. In fact, a recently published study on student's feelings after the pseudostuttering assignment reported that they showed higher anxiety, lower self-esteem, lower interpersonal skills, and a host of other negative traits following the assignment (Rami, Kalinowski, Stuart, & Rastatter, 2003). Those are just the effects of fake stuttering during ten telephone calls. Imagine what it is like when one cannot go back to normal speech but has to risk stuttering on every spoken word!

## Incidence and Prevalence

At any given time, approximately 1% of the people on this planet stutter (Bloodstein, 1995, p. 107). We describe this figure as being the "prevalence" of stuttering. On the other hand, the incidence of stuttering is 5% (Bloodstein, 1995, p. 116). That means that 5% of children show signs of stuttering at some point during their course of development. If 5% of children show signs of stuttering and the prevalence of the disorder in the general population is 1%, then there is an approximately 80% recovery rate from childhood stuttering. These figures themselves, and the fact that they appear to have remained stable over time, have numerous implications that require examination and contribute to our explanation of the pathology. It should be specified that these incidence and prevalence figures refer to "developmental" stuttering and no other form of the disorder. Developmental stuttering is the focus of this textbook and typically manifests in children between the ages of about 2 and 6 years (Bloodstein, 1995; Kalinowski & Saltuklaroglu, 2003). In contrast, the less common forms of stuttering, such as neurogenic stuttering (i.e., displaying overt stuttering following damage to the brain) or psychogenic stuttering (i.e., a sudden onset of overt stuttering symptoms for no apparent physical reason that may be related to psychological trauma) usually develop later in life, generally do not follow the same developmental course, and carry fewer of covert symptoms.

When we discuss recovery from developmental stuttering, we must be specific as to what recovery really means. We stress that total recovery should be defined by the complete removal of the signature overt (e.g., syllabic repetitions, part-word prolongations of speech sounds) and covert (e.g., avoidances, substitutions, and circumlocutions) stuttering events. Total recovery also entails producing speech that is natural sounding and, therefore, indistinguishable from the speech of those who do not stutter, as perceived by both the child and other listeners (Finn et al., 1997). Finally, the "truly fluent" (Dayalu & Kalinowski, 2002) speech of the recovered child must extend across all speaking situations over time, and not be restricted to contrived, repeated test environments with the same examiners (e.g., parents, or therapists).

Information regarding recovery should be provided via self-report if possible, because stuttering is "experiential" in nature and only the person who stutters can truly know when covert symptoms of the pathology are being extinguished. This definition is quite comprehensive and for good reason. We have known for decades that the overt symptoms of stuttering are highly amenable to short-term symptom reduction, especially via simple syllable prolongation (which may be a form of "controlled symptom substitution"), yet the pathology remains overwhelmingly resilient to long-term remission and complete recovery. The use of therapeutic techniques that may simply substitute one symptom for another (i.e., droned prolonged speech replaces overt stuttering) can be difficult to maintain over time and the speech production system has the tendency to return to its homeostatic state, which includes more natural sounding speech and more aberrant stuttering behavior. Numerous efficacy studies (Bloodstein, 1995, pp. 437–445), which have used nearly every method under the sun, have provided data that show substantial reduction or elimination of overt stuttering, often with a droninglike quality speech, as a consequence of therapy using permutations of prolonged speech. However, if those data were truly indicative of the ease with which stuttering could be remitted, there would be little need for further studies or the writing of this text. Thus, while reduction in overt stuttering measures obtained in the numerous efficacy studies may seem impressive, they may be misleading. They may only represent levels of temporary suppression of the overt symptoms and not true levels of long-term recovery. In other words, they may only represent the extent that the therapies in question can chip away at the tip of the iceberg. In the next chapter, we discuss the assessment of stuttering and provide our criteria for therapy efficacy.

Possibly the most interesting aspect of the stuttering epidemiology is the difference between incidence and prevalence rates, or the role of spontaneous recovery. Remember, that despite all our extensive history of therapeutic attempts, incidence and prevalence rates have not changed. About 80% of children who may be diagnosed with stuttering eventually recover, regardless of the presence or absence of therapy (Kalinowski & Saltuklaroglu, 2003). Spontaneous recovery from stuttering is an example of the wonders of Mother Nature. Those children who spontaneously recover from stuttering meet the criteria outlined above, showing no residual effects of stuttering. Also, Mother Nature appears to be capable of healing even severe cases of stuttering. In fact, though numerous longitudinal (i.e., time series) studies have followed stuttering children over time and attempted to decipher Mother Nature's recovery code, this has been to no avail. So far, the results are inconclusive and we believe that they will remain this way for some time, as the answer probably exists at a deeper neurological level. In other words, the stuttering behaviors we can observe are only the surface manifestations of a more deeply rooted pathology. We closely examine the relationship between the observable manifestations of stuttering and their "source" in a later section. No overt behavior or characteristic stuttering pattern (acoustic or otherwise) has ever emerged that differentiates children who will continue to stutter from those who will recover. Though it may be intuitive that milder cases will overcome the disorder and more severe cases will continue to stutter, Mother Nature does not appear to work so predictably (Yairi et al., 1996). However, if we assume that stuttering begins somewhere in the brain, then it may not be surprising that the overt or surface symptomatology does not provide any predictive basis for recovery. In other words we cannot subject children's overt stuttering behaviors to a "biopsy" and differentiate what is benign and what is malignant. However, generally speaking, the chances of recovery become less likely as the initial symptoms and their impact upon communication become ingrained over time.

With that said, Mother Nature does seem to have a time schedule for recovery. For example, Andrews et al. (1983) reported that 75% of 4-year olds, 50% of 6-year olds, and only 25% of 10-year olds would recover from stuttering by age 16. In addition, Yairi and Ambrose (1999) reported recovery schedules of children who began stuttering between the ages of two and five years. They found that the peak recovery periods were between one and three years post-onset. Thus, the trend seems to be that most recovery happens relatively quickly after the initial onset and the window of opportunity for recovery becomes smaller with age. Generally speaking, if stuttering persists past puberty, it will most likely become a chronic problem. To illustrate this, we recently conducted a study whereby we asked speech therapists treating children who stutter in the North Carolina public school systems about the number of stuttering children on their caseload that had truly recovered from stuttering. We received responses from 101 speech therapists who claimed a median recovery rate of 13.9%. We found this to be very low as many children being served in the school system were still within an age range that spontaneous recovery should play a role and boost recovery rates. However, it appeared that most children being treated for therapy in the North Carolina schools were simply beyond the age of natural recovery and therapy was doing little to help (Kalinowski et al., in press).

Does this mean that speech therapy has done little to help stuttering children? Before we answer that question, keep in mind that numerous efficacy studies have claimed a great deal of success in remitting stuttering in children using a variety of different methods. Johnson saw numerous children recover simply by telling parents to refrain from drawing attention to stuttering. Behavioral therapies have also shown very high rates of recovery (Craig et al. 1996; Culp, 1984; Onslow et al., 1994; Shine, 1984). We have argued that if all therapies work for helping children recover from stuttering, then no therapy is truly working. When methods that are opposite in both orientation and implementation can yield essentially the same results, there simply has to be another explanation. That explanation is most likely to be spontaneous recovery. Any claims of therapeutic success in the treatment of stuttering children may be jaded by the possibility of spontaneous recovery occurring during the period of intervention, which can often take place over an extended period shortly after the onset of stuttering. After all, when children begin to stutter, parents often do not wish to wait. Because of the desire to help their child, they generally seek immediate help. Considering that most children recover within two years or so, it seems highly likely that the time schedules of therapeutic intervention and spontaneous recovery will overlap. Thus, it is usually impossible to identify the role of therapy in the recovery of children who stutter. However, if we draw our attention back to the incidence and prevalence rates, we may conclude that therapy has yet to play a substantial role in recovery. At the same time, we do not wish to completely discount any positive effects from childhood stuttering therapy. We suspect that therapy can play a role in accelerating recovery in the lucky 80%. Similarly, it may push in the right direction some children who teeter on the edge between complete recovery and persistent stuttering and educate parents with regard to the nature of stuttering and how to best cope with its presence in their children.

The current trend in treating children who stutter is toward early identification and intervention. From a logical standpoint this makes sense for two reasons. First, the developmental nature of the pathology suggests that "nipping it in the bud" at its earliest stage would provide the best chance for complete recovery. Younger brains are more "plastic" than older brains. It takes time for speech and language to develop in children and for speech behaviors to become "hard-wired." Therefore, the chances of being able to make positive strides toward fluent speech seem to be higher if the agent responsible for inducing fluency is introduced earlier rather than later. As such, Onslow's Lidcombe program attempts to identify preschool children who are beginning to stutter and administer behavioral therapy to try to replace stuttered speech patterns with fluent ones as early as possible, so that the developing brain becomes hard-wired for fluency rather than stuttering. However, rather than administering standard therapy in the clinical environment, the Lidcombe program provides a twist. Instead of the speech therapists providing direct therapy to the stuttering children, speech therapists train parents and caregivers to administer the therapy so that the child may receive treatment more often and in more natural settings, so as to promote generalization and attain measures of stuttering beyond the clinical walls.

The Lidcombe program consists of two stages. The first stage is an attempt to remove all overt stuttering behaviors in the child. Parents and children attend a speech clinic, where the speech therapist teaches the parent to administer therapy using proper feedback and schedules of reinforcement. Parents learn to praise children for fluent speech and teach children how to "self-correct" stuttered speech. At the same time, parents begin to directly administer the therapy to their children. This stage continues until all overt stuttering behaviors are nearly or completely eliminated. Stage 2 of the program commences at this point. The second stage is a "maintenance" stage whereby parents continue to administer the therapy themselves with the goal of maintaining stutter-free speech for a year. Considering the history of relapse from previous therapy that has been observed, this is a noble goal. The need for long-term efficacy measures has been overlooked in the past and should now be considered essential in the evaluation of any therapy for stuttering.

The Lidcombe program has received a great deal of attention lately. It is being implemented across the globe and is backed by a number of studies supporting its use (Harrison et al., 2004; Jones et al., 2000; Kingston et al., 2003; Onslow, 2003; Onslow et al., 2001; 2002; Wilson et al., 2004; Woods et al., 2002). It is the therapy "du jour" for incipient stutterers and it may possibly be helping children recover from stuttering. However, before jumping on the Lidcombe bandwagon, we should throw out a few cautions with regard to this approach. First of all, given the rates and schedules of spontaneous recovery, the decreases in stuttering frequency observed under the Lidcombe program may be influenced by spontaneous recovery. The safest way to assess the efficacy of this treatment may be to examine the rates of total recoveries. Though as a group the Lidcombe program produces impressive levels of stuttering reduction, low levels of stuttering appear to remain in many children who undergo this program. As such, we may not be witnessing complete recovery within the treated group that exceeds levels of 80% and cannot, therefore, differentiate the therapeutic effects from natural recovery. Rather, we may simply be witnessing accelerations in the recovery schedule of those children already prone to recover. Simply put, for the Lidcombe to be considered truly effective, we should see a complete removal of all stuttering behaviors in over 80% of children treated. Second, from our reading of some of the Lidcombe studies, the exclusion criteria appear to be fairly loose. That is, a number of children are excluded from treatment based on reasons such as transportation problems, marriage breakups, aggressive behaviors, or mothers struggling to deliver treatment (Kingston et al., 2003). Thus, we wonder how inclusion of these "difficult" cases may have affected the data obtained. Although the idea behind these indirect forms of therapy appears sound, we continue to question whether simple parental reinforcements and reminders to "self-correct" can halt the course of an involuntary pathology that has baffled us for centuries. If it is possible, then the evidence will soon be clear in higher numbers of truly recovered stutterers. If it is not possible, the training of the parents to do direct therapy under the Lidcombe premises may yield the same results as Johnson's indirect parental counseling—about an 80% success rate. Finally, the criteria for recovery from stuttering are simple: an absence of part-word repetitions and prolongations, as well as covert behaviors, accompanied by natural-sounding speech that is indistinguishable from that of children who do not stutter and the self-identification of a normally fluent child.

## Onset and Development

It can often be difficult to determine when stuttering begins to manifest in a child and whether its onset is sudden or gradual. A number of factors may contribute to this difficulty. First, the overlap in overt behaviors associated with normal nonfluency and stuttering may make it difficult to differentiate the two disfluency types until truly stuttered forms are easily discernible from the more innocuous nonfluencies. Second, an initial diagnosis is often made by parents, who may wait for a period of time before reporting to a speech therapist or pediatrician. While we do not question any parent's ability to detect aberrant speech patterns in his or her child, a parent may only have a general idea as to when stuttered speech patterns began (Onslow, 1996). It may require a salient event such as a particular difficulty asking for a favorite toy or describing a game being played for a parent to distinguish between normal and impaired communication in their child. Third, subperceptual forms of stuttering may be present before a child displays overt stuttering behaviors such as part-word repetitions. Subperceptual stuttering refers to slight differences in the acoustics and kinematics in fluent speech productions that do not actually result in the surfacing of core suttering behaviors. We will examine subperceptual stuttering in more detail in the next chapter as it plays an important role in our definition of stuttering and how all stuttering behaviors emanate from the brain but may not all be overtly detectable. Fourth, the predisposition for stuttering may be present from birth, but actual stuttering behaviors may be suppressed during the early phases of language development due to the use of simple imitated forms. This point will be further elaborated upon. However, for now it is enough to say that before stuttering actually surfaces, it may be suppressed during the early phase of language acquisition by the same neural mechanism that may underlie the bulk of speech-related conditions that temporarily reduce stuttering at later stages of development.

## Development of Stuttering

It is generally agreed that the presence of part-word repetitions is the initial red flag for incipient stuttering (Bloodstein, 1995; Mansson, 2000; Silverman, 1996; Van Riper, 1971; Yairi et al., 1993; Zebrowski, 1995). These conspicuous behaviors may appear without warning; yet even if they are only displayed for a short period of time, they can evoke anxiety, apprehension, and fear in parents and other adults who may witness them (Ratner, 2004). The fear may not lie in the incipient behaviors themselves, for they typically are produced with little effort, flow freely, have little impact on communication, and may not even enter the child's awareness. Instead, the fear lies more in the knowledge that stuttering is a dynamic and progressive disorder, and that more advanced forms of the pathology may lie ahead if the child producing these easy incipient behaviors is among the prevailing 1% (Mansson, 2000) of the population who do not undergo the natural recovery processes. However, the progression of stuttering within any child can be unpredictable, heterogeneous, and nonlinear, as evident by the wide variety of outcomes and rates of progression. It is these characteristics that make it so insidious. Simply put, seemingly innocuous incipient stuttering behaviors may at almost any time be replaced by more severe forms that can become a true force to be reckoned with. As such, incipient stuttering behaviors often herald a future of impeded communication.

Although the progression of stuttering within any given child is unpredictable and may be unique, there seem to be some general group development trends. General developmental courses have been broken down into two stages (Bluemel, 1957), four phases (Bloodstein, 1960), and four tracks (Van Riper, 1971). Bluemel's categorization scheme is probably the simplest. He divides his two stages by the general severity of overt behaviors. As such his primary stage is generally characterized by easy, tension-free repetitions, whereas his secondary stage is characterized by more severe struggle behaviors (e.g., disturbed breathing), as well as stoppages in speech. This stage is also marked by the emergence of covert behaviors such as avoidances, substitutions, and circumlocutions. As one can see, this dichotomous breakdown lacks detail and leaves many holes in the progression of the disorder.

Bloodstein's phases are more descriptive. Unlike Van Riper's tracks, age does not directly factor into any but the first of Bloodstein's phases (which corresponds to 2 to 6 years of age), highlighting the variability in the developmental chronology. However, it should be noted that his first stage offers little to separate incipient stuttering behaviors from normal nonfluencies (Silverman, 2004). Bloodstein's phases are summarized as follows:

*Phase 1:*

- Stuttering is "episodic." It is not predictable and does not occur in all speech productions. However, it probably occurs most during times in which emotions are high (e.g., anger, excitement, anxiety, etc.).

- Repetitions are the dominant behaviors.

- Stuttering usually occurs at the beginning of an utterance and on function words.

- Lack of concern from the child. Whether or not children are aware of their stuttering, they tend to show little concern about it. As a result there are relatively few social or emotional penalties associated with this early stage.

- Typically associated with preschool ages (i.e., 2–6 years).

*Phase 2*

- Rather than being "episodic," the disorder now becomes "chronic," meaning that it can interrupt speech at almost any time.

- The child now sees himself or herself as a "stutterer." This means full awareness of their overt stuttering and recognition that their speech is different from that of other children.

- Despite his or her awareness of overt stuttering behaviors, the child does not appear to display any covert stuttering such as avoidances, substitutions, and circumlocutions.

- Although stuttering still occurs frequently on initial sounds, it can permeate an utterance at any position.

- Stuttering begins to be more frequent on nouns, verbs, adjectives, and adverbs, rather than prepositions, conjunctions, and pronouns.

- More frequent stuttering continues to be associated with situations of high emotion.

- Generally associated with the elementary school years.

*Phase 3*

- Stuttering becomes more severe in response to specific "stressful" situations, such as using the telephone, talking to a teacher or people of authority, answering questions in class.

- The child begins to associate stuttering with difficult sounds and may describe some words as being more difficult than others.

- Though most sounds, words, and situations are generally not avoided yet, covert behaviors such as substitutions and circumlocutions begin to surface.

- Generally associated with late childhood to early adolescence.

*Phase 4*

- ▓ By this stage, stuttering can permeate all aspects of life. Speaking situations are approached fearfully and with anticipation of stuttering.

- ▓ Salient fears exist of particular sounds, words, and speaking situations.

- ▓ Avoidances, substitutions, and circumlocutions are a way of life. They are done relatively automatically as compensatory strategies to get through any speaking situation.

- ▓ Generally characteristic of late adolescence and adulthood.

Van Riper's four tracks offer an account of four different ways that stuttering can manifest and develop from childhood to adulthood. His first track is very similar to Bloodstein's continuum of phases, which Van Riper suggests accounts for about 50% of all stuttering cases. Track 2 is associated with a later onset, yet begins with poorly articulated speech, gaps, revisions, as well as word and syllable repetitions. There is often little awareness and this changes little with age. Though the duration of disfluencies may increase, few covert behaviors develop. Silverman (2004) notes that this track may be associated more with cluttering than stuttering. Van Riper's third track can begin at any age after speech develops and is associated with a sudden onset, possibly caused by some trauma. The disfluencies are characterized by high levels of tension and silent postural fixations. As the disorder progresses, the overt behaviors become more severe with an increase in ancillary behaviors such as tremors and facial contortions. Not surprisingly, this track, characterized by severe overt stuttering behaviors, is also characterized by strong covert behaviors such as fears and avoidances. Van Ripers fourth track usually has a late but sudden onset. He describes the onset as being characterized by "unusual behaviors" that usually occur on the first word. These behaviors change little over the developmental course, although the loci may change. In addition, this track seems milder and results in few covert behaviors. For a full description of each track, see Van Riper (1971, pp. 116–117).

From our perspective, the most important point is that the pathology progresses. Instead of saying "muh, muh, muh name is . . . ," a child may begin to say "mmmmmy name is," as the disorder progresses from the easy incipient syllabic repetitions to more tension-filled audible prolongations. Later the child may say the same utterance, initiated with a long silent pause filled with visible tension in the lips and jaw, finally to blurt out "mmy name is . . . " Covert symptoms evolve to compensate for the persistence, development, and increased severity of the overt symptoms, but why do the overt symptoms progress from one form to another? Most textbooks simply describe the developmental course of stuttering without answering this question. However, this course can tell us a great deal about the pathology and we will attempt to explain it from our perspective.

First of all, rather than seeing the overt stuttering behaviors as the stuttering problem, we view them as the stuttering solution. What if these behaviors were produced by children to release the speech mechanism from whatever block was sent from the brain to hinder normal speech? Perhaps these involuntary oscillatory speech movements serve a function. Perhaps it is their manifestation that allows for an 80% recovery rate with or without treatment. However, if these behaviors are so powerful, then why stray from producing them and allow the pathology to progress? Surely Mother Nature would not play such a cruel joke. We suggest that in the 20% of children who do not recover, the pathology may have progressed to a more severe state faster than nature's recovery course allows for remission. Thus, in an attempt to generate a larger and more potent dose of Mother Nature's self-healing medicine, the pathology progresses from intermittent repetitive forms to more continuous forms. Interestingly, behavioral therapies that reduce stuttering have employed volitionally produced forms of both syllabic repetitions (e.g., "bouncing" [Johnson et al., 1959], "pseudostuttering" [Van Riper, 1982]) and prolongations (e.g., prolonged speech [Bothe, 2002; Onslow, 2003; Onslow et al., 1996]). So, what therapies have taught people to do is simply produce volitionally controlled analogs of stuttered events in order to reduce the chances of real stuttering occurring. As we discuss the neural mechanism thought to be responsible for powerful stuttering reduction, this paradoxic nature of behavioral stuttering management techniques will become clearer.

We also speculate as to why the pathology may then progress to "silent blocking." Perhaps it is due to a combination of at least two factors. The first is in line with the initial progression from repetition to prolongation. It may be to build up a large dose of acoustic energy which when finally released provides an explosion to release the neural block. The second factor may be related to the development of covert reactions to stuttering. Repetitions and prolongations are acoustically conspicuous, often producing negative reactions from listeners. They simply sound like disrupted speech that is produced with tension and struggle. However, silent blockages in the speech flow, especially during initiation, may be less conspicuous. The tension and struggle can be less visible during silent blockages. Therefore, in an attempt to reduce the conspicuous nature of overt stuttering, the development of silent blockages may represent attempts to internalize the manifestations of overt behaviors and keep them out of the realm of visibility to avoid reactions in listeners.

## Recovery from Stuttering

Another question that is often asked is whether recovery from stuttering can take place later in life, after Mother Nature closes her window of opportunity for recovery. If one looks on the Internet, there are many who claim to have recovered from stuttering and are willing to share their secret—often for a price. These charlatans aside, numerous accounts exist of others who claim that they are completely healed and do not suffer from any symptoms of stuttering. However, people define recovery in different ways, some more loosely than others. For many, if stuttering ceases to impede their lives and they are able to communicate effectively and comfortably, they may consider themselves recovered. There are also a select few who manage to master the use of therapeutic techniques in almost every speaking situation and may appear overtly fluent to almost everyone they speak to. Some of these folks may consider themselves completely recovered, although it is difficult to measure the effort required to continuously monitor speech production while using therapeutic techniques at all times.

However, if we recall our definition of recovery, we suspect that complete recovery from stuttering, beyond what is found in Mother Nature's schedule, is almost nonexistent. Even if a person who stutters at some point later in life is able to achieve relatively spontaneous, natural-sounding, and effort-free speech that is perceptually stutter-free, it is still difficult to shed the emotional baggage associated with stuttering. Even after achieving some degree of fluency, situational fears can still exist, as well as the use of avoidances, substitutions, and circumlocutions. Anyone who does not achieve recovery from stuttering at an early age is likely to be scarred from it at some level and suffer some consequences of stuttering for the rest of their lives.

## Problems with Definitions

As we discussed in the previous chapter, the field of stuttering has observed the rise and fall of various paradigmatic approaches. Under each dominant paradigm the disorder of stuttering has been etiologically defined (i.e., with regard to its source) in a different way, and therefore treated in a different way. For those in need of treatment for stuttering, the adopted viewpoint is of little importance so long as the treatment provides some form of relief. However, at any given time the availability of therapeutic options remains dependent on the existing paradigmatic viewpoint. Simply put, the way that any disorder is viewed by the scientific population is instrumental in deciding what treatment options are available to those seeking help. For example, Travis saw the disorder as a problem with cerebral dominance and tried to correct it by exploring changes in handedness. The psychoanalysts saw the disorder as resulting from deep unresolved conflicts and spent countless hours attempting to resolve these conflicts by reaching an emotional catharsis. Johnson believed the disorder only existed in the ear of the listener and that stuttering was caused by labeling and the attention drawn to aberrant speech. It followed that he advocated an indirect hands-off approach. Johnson could see problems where they may not even have existed, which is also why his indirect methods of treating children achieved similar success rates to the direct methods that would follow. Both the learning theorists and those championing the notion of compromised speech motor dynamics advocated direct behavioral speech retraining for the unlearning of poor speech habits and to correct a temporal motor deficit, respectively. The pattern is clear. Orientation toward the pathology directly impacts the treatment modality.

Silverman (1996) made an astute comparison when describing how the various definitions of stuttering have failed to capture the complete essence of the disorder. He compared the various definitions of stuttering to the parable of the "blind men of Indostan" who tried to accurately describe an elephant. Each blind man independently touched a different part of the great beast and provided a description of the animal based on the small area that he was able to touch. The point is that each man was correct in his own way, but failed to provide a description that captured the true essence and enormity of the animal. The descriptions of stuttering suffer from the same shortcomings. Each one describes a part of the disorder, yet none of them manage to clearly explain all of the phenomena associated with stuttering.

To discuss every definition of stuttering propagated would be exhausting and serve little purpose. However, a few definitions of stuttering should be discussed to show how each one does capture a portion of the pathology. For example, even Johnson's (1955) definition of an " . . . anticipatory, apprehensive, hypertonic avoidance reaction" had its merits as it captures the notion of covert behaviors and word fears. The WHO (1977) and DSM-IV definitions all capture the involuntary essence of stuttering. Wingate's standard definition (1964) of "repetitions and prolongations" draws attention to the overt behaviors, although, it is limited even in that area. Perkins (1984, 1990) describes the speech disruptions as resulting in a "loss of control," providing a sense of the experiential nature of the disorder, that nonstutterers cannot appreciate. Finally, Cooper and Cooper (1985) describe stuttering as a "clinical syndrome," a notion that we also embrace, considering the scope of the grasp that stuttering can wield over a person's life.

Thus, each of these definitions has its merits, yet individually may not possess the explanatory power to cover the full scope of the disorder. In our description of paradigm shifts, we stated that for one paradigm to supplant another, it must be logical, scientifically based, and have more explanatory power than its predecessor. Perhaps the main problem with previous definitions of stuttering and a reason that they only encompass a portion of the disorder is that they generally fail to separate causes of stuttering from effects of stuttering. We return to our analogy of a fever. A fever occurs in the body when there is an infection that needs to be fought. Simply put, the fever occurs as a symptom, result, or effect of the infection. The fever itself is not the cause of disease. In stuttering, what if previous definitions were simply descriptions of the wide range of symptoms, results, or effects of the deeper stuttering pathology?

Without making any specific assumptions, one thing that we can be fairly sure of is that the developmental origin of stuttering lies somewhere in the brain. This is a very broad statement, as intended. In fact, this description is appropriate for describing numerous communication, psychological, cognitive, neurological, and emotional disorders. However, its implications for stuttering are far-reaching. We have been looking for an explanation of stuttering that can explain all the above descriptions of the pathology. Explaining the manifestations of overt behaviors, their structure, the development of the pathology, ancillary behaviors, covert behaviors, spontaneous recovery, adaptation and consistency effects, differences in the speech of those who stutter from "normals," as well as all the means of inhibiting stuttering may be a tall order. However, we will attempt to provide a perspective that accounts for as many of the stuttering phenomena as possible and one that can serve as a viable model for implementing efficacious therapeutic procedures.

# References

Adams, M. R. (1977). A clinical strategy for differentiating the normally non-fluent child and the incipient stutterer. *Journal of Fluency Disorders, 2,* 141–148.

American Psychiatric Association. (1994). *Diagnostic and statistical manual of mental disorders* (4th ed.). Washington, DC: Author.

Andrews, G., Craig, A., Feyer, A. M., Hoddinott, S., Howie, P., & Neilson, M. (1983). Stuttering: A review of research findings and theories circa 1982. *Journal of Speech and Hearing Disorders, 48*(3), 226–246.

Andrews, G., & Harris, M. (1964). *The syndrome of stuttering. Clinics in developmental medicine,* No. 17. London: Spastics Society of Medical Education and Information Unit in association with Wm. Heinemann Medical Books.

Armson, J., & Kalinowski, J. (1994). Interpreting results of the fluent speech paradigm in stuttering research: Difficulties in separating cause from effect. *Journal of Speech and Hearing Research, 37*(1), 69–82.

Bloodstein, O. (1960). The development of stuttering: II. Developmental phases. *Journal of Speech and Hearing Disorders, 25,* 219–237.

Bloodstein, O. (1995). *A handbook on stuttering* (5th ed.). San Diego, CA: Singular Publishing Group, Inc.

Bluemel, C. S. (1957). *The riddle of stuttering.* Danville, IL: Interstate Publishing.

Bothe, A. K. (2002). Speech modification approaches to stuttering treatment in schools. *Seminars in Speech and Language, 23*(3), 181–186.

Brown, S. F. (1945). The loci of stutterings in the speech sequence. *Journal of Speech Disorders, 10,* 181–192.

Comings, D. E, Wu, S., Chiu, C., Ring, R. H., Gade, R., Ahn, C., MacMurray, J. P., Dietz, G., & Muhleman, D. (1996). Polygenic inheritance of Tourette syndrome, stuttering, attention deficit hyperactivity, conduct, and oppositional defiant disorder: The additive and subtractive effect of the three dopaminergic genes—DRD2, D beta H, and DAT1. *American Journal of Medical Genetics, 67*(3), 264–288.

Cooper, E. B., & Cooper, C. S. (1985). Clinician attitudes toward stuttering: A decade of change (1973–1983). *Journal of Fluency Disorders, 10,* 19–33.

Craig, A., Hancock, K., Chang, E., McCready, C., Shepley, A., McCaul, A., Costello, D., Harding, S., Kehren, R., Masel, C., & Reilly, K. (1996). A controlled clinical trial for stuttering in persons aged 9 to 14 years. *Journal of Speech and Hearing Research, 39*(4), 808–826.

Culp, D. M. (1984). The preschool fluency development program: Assessment and treatment. In M. Peins (Ed.), *Contemporary approaches in stuttering therapy* (pp. 39–71). Boston: Little, Brown.

Dayalu, V. N. & Kalinowski, J. (2002). Pseudofluency in adults who stutter: The illusory outcome of therapy. *Perceptual and Motor Skills, 94,* 87–96.

Dayalu, V. N., Kalinowski, J., Stuart, A., Holbert, D., & Rastatter, M. P. (2002). Stuttering frequency on content and function words in adults who stutter: A concept revisited. *Journal of Speech Language and Hearing Research, 45*(5), 871-878.

Dayalu, V. N., Saltuklaroglu, T., Kalinowski, J., Stuart, A., & Rastatter, M.P. (2001). Producing the vowel /a/ prior to speaking inhibits stuttering in adults in the English language. *Neuroscience Letters, 306*(1-2), 111–115.

Eisenson, J. (Ed.). (1958). *Stuttering: A symposium.* New York: Harper & Row, Publishers.

Finn, P., Ingham, R. J., Ambrose, N., & Yairi, E. (1997). Children recovered from stuttering without formal treatment: Perceptual assessment of speech normalcy. *Journal of Speech Language and Hearing Research, 40*(4), 867–876.

Fox, P. T., Ingham, R. J, Ingham, J. C., Hirsch, T. B., Downs, J. H., Martin, C., Jerabek, P., Glass, T., & Lancaster, J. L. (1996). A PET study of the neural systems of stuttering. *Nature, 382*, 158–161.

Guntupalli, V. K., Kalinowski, J., Nanjundeswaran, C., Saltuklaroglu, T., & Everhart, E. (under review). Psychophysiological responses of adults who do not stutter while listening to stuttering. *International Journal of Psychophysiology.*

Harrison, E., Onslow, M., & Menzies, R. (2004). Dismantling the Lidcombe program of early stuttering intervention: Verbal contingencies for stuttering and clinical measurement. *International Journal of Language and Communication Disorders, 39*(2), 257–267.

Hood, S. B (Ed.) (1997). *Stuttering words* (3rd. ed). Memphis, TN: Stuttering Foundation of America.

Howell, P., Au-Yeung, J., & Sackin, S. (1999). Exchange of stuttering from function words to content words with age. *Journal of Speech, Language and Hearing Research, 42*(2), 345–354.

Hubbard, C. P., & Prins, D. (1994). Word familiarity, syllabic stress pattern, and stuttering. *Journal of Speech and Hearing Research, 37*(3), 564–571.

Hulstijn, W., Pascal, H. H. M., Leishout, V., & Peters, H. F. M. (1991). On the measurement of coordination. *Speech motor control and stuttering* (pp. 211–230). Amsterdam–Oxford–New York: Excerpta Medica.

Johnson, W. (1959). *The onset of stuttering: Research, findings and implications.* Minneapolis: University of Minnesota Press.

Johnson, W., & Knott, J. R. (1937). Studies in the psychology of stuttering: I. The distribution of moments of stuttering in successive readings of the same material. *Journal of Speech Disorders, 2*, 17–19.

Jones, M., Onslow, M., Harrison, E., & Packman, A. (2000). Treating stuttering in young children: Predicting treatment time in the Lidcombe Program. *Journal of Speech Language and Hearing Research, 43*(6), 1440–1450.

Kalinowski, A., Kalinowski, J., Stuart, A., & Rastatter, M. P. (1998). A latent trait approach to the development of persistent stuttering. *Perceptual and Motor Skills, 87*, 1331–1358.

Kalinowski, J., Dayalu, V. N., Stuart, A., Rastatter, M. P., Rami, M. K. (2000). Stutter-free and stutter-filled speech signals and their role in stuttering amelioration for English speaking adults. *Neuroscience Letters, 293*(2), 115–118.

Kalinowski, J., & Saltuklaroglu, T. (2003). Choral speech: The amelioration of stuttering via imitation and the mirror neuronal system. *Neuroscience and Biobehavioral Reviews, 27,* 339–347.

Kalinowski, J., Saltuklaroglu, T., Dayalu, V. N., & Guntupalli, V. K. (in press). Is it possible for speech therapy to improve upon natural recovery rates in children who stutter? *International Journal of Language and Communication Disorders, 40,* 1–10.

Kidd, K. K. (1977). A genetic perspective of stuttering. *Journal of Fluency Disorders, 2,* 259–269.

Kidd, K. K., Heimbuch, R. C., & Records, M. A. (1981). Vertical transmission of susceptibility to stuttering with sex- modified expression. *Proceedings of the National Academics of Sciences USA, 78,* 606–610.

Kidd, K. K., Kidd, J. R., & Records, M. A. (1978). The possible causes of the sex ratio in stuttering and its implications. *Journal of Fluency Disorders, 3,* 13–23.

Kingston, M., Huber, A., Onslow, M., Jones, M., & Packman, A. (2003). Predicting treatment time with the Lidcombe program: Replication and meta-analysis. *International Journal of Language and Communication Disorders, 38*(2), 165–177.

Klein, J. F., & Hood, S. B. (2005). The impact of stuttering on employment opportunities and job performance. *Journal of Fluency Disorders, 29*(4), 255–273.

Lutchmaya, S., Baron-Cohen, S., Raggatt, P., Knickmeyer, R., Manning, J. T. (2004). 2nd to 4th digit ratios, fetal testosterone and estradiol. *Early Human Development, 77*(1–2), 23–28.

Mansson, H. (2000). Childhood stuttering—Incidence and development. *Journal of Fluency Disorders, 25*(1), 47–57.

McClean, M. D., Kroll, R. M., & Loftus, N. S. (1991). Correlation of stuttering severity and kinematics of lip closure. *Speech motor control and stuttering* (pp. 117–122). Amsterdam–Oxford–New York: Excerpta Medica.

Meyer, B. C. (1945). Psychosomatic aspects of stuttering. *Journal of Nervous and Mental Disease, 101,* 127–157.

Montgomery, B. M., & Fitch, J. L. (1988). The prevalence of stuttering in the hearing impaired school age population. *Journal of Speech and Hearing Disorders, 53*(2), 131–135.

Neeley, J. N., & Timmons, R. J. (1967). Adaptation and consistency in the disfluent speech behavior of young stutterers and non stutterers. *Journal of Speech and Hearing Research, 10,* 250–256.

Onslow, M. (1996). *The behavioral management of stuttering.* San Diego, CA: Singular Publishing Group.

Onslow, M. (2003). Evidence-based treatment of stuttering: IV. Empowerment through evidence-based treatment practices. *Journal of Fluency Disorders, 28*(3), 237–244.

Onslow, M., Andrews, C., & Lincoln, M. (1994). A control/experimental trial of an operant treatment for early stuttering. *Journal of Speech and Hearing Research, 37*(6), 1244–1259.

Onslow, M., Costa, L., Andrews, C., Harrison, E., & Packman, A. (1996). Speech outcomes of a prolonged-speech treatment for stuttering. *Journal of Speech and Hearing Research, 39*(4), 734–749.

Onslow, M., Menzies, R. G., & Packman, A. (2001). An operant intervention for early stuttering. The development of the Lidcombe program. *Behavior Modification, 25*(1), 116–139.

Onslow, M., Stocker, S., Packman, A., & McLeod, S. (2002). Speech timing in children after the Lidcombe program of early stuttering intervention. *Clinical Linguistics and Phonetics, 16*(1), 21–33.

Perkins, W. H. (1984). Stuttering as a categorical event: Barking up the wrong tree—Reply to Wingate. *Journal of Speech and Hearing Disorders, 49*, 431–434.

Perkins, W. H. (1990). What is stuttering? *Journal of Speech and Hearing Disorders, 55*, 370–382.

Peters, T. J. & Guitar B. (1991). *Stuttering: An integrated approach to its nature and treatment.* Baltimore, MD: Williams & Wilkins.

Rami, M. K., Kalinowski, J., Stuart, A., & Rastatter, M. P. (2003). Self perceptions of speech language pathologists-in-training before and after pseudostuttering experiences on the telephone. *Disability and Rehabilitation, 5*(9), 491–496.

Ratner, N. B. (2004). Caregiver-child interactions and their impact on children's fluency: Implications for treatment. *Language Speech and Hearing Services in School, 35*(1), 46–56.

Saltuklaroglu, T., & Kalinowski, J. (in press). How effective is therapy for childhood stuttering? Dissecting and reinterpreting the evidence in light of spontaneous recovery rates. *International Journal of Language and Communication Disorders.*

Saltuklaroglu, T., Kalinowski, J., & Guntupalli, V. K. (2004). Towards a common neural substrate in the immediate and effective inhibition of stuttering. *International Journal of Neuroscience, 114*, 435–450.

Sheehan, J. G. (1958) In J. Eisenson (Ed.), *Stuttering: A symposium* (pp. 121–166). New York: Harper & Row, Publishers.

Shine, R. E. (1984). Assessment and fluency training and the young stutterers. In M. Peins (Ed.), *Contemporary approaches in stuttering therapy* (pp. 173–211). Boston: Little, Brown.

Shulman, E. (1955). Factors influencing the variability of stuttering. *Stuttering in children and adults* (pp. 207–217). Minneapolis, MN: University of Minnesota Press.

Silverman, F. H. (1996). *Stuttering and other fluency disorders* (2nd ed.) Englewood Cliffs, NJ: Prentice-Hall.

Silverman, F. H. (2004). *Stuttering and other fluency disorders* (3rd ed). Long Grove, IL: Waveland Press Inc.

Sommer, M., Koch, M. A., Paulus, W., Weiller, C., & Buchel, C. (2002). Disconnection of speech-relevant brain areas in persistent developmental stuttering. *Lancet, 360,* 380–383.

Van Riper, C. (1971). *The nature of stuttering.* Englewood Cliffs, NJ: Prentice-Hall, Inc.

Van Riper, C. (1982). *The nature of stuttering* (2nd ed). Englewood Cliffs, NJ: Prentice-Hall, Inc.

Williams, D. E., Silverman, F. H., & Kools, J. A. (1968). Disfluency behavior of elementary school stutterers and nonstutterers: The adaptation effect. *Journal of Speech and Hearing Research, 11,* 622–630.

Williams, D. E., Silverman, F. H., & Kools, J. A. (1969). Disfluency behavior of elementary-school stutterers and non-stutterers: Loci of instances of disfluency. *Journal of Speech and Hearing Research, 12,* 308–318.

Wilson, L., Onslow, M., Lincoln, M. (2004). Telehealth adaptation of the Lidcombe program of early stuttering intervention: Five case studies. *American Journal of Speech Language Pathology, 13*(1), 81–93.

Wingate, M. E. (1964). A standard definition of stuttering. *Journal of Speech and Hearing Disorders, 29,* 484–489.

Wingate, M. E. (1966). Stuttering adaptation and learning. II. The adequacy of learning principles in the interpretation of stuttering. *Journal of Speech and Hearing Disorders, 31*(3), 211–218.

Wingate, M. E. (1982). Early position and stuttering occurrence. *Journal of Fluency Disorders, 7,* 243–258.

Wischner, G. J. (1950). Stuttering behavior and learning: A preliminary theoretical formulation. *Journal of Speech and Hearing Disorders, 15,* 324–335.

Woods, S., Shearsby, J., Onslow, M., & Burnham, D. (2002). Psychological impact of the Lidcombe program of early stuttering intervention. *International Journal of Language and Communication Disorders, 37*(1), 31–40.

World Health Organization. (1977). *Manual of the international classification of diseases, injuries and the causes of death* (Vol. 1). Geneva: Author.

Yairi E. (1981). Disfluencies of normally speaking two-year-old children. *Journal of Speech and Hearing Research, 24*(4), 490–495.

Yairi, E., & Ambrose, N. (1992). A longitudinal study of stuttering in children: A preliminary report. *Journal of Speech and Hearing Research, 35*(4), 755–760.

Yairi, E., & Ambrose, N. G. (1999). Early childhood stuttering I: Persistency and recovery rates. *Journal of Speech Language and Hearing Research, 42*(5), 1097–1112.

Yairi, E., Ambrose, N. G., & Niermann, R. (1993). The early months of stuttering: A developmental study. *Journal of Speech and Hearing Research, 36*(3), 521–528.

Yairi, E., Ambrose, N. G., Paden, E. P., & Throneburg, R. N. (1996). Predictive factors of persistence and recovery: Pathways of childhood stuttering. *Journal of Communication Disorders, 29*(1), 51–77.

Zebrowski, P. M. (1995). The topography of beginning stuttering. *Journal of Communication Disorders, 28*(2), 75–91.

# 3

# Searching for an Invariant to Define Stuttering:

## What Is Necessary and Sufficient for Stuttering and How Do We Assess Its Impact?

> *"The eye sees only what the mind is prepared to comprehend."*
>
> —*Henri Bergson*

It is probably fair to say that almost everyone who has ever studied stuttering has attempted to find the "invariant" in stuttering. A pathologic invariant is simply an entity that is found in every case of the disorder and, hence, may be causally linked to its occurrence. One important criterion for causality is "temporal precedence." That is, for a factor to be considered causal to pathology, it must always occur before (i.e., temporally precede) it. Throughout history, a list of entities has emerged as the possible invariants in stuttering. These have included evil spirits, punishment, enlarged tongues, competing hemispheres, blood chemistry, handedness (Travis, 1931), neuroses, bad habits, and paternal mistreatment (Johnson, 1942). However, in each of these cases, two basic problems exist when trying to establish "invariance" to stuttering. First, the definitions of each are nebulous at best. It can be difficult to define the onset of stuttering and even more so "evil spirits" or even what may be considered an "enlarged tongue." Secondly, none of these factors can be proven to temporally precede cases of stuttering so as to be assigned causality.

Nonetheless, at one time or another, all have been candidates for the invariant in stuttering. That is, they have been considered necessary and/or sufficient in accounting for occurrences of stuttering symptoms. By "necessary," we mean that it needs to be there in every case of stuttering. By "sufficient," we mean that this factor alone is enough to precipitate every stuttering event. For example, the HIV virus is both necessary and sufficient to cause AIDS. Though we may not know the true origin of the HIV virus, we still know that every case of AIDS coincides with its presence. Conversely, if we consider how conception occurs, both a sperm and an egg are necessary, but neither one individually is sufficient. If we ask what is necessary and sufficient for stuttering to occur, the answer is not so clear. Though speech-language pathologists often require the presence of overt stuttering behaviors to diagnose stuttering and chart the course of remediation, it should now be clear that covert avoidance strategies are often used to hide the overt stuttering behaviors. In addition, overtly stuttered speech patterns may be masked by the use of therapy techniques (e.g., droning—via prolonged speech patterns). That is, perhaps therapy procedures replace individual stuttering events with long prolongations produced across entire utterances. If so, can such tenuous and unnatural speech patterns be considered fluent? Obviously, the invariant in stuttering is not found in the disrupted speech patterns themselves.

For another perspective, we may also turn the question around and ask, what is fluent speech? Until not too long ago, it was simply the absence of repetitions and struggle behaviors. Even today this criterion is acceptable by some therapies; namely, those that attempt to "shape" fluent speech in those who stutter. However, finding invariants for both stuttering and fluency is a more complex matter. Whereas stuttering is considerably more than the presence of repetitions, prolongations, and overt struggle behaviors, fluency is considerably more than the absence of these behaviors (Guntupalli, Kalinowski, & Saltuklaroglu, in press). Anyone who stutters knows that simply removing overtly disruptive behaviors does not make speech fluent, and any normally fluent person knows that one or two occurrences of slight nonfluency does not make him or her a "stutterer." Overt stuttering behaviors are simply not the invariants in the disorder. With this in mind, many have traveled the scientific path in search of the stuttering invariant. Once it became accepted that stuttering could best be attributed to organic or physiologic deficits, scientists in the speech motor paradigm (e.g., Adams, Agnello, Watson, Alfonso, etc.) began to examine dynamic control in the speech motor periphery (e.g., lungs, larynx, and articulators). Later, the search for invariants moved higher toward the brain. To better understand our model of stuttering and how it arose, it is necessary for students to have a brief understanding of the search for an organic invariant in stuttering.

## Separation of Causes and Effects of Stuttering

Although psychologic and environmental factors may exacerbate occurrences of stuttering once the pathology has developed, they do not appear to be accountable for its origin. Thus, when searching for an organic invariant, the speech motor periphery became the primary target for examination, as this was where the manifestations of the disorder occurred. Thus, it was assumed that the proximal (i.e., visible) disturbances might also be sources of causal agents in the disorder. This is similar to a criminal investigation during which detectives begin their examination with those closest to the scene of the crime to determine if they were the culprits responsible or just other victims who happened to be near. Medical investigations work in the same manner, beginning by examining the site of lesion and then working outward until the true distal etiology of pathology is known.

As we have previously outlined, numerous hypotheses have been offered to explain stuttering. To those espousing them, these hypotheses made logical, intuitive, and coherent sense. When scientifically scrutinized, however, their underlying notions are wanting at best or simply untestable, leaving us in a conundrum. Factors such as evil spirits, punishment for sin, neuroses, internal conflicts, and overly perfectionist parents have all been largely discredited as causal agents in stuttering. Even the iconic statuses of people like Freud and Johnson could not carry their theories without the evidence to bolster them. Though Johnson seemed to be onto something special, achieving about 80% recovery in children, his notions of parental labeling could not prove to be an invariant in the disorder, especially considering that his explanations were made in a "post hoc" (after the fact) manner. That is, only after children continued to stutter were the parents blamed for the critical manner in which they interacted with them, removing any element of predictive validity from Johnson's approach and, at the same time, discrediting his search for an invariant.

Early organic factors such as the notion that those who stutter had enlarged tongues have also been discredited. Oral surgeons such as Dieffenbach removed V-shaped wedges from the tongues of persons who stuttered in attempts to make the tongue more flexible and better fit the oral cavity (Lebrun & Bayle, 1973). Initial results looked promising. The use of novel speech patterns imposed by the sensitivity of the wound produced reduced levels of stuttering, and the oral surgeon was hailed a miracle worker. Sadly, after the tongue healed, stuttering usually returned, again discrediting any notion that the stuttering invariant was the enlarged tongue. This was an early attempt to uncover an organic invariant in stuttering. Travis' (1931, p. 338) competing hemispheres hypothesis was another organic theory of stuttering invariance that yielded little therapeutic efficacy. However, the notion of an organic invariant would later resurface and play a large role in the way scientists have viewed and therapists have treated the disorder.

From the 1970s and until the early 1990s, the speech motor dynamics paradigm in stuttering prospered. Marcel Wingate's "vocalization hypothesis" (Wingate, 1969) and Martin Adams' empirical work (Adams, 1985) on voicing frequency and laryngeal reaction times in persons who stutter drove the bedrock of this "rush to larynx." Wingate's theory, though nebulous, inferred laryngeal behavior as an agent in stuttering and enumerated conditions that changed laryngeal behavior as ameliorative agents (e.g., singing, whispering). Adams and his colleagues made a case for laryngeal differences in people who stutter and spread beyond the laryngeal mechanism to respiratory and articulatory systems. As the "source" of acoustic energy for speech, the larynx seemed an obvious choice for examination. Differences found between stuttered and nonstuttered speech at the laryngeal level were thought to illuminate the nature of the disorder. Both these researchers were probably correct in looking at vocal "gestures" but the final or distal "object" of these laryngeal manipulations would lie outside the physical speech production mechanism per se. In other words, although behaviors of the larynx may be quite different during stuttering and fluent speech, perhaps they are different simply because the speech is fluent or stuttered and these laryngeal behaviors may not be causal invariants in stuttering. Nevertheless, the hunt was on for differences between persons who stutter and those who did not.

Everybody knew that stuttered speech was acoustically (with respect to its sound) and kinematically (with respect to the movements of the articulators) different from fluent speech. Stuttered speech contains repetitions, prolongations, dysrhythmic phonations, as well as numerous other overt struggle behaviors that are absent in fluent speech of normal speakers. We do not need technologic advances (e.g., cinefluourography, EMG [electromyograpy], EMMA [electromagnetic midsagittal articulometry], X-ray microbeam, etc.) to continuously remind us that the speech periphery in those who stutter is operating in a different manner from normal speakers. But, the question still remained: is it working in an invariantly different manner? That is, are all stuttering events common in some overt, physiologic way that signals an etiologic or causal agent.

Although it appeared clear to most that the observed differences between stuttered and fluent speech were simply the effects of stuttering rather than causes of it, scientists looked for a "stuttered invariance" to signal a causal agent in the pathology. Zimmermann (1980) showed evidence of differences in interarticulator positioning in people who stuttered prior to moments of repetitive stuttering or silent postural fixations, but not for all participants. Freeman and Ushijama (1978) used electromyography (EMG) to show that stuttering was associated with higher levels of laryngeal muscle activity relative to fluent speech. They showed different relationships between abductor and adductor muscles that were interpreted by the authors to show "a laryngeal component in stuttering," but again the invariant was intermittent. For example, participant DM showed cocontraction of the posterior cricoarytenoid (PCA) and the lateral cricoarytenoid (LCA) occurring during stuttering. This was the first real physiologic sign of difference between these two groups and it was dramatic. The PCA is an abductor and the LCA is an adductor of the vocal fold and they are not supposed to be working in opposition. In an acoustic analysis of stuttered speech, six of ten stuttering participants showed rhythmic spectral oscillations between frequencies of 5 and 12 Hz that were not observed in any of the nonstuttering control group. Not surprisingly, these spectral oscillations occurred during stuttering events and also generally coincided with frequencies of oscillation in muscles of the jaw, lip, and neck (ancillary stuttering) that were reflected in high levels of muscle activity found in EMG data. High amplitude gains and increases in frequency for EMG data are typically observed in those who stutter severely and are characteristic of tense, struggle-filled oscillations found in severe blocks. Simply put, the more the speech system is pushed via long block, the more likely it is that the system will produce behaviors that result in higher EMG amplitudes. However, these behaviors may not be present in milder cases of stuttering in which participants may produce EMG amplitudes that vary little from normally fluent speakers. As such, they cannot be considered a necessary invariant in stuttering. In other words, when examining behaviors of the speech musculature associated with stuttering, the use of severe participants can produce events that are so different from normal speech production that they may have appeared to be revealing something important about the pathology. However, the high oscillatory behaviors that are seen in the EMG data simply show what occurs when severe stutterers struggle with speech production. Instead of revealing an invariant in stuttered speech, this study simply employed measures that effectively captured severe levels of stuttering. Even more compelling was that, even for participant DM, all signs of aberrant EMG activity were removed when he produced fluent speech while under choral (speaking in unison with another speaker) conditions. The use of choral speech to eliminate all signs of stuttering has also been used in brain imaging studies and constitutes a problem for those seeking an omnipresent invariant (Fox et al., 1996). That is, if the simple presence of an additional acoustic speech signal can eliminate all evidence of stuttering without any imposed motoric manipulations to speech, then it is highly unlikely that any invariant exists in any of the observable mechanical processes of speech production. In subsequent chapters we continue to examine the magic of choral speech as we look at possible invariants in the "inhibition" of stuttering.

Other works have examined the "moment of stuttering" and variable findings have also been found. For example Smith et al. (1996) found that moments of stuttering were not associated with high levels of laryngeal muscle activation. In an earlier study Smith et al. (1993) found that only some participants in the study showed the presence of tremorlike oscillations in both orofacial and laryngeal muscles which the authors suggested may have become "entrained" via autonomic activity. When these data are examined with the Freeman and Ushijama (1978) study, we see that a great deal of variability can exist in the functioning of laryngeal muscles during stuttering, and that it is highly unlikely that a laryngeal invariant in stuttering will be found. For the most part, we have yielded to the idea that an invariant will likely not be found here and that most findings are reflections of stuttering severity, developmental history of stuttering, and therapy effects. Thus, this line of studies made use of the latest in technology and simply highlighted what was perceptually evident to anyone observing—that stuttered and fluent speech are indeed different but that they are different in different ways for various participants and there is no invariant in the stuttering event per se.

It became obvious that comparisons between stuttered and fluent speech were analogous to comparing apples and oranges. They were clearly different entities and the search for an acoustic or kinematic "stuttered" invariant would prove to be futile. Therefore, in an attempt to compare apples with apples, the next logical step was to examine the perceptually fluent speech (as defined by an absence of overt stuttering, though not necessarily normal sounding speech) of those who stutter with the speech of normally fluent speakers. The speech motor dynamics paradigm focused on uncovering the organic factors by examining the perceptually fluent speech of those who stuttered and those who did not with the goal of trying to find a consistent or "invariant" difference that might be linked to stuttering. Acoustic measures were used initially and most frequently because they were accessible and easily interpretable. However, these were not direct measures of the speech production system and were limited in their scope (Armson & Kalinowski, 1994). Investigators became more aggressive in their assault on speech production mechanism and indirect measures became inadequate. As such, studies began to make use of direct spatial and temporal measures (duration, displacement, velocity, acceleration, jerk of the lip, tongue jaw, etc.) of speech production, which were obtained via respiratory inductive plethysmography (Respitrace), optoelectronic position tracking system (Selspot) of articulators, X-ray microbeam tracking of articulators, electroglottography (EGG), photoglottography (PGG), and so forth. A series of acoustic studies failed to reveal differences between the fluent speech of those who stuttered and those who did not, with respect to pause time (Few & Lingwall, 1972), voice onset time (Borden, Baer, & Kenny, 1985; Zebrowski, Conture, & Cudahy, 1985), acoustic reaction time (Cullinan & Springer, 1980; Watson & Alfonso, 1987), segment duration (Healey & Adams, 1981; Zebrowski 1991), and articulatory rate (Gronohovd, 1977; Healey & Adams, 1981; Perkins, 1975). Furthermore, a number of kinematic studies examining movement duration, amplitude, and velocity failed to yield differences between stutterers and nonstutterers (e.g., Caruso et al., 1988; Conture, Colton, & Gleason, 1988; Goldsmith, 1983). However, it should be noted that all these studies employed either mild stutterers or children who stuttered but had less developmental history of stuttering, a factor that is discussed in the next section. That is, they probably had "less" of the pathology, making it difficult to detect differences, if any were present, in their overtly fluent speech as compared to normally fluent speakers. In the next section, we discuss how having "more" or "less" of the stuttering pathology can influence the nature of speech that is otherwise perceptually fluent.

Although these studies appeared to suggest that perceptually fluent speech was essentially produced in the same manner, regardless of who produced it (e.g., stutterer or nonstutterer), a number of other studies seemed more compelling as they revealed differences in the perceptually fluent speech of the two populations. For example, in the acoustic domain, it was found that the perceptually fluent speech of persons who stuttered when compared to the fluent speech of normally fluent speech of nonstutterers demonstrated increased pause times (Love & Jeffress, 1971), longer voice onset times (Agnello, 1975; Healey & Gutkin, 1984; Hillman & Gilbert, 1977), longer reaction time for initiating phonation (e.g., Adams & Hayden, 1976; Cross & Luper, 1983; Starkweather, Hirschman, & Tannenbaum, 1976; Watson & Alfonso, 1987), longer segment durations (Colcord & Adams, 1979; DiSimoni, 1974; Starkweather & Meyers, 1979), and slower articulation rates (Borden, 1983; Ramig, Krieger, & Adams, 1982). In addition, kinematic studies (i.e., studies examining movement) have shown differences in articulator placement and sequencing in those who stutter relative to normally fluent speakers (Story, Alfonso, & Harris, 1996; Zimmermann, 1980). Watson and Alfonso (1987) found different coordination patterns for respiration and phonation at the onset of phonation during an acoustic reaction time task. A stuttering group initiated the muscular process of exhalation prior to vocal fold adduction, whereas in the normal control group, this sequence was reversed. Differences between stuttering and nonstuttering groups for articulator sequencing have also been found by Caruso et al. (1988), Story, Alfonso, and Harris (1996) and McClean et al. (1990), who used a group of "treated" stutterers. In addition to reversals in articulatory sequencing, McClean et al. (1990) showed that treated stutterers exhibited longer times to reach peak velocity in the movements of the upper lip, lower lip, and jaw during productions of the nonsense word "sappaple." These findings were corroborated by Pindzola (1986), who found lower velocities in articulator movement in fluent vowel-consonant-vowel productions of those who stuttered relative to a nonstuttering group. It should be noted, that compared to the studies that did not reveal differences in the fluent speech of stutterers and nonstutterers, these studies made use of relatively severe stuttering groups, in which any differences were more readily apparent or more influenced by the presence of the stuttering pathology.

Findings such as these led scientists to believe that those who stutter had diminished motor capacities for speech production, as shown by statements such as those made by Adams (1985), "the speech production abilities of those who stutter are inherently inferior to those of normal speakers" (p. 186), and Caruso et al. (1988) when they suggested that stuttering occurs due to "a specific impairment in multiple movement coordination associated with the sequencing of those movements" (p. 439). In other words, the manner in which people who stuttered produced their fluent speech was temporally (takes more time) and spatially (smaller ranges of movements) different from normally fluent speakers, resulting in slight differences in the speech acoustics of the perceptually fluent speech of those who stutter relative to normal nonstutterers. Thus, it was suggested that these differences might indicate an ever-present chronic pathology that could explain overt intermittent unstable speech acts (e.g., repetitions and prolongations). However, the problem separating cause and effect arose. Kalinowski and Armson, et al. (1994) examined the bulk of studies that found differences between the fluent speech samples of stutterers and nonstutterers and concluded that even the fluent speech of those who stutter cannot be free of the influence of stuttering. They outlined four possible ways that some component of stuttering can contaminate fluent speech samples in those who stutter.

## 1. Sample Context

When we count stuttering for assessment purposes, we tend to view stuttered and fluent syllables as dichotomous or categoric events—either stuttered or fluent. However, this categoric distinction does not appear to be appropriate. Even though some syllables or words may appear perceptually fluent, they may be influenced by the stuttering on adjacent words or syllables. For example, Knox (1975) and Vishwanath (1989) both showed that the durations of words spoken fluently were shorter when they preceded fluent speech than when they preceded stuttered speech. In other words, it appeared that those who stutter may have intentionally or unintentionally been "slowing down" in anticipation of the upcoming stuttering event. A person who stutters may persistently "slow down" when stuttering in anticipation of stuttering, yet it may be exaggerated when a significant stuttering moment occurs. Therapeutically, this certainly is a helpful strategy and, once used, may become self-taught and consistently implemented. Thus, it is not surprising that it was found in these studies.

This influence of stuttering on otherwise perceptually fluent speech productions is known as "subperceptual stuttering" and has been made apparent in a number of other studies. Subperceptual forms of stuttering are captured by sophisticated measurement tools and may be indiscernible to the ear or eye. They simply reflect stuttering at deeper levels of the speech production system (i.e., acoustic, kinematic, and neuromuscular levels). Freeman (1984) acknowledged the existence of subperceptual forms of stuttering, stating that, "stuttering is a problem of frequently occurring physiological blocks, only a percentage of which result in listener identified disfluencies" (p. 111). Furthermore, Alfonso (1990) suggested that even if an utterance produced by a person who stutters is deemed fluent by an experienced listener, a deeper analysis at the kinematic or neuromuscular level may reveal evidence of disfluent features (e.g., subperceptual forms of stuttering). Other evidence exists to support these statements. For example, acoustic subperceptual stuttering has been revealed in the presence of isolated pitch pulses before continuous phonation (Watson & Alfonso, 1987). In this study, these researchers elected to eliminate 22% and 27% of "perceptually fluent" in mild and severe stutterers, respectively, on a phonatory reaction time task. The tokens discarded may be considered evidence of inaudible, subperceptual stuttering. This type of evidence has also been seen at a kinematic level. For example, Story (1990) found aberrant respiratory and laryngeal activity before the production of fluent utterances in stuttering subjects. In addition, while conducting research at a neuromuscular level, Freeman and Ushijima (1978) uncovered evidence of discoordination in the muscles of the larynx in those who stutter prior to the initiation of perceptually fluent speech that was similar to the activity observed prior to the initiation of stuttered speech. These findings were considered physiologic evidence of stuttering behaviors that were inaudible or visibly apparent

(Freeman, 1984). It is impossible for observers to quantify all stuttering behaviors found below the surface level of speech production, no matter how sophisticated the measurement tool they use. Persons who stutter can sense a physiologic block in any or all the respiratory, laryngeal, and articulatory speech subsystems that may or may not "jump out" in the kinematic or acoustic signals. These differences may simply be longer durations, smaller amplitudes, rearranged peaked velocities, and a host of other measures that suggest difficulties in the temporal and spatial parameters of speech, even when perceptually fluent. Boberg (1981) also made reference to subperceptual stuttering when discussing relapse from therapy. He used the term "microstuttering" to describe the tiny blockages in speech that the stutterer feels but do not come to the surface as "countable" stuttering behaviors. Thus, evidence of these subperceptual "microstutters" provide additional support for the tenuous and unstable nature of post-therapeutic speech.

## 2. Treatment History

Behavioral therapies for stuttering attempt to retrain the speech motor system to produce stutter-free speech. This is often accomplished by continued practice of novel speech patterns that vary considerably from normal. Rather than being produced "automatically" and naturally, therapeutic speech has learned, methodical quality that is often overtly characterized by "droning" as a result of slow movements from one articulatory trajectory to another. The purpose of slowing down speech is to slow it to a rate where "fluent behaviors" can be inserted into the production stream and stuttering behaviors can be removed. It is believed that normal speech rates make this difficult and that a dramatic slowing process is necessary for the integration of new fluency-generating behaviors. Perceptually, this speech sounds unnatural to the listener and can feel unnatural to the person producing it. Droned speech may also be different from normal speech in the coordination of laryngeal and respiratory movements, articulatory pressures, and relative proportions of voicing during speech. Thus, it may not be surprising that after intensive therapies that attempt to ingrain these speech characteristics into the peripheral motor systems of those who stutter, acoustic and kinematic differences are found between the fluent therapeutic speech of stutterers when compared to the fluent speech of normals. For example, after treatment stutterers showed increased voice onset time (Metz, Onufrak, & Ogburn, 1979; Shenker & Finn, 1985), longer duration of vowels (Mallard & Kelley, 1982; Mallard & Westbrook, 1985; Metz et al., 1979; Metz, Samar & Sacco, 1983; Onufrak, 1980; Ramig, 1984; Robb, Lybolt, & Prince, 1985; Samar, Metz, & Sacco, 1986; Story, 1990), and increased proportion of voiced segments (Franken, 1987). All these acoustic differences are thought to contribute to the unnatural quality that has been attributed to post-therapeutic speech (Franken, Boves, Peters, & Webster, 1992; Kalinowski, Noble et al., 1994; Martin, Haroldson, & Tilden, 1984; Runyan & Adams, 1979; Runyan, Bell, & Prosek, 1990). As stated, McClean et al. (1990) found that, relative to normal speakers, treated stutterers showed reversals in articulatory sequencing when producing the word "sappple." These reversals were thought to be a direct result of the therapy. Thus, it appears that even when instructed not to use therapeutic strategies, the effects of therapy may influence the speech of those who stutter. Armson and Kalinowski (1994) perhaps best summarize the effects of therapy on the fluent speech of those who stutter by stating:

> Simply put, pervasive alterations occur as a result of an overgeneralized use of stuttering prevention strategies. Therefore, alterations in the fluent speech characteristics of stutterers after treatment should be considered to be a contaminating effect, related specifically, though indirectly, to episodes of stuttering (p. 74).

## 3. Stuttering Severity

Considering that "severe" stutterers generally exhibit more frequent and longer disruptions of speech than their milder counterparts, we also may expect fluent speech productions of more severe stutterers to exhibit higher levels of subpercetpual stuttering. McClean et al. (1990) examined this notion in a kinematic study. They found that severe stuttering was associated with longer movement durations and velocities than mild stuttering. The higher movement durations of severe stutterers was also corroborated by Samar et al. (1986). Interestingly, in both these studies, the longer durations and velocities of the severe stutterers were similar to those found in stutterers who had undergone treatment (e.g., McClean et al., 1990), again lending support to the notion of contamination by therapy.

Acoustic reaction time studies also provide evidence of higher subperceptual stuttering levels related to more severe stuttering. Armson and Kalinowski (1994) re-examined a large body of literature that demonstrated increased acoustic reaction times of stutterers relative to nonstutterers. Of the 23 studies examined that were conducted between 1976 and 1992, seven failed to provide information regarding stuttering severity. In the other 17 studies, these authors noted a disproportionate use of moderate and severe stutterers as compared to mild stutters. They speculated that the "overuse" of more severe stutterers helped increase the difference in acoustic reaction times between the two populations. In other words, moderate and severe stutterers were more likely to stutter during an acoustic reaction time task, thus increasing the latency of their responses. The authors also speculated that if milder subjects were used, the amount of difference between the two populations might be considerably less, perhaps even to the point of failing to achieve statistical significance. The notion of using severe stutterers is not all that illogical. It operates on the assumption that those who stutter more have more of the pathology and the causation will more likely be found in these individuals. The illogical nature of this premise is that it excludes all the rest of those who stutter and fail to exhibit the differences under observation.

## 4. Developmental History

In the previous chapter we discussed the development of stuttering, how it progresses from incipient to advanced forms, and the series of compensations that may develop along the way. Thus, it may be speculated that incipient stuttering is the "purest" form of the pathology, in which stuttering is predominantly characterized by syllabic repetitions and is relatively free from covert behaviors and other reactionary compensations. With this in mind, it has been suspected that studying the fluency of children may provide information on inherent capacities of those who stutter to produce fluent speech (Conture et al., 1988; Stromsta, 1986). However, as with the data obtained from adults who stutter, data from the fluent speech of children who stutter has provided mixed findings. Upon analysis of a number of these studies (e.g., Conture, Rothenberg, & Molitor, 1986; Cross & Luper, 1979; Cullinan & Springer, 1980; Healey & Adams, 1981; McKnight & Cullinan, 1987; Murphy & Baumgartner, 1981; Till, Reich, Dickey, & Seiber, 1983; Winkler & Ramig, 1986; Zebrowski et al., 1985), Armson and Kalinowski concluded that the likelihood of significant differences in the fluent speech of stuttering and nonstuttering children increases with age. That is, in preschool or early school-age populations, where stuttering is at its incipient stages, the fluent speech of stuttering children is likely to be perceptually, acoustically, and kinematically indistinguishable from the speech of nonstutterers. As the pathology develops with age and fluent speech becomes contaminated with the possibility of stuttering, as well as anticipatory reactions and compensations for stuttering, acoustic and kinematic differences in otherwise perceptually fluent speech are more likely to be found between the fluent speech of stuttering and nonstuttering children.

In summary, the influence of stuttering may permeate speech acoustics and kinematics as a function of at least four factors, as outlined above. As such, if stuttering can permeate speech acoustics and kinematics, which are representative of articulatory, respiratory, and laryngeal functioning, then the source of stuttering cannot be in these areas and the speech motor paradigm is essentially flawed due to its failure to separate causes and effects of stuttering. After seven years working on a doctoral dissertation from within this paradigm, the first author (JK) made this realization. The Armson and Kalinowski (1994) treatise followed and brought this issue into the research spotlight. Since then, though the occasional publication surfaces (e.g., McClean et al., 2004), research from this standpoint has diminished because of the difficulties that arise in separating causes and effects of stuttering.

# Stuttering and the Brain

Failure to find anything causal to stuttering in the motor periphery led back to examinations of the brains of those who stutter. In the 1990s modern brain imaging techniques (e.g., positron emission tomography [PET], functional magnetic resonance imaging [fMRI], and magnetoencephalography [MEG]) that allow scientists to take pictures of the brain and relate them to cerebral anatomy and physiology became more readily available to examine a variety of disorders (e.g., Parkinson's disease, schizophrenia, Huntington's disease, personality disorders, Tourette's syndrome, etc.). The problems separating causes and effects of stuttering in the "fluent" speech paradigm began to lead the focus of investigation away from the speech periphery and up to higher centers of control in the brain. Thus, the notion was furthered that stuttering had to be a result of some aberrant functioning of the brain during speech production (Braun et al., 1997, Fox et al., 1996, Wu et al., 1997) and, therefore, the timing was right for stuttering to become a prime candidate for investigation using brain imaging techniques.

During speech tasks, numerous differences in the cerebral activation patterns of those who stutter and normally fluent speakers have been revealed. For example, studies have found stuttering to be associated with increased activity in motor regions such as the supplementary motor area and superior lateral premotor cortex with right lateralization (Fox et al., 1996), left anterior cingulate and inferior prefrontal cortex (De Nil et al., 2000), right frontal operculum (Preibisch et al., 2003), frontomotor areas, parietal, temporal, limbic, and insular areas of the right hemisphere (Neumann et al., 2003). Further, suppression or deactivation relative to normal speakers has been found in the primary auditory association areas, left inferior frontal cortex (Fox et al., 1996, Ingham et al., 2000), posterior regions of the brain (Braun et al., 1997), and precentral gyrus (Preibisch et al., 2003). In summary, regions of the brain that are considered responsible for helping to coordinate speech production, as well as those that are involved in processing speech and language, show different patterns of neural activity when someone stutters relative to normal speakers.

The leap that some have made in interpreting these types of findings is that the observed differences in neurophysiology may be causal to stuttering. In the first chapter we stated that the separation of cause and effect would be a theme throughout this text. When interpreting data from brain imaging, this separation becomes paramount. Aside from the differences found between stutterers and fluent speakers during speech tasks, a number of other findings related to brain imaging and stuttering should be mentioned that detract from the likelihood that the aberrant activation patterns associated with stuttering are causal to the pathology.

First, when people who stutter and normally fluent people are silent, no differences are noted in the cerebral functioning of the two groups, indicating that any observed differences are related to the execution of speech. Second, an unpublished study presented at the 2002 American Speech and Hearing Association (ASHA) convention revealed that normally fluent speakers who produced pseudo- or fake stuttering behaviors elicited similar patterns of cerebral activation to people who stutter when stuttering (Ingham, 2002). Third, Ingham et al. (2000), found that the similar aberrant patterns of neural activity could be obtained when people who stutter simply thought about stuttering. They did not have to be stuttering per se, but men- tally going through the process of stuttering was sufficient to elicit aberrant neural patterns. In other words, the brain may produce these types of aberrant activations simply upon the self- perception of stuttering. If actual overt stuttering is not required to produce these patterns of activation, then it is likely that these types of activations are associated with the effects rather than the causes of stuttering. Fourth, a number of imaging studies (e.g., Fox et al., 1996; Ingham et al., 2000; Wu et al., 1995) have clearly shown that when those who stutter speak completely fluently, such as when speaking in unison with another speaker (more on this "choral speech" phenomenon later), their brain activation patterns become relatively normalized and are almost indistinguishable from those of normally fluent speakers. In other words, when speaking fluently pathologic signs of neuro- logic activation are virtually eliminated, again suggesting that aberrant neural activity is an effect rather than a cause of stuttering.

The studies described above are neurophysiologic studies, meaning that they relate to cerebral functioning. Another research group, based out of Tulane University has sought to investigate differences in cerebral anatomy between stutterers and nonstutterers. Foundas, Bollich, Corey, Hurley, and Heilman (2001) used MRI to determine differences in anatomy around the sylvian fissure (specifically an area called the planum temporale that runs deep from the posterior of the sylvian fissure) that are associated with speech and language. Foundas' group later found evidence of asymmetries in the prefrontal and occipital lobes of those who stutter (Foundas et al., 2003). This finding has been corroborated by Jancke, Hanggi, and Steinmetz (2004), who also found evidence of anatomic differences in perisylavian and prefrontal areas as well as sensorimotor areas of the brain. Interestingly Foundas' group has gone on to relate some of their findings with respect to atypical planum temporale development to positive responses to delayed auditory feedback (DAF) for reducing stuttering. DAF is examined in depth in subsequent chapters. It changes the timing schedule on which a person hears his or her own speech (creating the illusion of a second speaker). Foundas et al. (2004) have suggested that positive responses to DAF may somehow compensate for aberrations in planum temporale development.

The anatomic differences described above are both interesting and compelling. However, as with the physiologic studies, the separation of cause and effect still cannot be made (Jancke, Hanggi, & Steinmetz, 2004). It does not seem surprising to us that the brains of those who stutter not only show differences in function, but structural differences due to years of stuttering. This factor seems especially possible considering that the studies examining anatomic differences were all conducted on adults. It is possible that repeated communication failures, struggle, and use of compensatory behaviors over the years may have led to the observed anatomic differences.

So where do we stand now? The confluence of evidence suggests that origin of stuttering and the invariant in stuttering has to be found somewhere in the brain, simply because it appears to be nowhere else and the brain is the highest center of speech production. However, regardless of where the origin lies, current brain imaging techniques do not appear to be powerful enough to shed sufficient light on the nature of the stuttering brain. The author (JK) once made an analogy regarding the current state of brain imaging technology: trying to understand the workings of the human brain by using current imaging methods is like trying to understand human civilization by taking pictures of the earth from outer space. Simply put, we still do not have the combined spatial or temporal resolution to pinpoint stuttering to a specific pattern of neuronal activation. However, that may only be the start of our problems. Considering the complexity of the human brain, and its capacity for overlapping functions and parallel processing, we may be years away from understanding how even normal speech is produced and perceived at a neural level. Some speculate that stuttering may also be related to aspects of language development (Dworzynski & Howell, 2004; Melnick, Conture, & Ohde, 2003; Natke et al., 2004; Nippold, 2004; Watkins & Johnson, 2004; Weiss, 2000), although this relationship also remains unclear considering that our understanding of language development is hindered by many of the same factors that hinder our understanding of speech production and stuttering. However, when we discuss the mechanism that is thought to inhibit stuttering, we will discuss a possible relationship of stuttering and its inhibition to language development.

## Our Model

In light of the data and arguments presented above, we consider the origin of stuttering to occur at a central neurologic level. By addressing the nature of stuttering and by using deductive reasoning, we have concluded that the most parsimonious means of accounting for stuttering is via the occurrence of a "central involuntary block." That is, stuttering occurs in the brain (i.e., centrally), it is not under volitional control (i.e., involuntary), and it disrupts the flow of speech (i.e., a block). We make no assumptions as to the origin of the block although the predisposition for it appears to be present from birth and may be influenced by both genetic and environmental factors. It could be that it occurs due to some slight chemical imbalance of neuronal misfiring that we have yet to detect. It seems most likely that any precipitating events come together during a critical period of time during linguistic development to produce a neural "hitch" in the speech-producing mechanism. However, due to the rapid development and plasticity of children's brains, we cannot say how long these precipitating events may be present. The neural hitch or involuntary block seems to be most effectively overcome during this incipient stage of stuttering by the involuntary production of repetitious speech behaviors that somehow help heal up to 80% of children afflicted with this brief neural imperfection. However, with the continued use of this mechanism and increasing severity of the block in those children who do not recover, this healing mechanism seems to run "amuck,"The after-effects of the initial neural hitch become hardwired into the speech production mechanism as ingrained patterns of stuttering, hence, becoming the pathologic condition.

Regardless of our speculations as to its origin, we have no way to know for sure where or how stuttering originates. Neither do we have any means of knowing whether the neural block is due to relative increases or decreases in activation levels in areas of the brain. All we can be sure of regarding the block is, whatever forces are at work to create it, the cumulative effect is a disruption in speech, and all the other phenomena that comprise the syndrome of stuttering. By using the notion of a central involuntary block, we describe a theoretical factor that can be both necessary and sufficient for the manifestation of all stuttering symptoms and many phenomena associated with the removal or inhibition of its symptoms. A morbid though compelling analogy is comparing stuttering to what is necessary and sufficient to cause every human death. The only thing both necessary and sufficient to cause every human death is lack of oxygen to the brain. Numerous factors (observable or invisible) may contribute to the anoxic condition, but death is the invariable result. In stuttering, we still do not know the contributing factors, but the central involuntary block can be analogous to the lack of oxygen, in that its occurrence is necessary and sufficient to begin and advance the stuttering syndrome. As such, the model

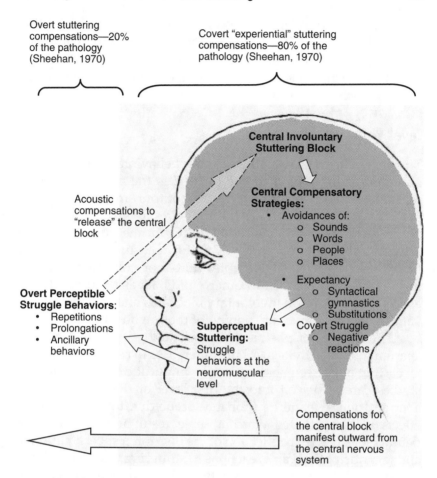

**Figure 3–1.** A minimalist model of stuttering.

displayed in Figure 3–1 may provide a parsimonious explanation of stuttering behaviors.

This "minimalist" model operates by assuming that a simple central involuntary neural block is responsible for all symptoms of stuttering and that all the observed phenomena associated with stuttering (e.g., overt and covert behaviors) are merely symptoms of or compensations for the centrally originating neural blockage. We have outlined three "levels" at which stuttering symptomatology can manifest. By placing the truly invisible behaviors at level 1 and the truly visible behaviors at level 3, this model also accounts for the subperceptual stuttering behaviors described above at level 2, somewhere between the overt and the covert. As such, the levels of stuttering emanating from the central block are as follows:

## Level 1

This level encompasses all stuttering behaviors that cannot be observed using the naked eye (or ear, as the case may be), or sensitive equipment that measures output from the speech periphery such as Respitrace (for measures of lung displacement and volumes), electromyography (EMG, for measures of muscle activity), photoglottography (PGG, for measures of vocal fold functioning), electropalatography (EPG, for collecting articulatory data), and so forth. In other words, level 1 represents the effects that the central involuntary block has on the cerebral activations and cognitive functioning of those who stutter.

The first set of phenomena associated with level 1 are the aberrant neural activities. All the differences in cerebral activation levels that have been observed in the multitude of neuroimaging studies can be placed into the first level of this model. These aberrant neural patterns probably occur due to the combined effects of at least three factors: (a) direct result of the involuntary neural blockage, (b) a reflection of the disrupted speech patterns, and (c) anticipations and reactions to stuttering. As such, as well as the possibility of activation patterns being directly affected by the neural block, aberrant activations are probably also the neural reflections of overt and covert stuttering events. For example, using MEG, Salmelin, Schnitzler, Schmitz, and Freund (2000), found that on a single-word production task, cerebral activation in normal speakers began in the left inferior frontal cortex (an area of articulatory programming) and then spread on the left lateral central sulcus and dorsal premotor cortex (areas of motor preparation). However, in stutterers the activation sequence occurred in reverse and was slightly out of temporal synchrony as compared to the nonstutterers. This suggests that possibly because of anticipated initiation difficulties due to stuttering, those who stutter began to prepare their speech periphery for production before developing the articulatory plan to produce the intended word. Thus, this observed difference in neural activity probably reflects a covert compensation for anticipated stuttering.

Another stuttering phenomenon that falls into level 1 is the presence of the covert behaviors themselves, or the "experiential" components of stuttering. As mentioned before, these include avoidance of sounds, words, people, places, and situations; and circumlocutions, substitutions that are constantly employed and constitute an ongoing series of "syntactic gymnastics." These events do not occur as a direct result of the involuntary block, but are cognitive strategies that develop to compensate for it and possibly postpone another occurrence of the block. These are also considered symptoms of the block, albeit later developing and covert in nature, or indirectly manifesting symptoms. For example, after numerous negative reactions from others to overt behaviors, people who stutter refrain from ominous tasks such as using the telephone or speaking with strangers, ordering in a restaurant, and so forth (Kalinowski et al., 1998; Woolf, 1967). The continuous "scanning ahead" in search of potential "landmine" words that can be replaced by easier words is another example of covert syntactic gymnastics. In other words, all the behaviors that the person who stutters employs either consciously or subconsciously to reduce the frequency of overt stuttering can be considered level 1 compensations for stuttering. Perkins (1971) aptly described these covert compensations by stating, "from outside looking in, stuttering can be quite different from the inside looking out."

Also falling under the level 1 umbrella are covert struggle behaviors such as the "loss of control" and the negative reactions to stuttering. Covert struggle represents the degree of mental effort exerted when stuttering, when seeking a way to avoid overt stuttering (e.g., approach-avoidance conflicts toward speaking situations), as well as the effort expended trying to maintain the façade of normalcy during speech production. The struggle to achieve normalcy can be associated with the effortful and tenuous use of therapeutic methods, as well as attempts to make the resultant speech sound natural without allowing overt stuttering to surface. Negative reactions to stuttering are exactly that—the negative emotions that people who stutter invariably experience when their speech failures are out of their control, destined to occur and recur, and evoke the strange, humiliating, and condescending reactions from others. In other words, it is these negative reactions that, over time, wear down the person who stutters and create the shell of communicative handicap in which they often live. Thus, all covert behaviors represent the "experiential nature" of the disorder, from the perceived loss of control to the negative emotions and compensations that are required for everyday dealings with stuttering.

## Level 2

As described above Armson and Kalinowski's (1994) treatise examined the impact of subperceptual forms of stuttering on acoustic and kinematic studies of speech production, casting a long shadow on the speech motor dynamics paradigm. Thus, in those who stutter there is an omnipresent possibility of perceptually fluent speech being contaminated by subperceptual stuttering. The presence of subperceptual stuttering adds another level to our model. Subperceptual stuttering events are those acoustic and kinematic phenomena that, by their nature, transcend the boundaries of the truly overt, yet are still invisible without the use of sensitive measuring equipment. By including subperceptual stuttering in this model, it becomes clear that the central involuntary block precipitates a continuum of disruptive events that begin in the central nervous system and manifest outward toward the motor periphery. That is, instead of categorizing stuttering symptoms into simply overt and covert behaviors, we now realize that the continuum of symptoms really represent a complete syndrome that handicaps communication before speaking, while speaking, and after speaking.

## Level 3

The 20% of the pathology, which is analogous to Sheehan's (1970) "tip of the iceberg," is found at the third and final level of our model. These overt behaviors consist of core speech disruptions (e.g., repetitions, prolongations, silent postural fixations), and ancillary behaviors (e.g., eye rolling, fist pounding, facial grimacing, jaw clenching, finger tapping, foot stomping, etc.)

and are the most easily countable, demarcated, and categorized. Thus, they have received the greatest attention from clinicians trying to eliminate stuttering behaviors. Counting the overt frequency of stuttering behaviors is the benchmark tool for assessing the efficacy of treatment protocols for stuttering (Bloodstein, 1995) because it is their presence that alerts speech-language pathologists to the presence of a communicative pathology. A significant reduction in overt stuttering behaviors is often accompanied by a decrease in other overt struggle and ancillary behaviors and is, thus, considered by many a sign of "improvement" (Saltuklaroglu & Kalinowski, 2002). Typically, clinicians count the number of repetitions, prolongations, and postural fixations based on their perceptual judgments, often made after multiple viewings of videotaped assessments of standardized stuttering tests, such as the Stuttering Severity Instrument (Riley, 1994). Specifically, a syllable/word is considered "stuttered" if a part-word repetition or prolongation exceeds a perceptually self-imposed threshold. In other words, the unit of speech being counted is considered to be stuttered only when "normalcy" is broken by "distinctive perceptual elements of repetitions and prolongations."

One element that distinguishes the current model from other models of stuttering is that this model allocates a necessary function to the overt behaviors. Even though people stutter, at some point they resume speaking fluently, meaning that somehow the involuntary block impeding speech has been overcome or inhibited. The current model suggests that the role of overt stuttering behaviors is to release the central involuntary block and allow fluent speech to be reinstated. Thus, contrary to how many others have viewed the disorder (e.g., the psychoanalytic, Johnsonian, and behavioral schools), we choose an orientation in which repetitions and other overt stuttering behaviors are the "solution" to a central involuntary pathology. Logically speaking, this makes sense as even in the most severe cases, stuttering is an intermittent pathology and the speech of those who stutter is a canvas of interwoven fluent and stuttered utterances. Hence, though involuntarily produced, acoustically noticeable repetitions and prolongations may actually engage the same neural mechanism for "inhibiting" stuttering and improving fluency levels as therapeutic methods and other methods that are commonly known to reduce stuttering (such as choral speech). This mechanism is discussed in detail later. However, it should be noted that it is probably the continued engagement of this mechanism during the incipient stages of stuttering that allows for spontaneous recovery in up to 80% of stuttering children. The only down side of producing overt stuttering behaviors to engage this mechanism is that they are highly conspicuous and impede the normal flow of communication, resulting in the syndrome we observe.

## The Assessment of Stuttering

### General Concerns

It is necessary for any professional administering therapy for stuttering to have an adequate battery of assessment tools. Without conducting assessments, it is impossible to determine the impact of any therapeutic intervention. Thus, assessment is necessary for accountability and proof of clinical effectiveness. When attempting to assess the presence of any pathologic condition and/or its impact on life, it is imperative to use tools that are both valid and reliable. A valid tool is one that actually measures what it claims to be measuring, whereas a reliable tool is one that yields consistent results when administered by different people and across a variety of settings. In the field of stuttering, finding tools that provide both valid and reliable measures has not been an easy task due in part to the disorder's dynamic and heterogeneous nature. Bloodstein (1995) clearly states, " . . . the assessment of results of therapy is a process fraught with opportunities for error and self-delusion" (p. 439). In his textbook, he reviews 162 studies investigating the efficacy of therapeutic interventions for stuttering over the last 70 years that have used a vast array of therapeutic protocols, including drug therapies (e.g., haloperidol, chlorpromazine, reserpine, meprobamate, etc.), behavioral therapies that involved the modification of peripheral speech subsystems (e.g., slowed speech, prolonged speech, syllable-timed speech, gentle phonatory onsets, light articulatory contacts, regulated breathing, etc.), cognitive-behavioral therapies (e.g., rational emotive therapy, assertion training, verbal reward, punishment, etc.), psychotherapies (e.g., relaxation, systematic desensitization, group psychotherapies, psychotherapy with parent and child, etc.), psychoanalytic therapies (e.g., regression, free association, hypnosis and role-training, etc.), the use of bulky auditory masking devices, and other "fluency aids" that used delayed auditory feedback and electronic metronomes. This list is not exhaustive, yet it highlights the broad range of therapeutic protocols used. Surprisingly, almost all were found to be effective in the treatment of stuttering, according to the published reports. In fact, approximately 95% of the 162 studies found significant reductions in overt stuttering behaviors (e.g., repetitions and prolongations). Thus, nearly every treatment study reviewed was seemingly effective based on a typical criterion of reducing the frequency of stuttering events to less than 2 or 3% stuttered syllables. However, if stuttering were as easily amenable to long-term remission as the data from these studies suggest, speech-language pathologists and others treating the disorder would have a much easier time prescribing and implementing therapeutic protocols. To us, it seems apparent that though numerous methods may provide some immediate reduction in the frequency of overt stuttering, it is doubtful that all of them (or any of them) can be truly effective for achieving long-term relief. Put simply, if every therapy appears to show clinical effectiveness, then it is most likely that our assessments of clinical intervention are missing their mark, especially considering that many of the protocols used were completely opposite in both theoretical orientation and method of implementation (Dayalu & Kalinowski, 2002).

The notion of valid and reliable assessment procedures has also recently been brought to light by a number of researchers, predominantly from behavioral backgrounds, who have recently published a series of articles under the general heading of "Evidence-based treatment of stuttering" (e.g., Bothe, 2003; Finn, 2003; Ingham, 2003; Langevin & Hagler, 2003) that have also been compiled into a similarly titled textbook. One would assume there should be no debate as to the necessity of "evidenced-based" protocol in stuttering therapy, or in any other. However, the question arises as to what constitutes adequate evidence for promoting a therapeutic approach in stuttering. It seems that evidentiary validity (e.g., clinic-based measurements) is often-times in question. According to Bothe, therapeutic change cannot be monitored if starting points are not accurately measured and, thus, without knowing the starting point, the impact of therapy cannot be determined. It is inferred that traditional stuttering therapy has lacked rigor, standardization, and quantification. Bothe states that traditional therapy is analogous to a "quasi religious knowledge that was taught by great teachers and perpetuated unchanged in the next generation" (p. 7). She continues to state that failure to focus on detailed and precise counting of overt manifestations is the great demarcation point of evidenced-based therapy over traditional stuttering therapy and points to the inherent flaws in traditional therapies. In other words, if detailed record keeping is not inherent in therapy then success or failure of therapy is unknown. Although we concur with the general notion of the need for good data keeping and monitoring of progress, we believe that determining the impact of therapy is really a much trickier business than one would think from simple first observation. If we simply adhered to the behavioral philosophy whereby stuttering events are counted and therapy efficacy could be optimally measured by carefully recorded objective observations of decreases in stuttering frequency across a variety of speaking situations, then the assessment procedure would still be relatively simple. However, in our model, we consider that overt behaviors only constitute about 20% of the stuttering pathology. Hence, how do we gain access to the other 80%, what important factors may we be ignoring when we place our faith in these overt measures of stuttering frequency, and how does this impact the validity of the assessment? We will provide information on the nature of frequency counting procedures and attempts to access the covert "experiential" nature of the pathology, as well as providing our take on conducting valid assessments of stuttering.

## Frequency Counts of Stuttering

Perceptually demarcated overt stuttering behaviors include repetitions, prolongations of speech sounds, and postural fixations. These observable events typically receive the greatest attention from speech-language pathologists as they appear to be countable and are indicators of disrupted speech. Thus, counting overt stuttering behaviors is the benchmark tool for assessing the efficacy of treatment protocols for stuttering (Bloodstein, 1995). Assessment batteries typically employ a standardized test such as the Stuttering Severity Instrument (SSI-3) that counts the frequency of overt behaviors (Riley, 1994). Using the SSI-3 as an example, those who stutter are asked to perform a reading task and a spontaneous speech task (e.g., picture description). During these two speaking tasks, clinicians attempt to collect about 300 syllables of speech output. Nonreaders are only asked to complete the picture description task. The speech tasks are usually videotaped so that clinicians can then watch the tape, transcribe the speech output, and count the number of stuttering events. A proportion of stuttered syllables (%SS) is then obtained by dividing the number of stuttered syllables by the number of total number of syllables in the speech output. It should be noted that in the past others have calculated percentage of stuttered words, stuttered words per minute, and stuttered events per utterance. However, Perkins (1981) stated the syllable is the basic physiologic unit of speech and should be used when assessing fluency. Costello and Ingham (1984) also noted that syllable counts provide more accurate descriptions when stuttering occurs on more than one syllable in a word.

In addition to calculating stuttering frequency, the SSI-3 also requires clinicians to measure (i.e., time) the three longest "blocks" (i.e., stuttering events) to the nearest 1/10th of a second, a task which given the nature of speech and stuttering is likely to yield measures that are even less reliable than the frequency counts. Lastly, clinicians are asked to assess "physical concomitants" or ancillary behaviors such as distracting sounds, facial grimaces, and head and extremity movements, and subjectively decide their distractive impact on communication. The frequency counts, timing of the blocks, and assessment of physical concomitants are assigned scaled scores which are combined to determine a "severity rating" (i.e., very mild to very severe). It is this severity rating that is often entered into clinical reports, with the intention of providing others with a general picture of how stuttering manifests in a particular individual. However, there are numerous concerns with regard to measuring overt behaviors and the determination of overall severity levels.

## *Frequency Counts of Stuttering Address Only a Small Portion of the Pathology*

First, demarcated visible and audible overt behaviors only constitute a small portion of the stuttering syndrome (see Figure 3–1) and, thus, counting these behaviors can estimate only the most salient or countable portion of the syndrome (Sheehan, 1970; Van Riper, 1982). In other words, removing these discrete events from the speech of those who stutter is analogous to skimming the cream from whole milk in an attempt to remove the fat. Although the cream at the surface is easily accessible, it only constitutes a small percentage of the fat product contained in whole milk. Skimming is easy and fast, yet it fails to remove all the fat from the milk. Similarly, by only addressing overt stuttering behaviors, much of the syndrome remains unaddressed. Even if the overt behaviors are almost completely eliminated over the course of an intervention period, without addressing the remaining 80% of the disorder, it is impossible to determine the true impact of the intervention. Even though procedures such as pre and post administration of the SSI may yield what appear to be evidence of therapeutic efficacy, stuttering may be continuing to loom beneath the surface, like a pot of boiling water waiting to bubble over.

## *Reliability of Counting Overt Stuttering Behaviors*

As stated, the counting of stuttered syllables is not a reliable process. First of all, when presented with the same samples of stuttered speech, experienced judges from various research centers have found poor levels of interjudge agreement when counting the number of stuttered syllables, suggesting that considerable variability exists as to what is being counted, even among the so-called experts in the field (Cordes & Ingham 1995; Ham 1989; Kully & Boberg 1988). Most research experiments that count stuttered syllables employ both inter- (between) and intra- (within) judge reliability using statistical measures such as Cohen's kappa. Using this measure, a perfect reliability score would be 1.00. However, to the best of our knowledge, neither inter- or intrajudge reliability in stuttering counts ever reaches 1.00. It is generally accepted that reliability scores over 0.75

represent excellent agreement, and we strive to achieve at least this level of reliability in all experimental procedures. One may expect that it would not be difficult, especially when frequency counts are made by the same person (intrajudge) or when two people with essentially the same training and background make comparisons of their counts. However, the fact that perfect reliability is seldom achieved even in optimal settings may always cast doubt on the use of frequency counts, especially when little change is evident in pre-post counts of stuttered syllables, as may be the case in some overtly mild stutterers.

Ingham et al. (1993a, 1993b) suggested the use of time interval measurement for the purposes of improving intra- and interjudge reliability. Under this procedure, one-minute speech samples were divided into 15 intervals of four seconds each. Each four-second speech segment was interspersed between five-second silences and presented randomly to judges who were asked to decide whether stuttering was present or absent in each sample. By simplifying the task of counting stuttering, an increase in reliability was achieved. However, this type of gross simplification also denied the nature of coarticulatory encoding and the gestural nature of the speech (Liberman & Mattingly, 1985), which is discussed in chapter 5. Thus, any attempt to split a continuous speech signal into discrete, short time intervals of speech (i.e., 1 s, 2 s, 3 s, 4s, 5 s, 6 s, 8 s, 10 s, 15 s) can be misleading. Another shortcoming when allocating a set time interval of speech is that numerous stuttering events may occur in any interval that may only be counted as a single stuttering event. Conversely, a single stuttered event (albeit one of longer duration) may transcend from one speech segment into the next. Thus, an undercount or overcount of stuttering events is inherently inevitable in such time interval procedures. By employing this form of simplification, we may lose valuable information, creating insufficient payoff for the effort expended. Now, many behaviorists use technologies like Noldus™ to increase sensitivity of measure. However, the time interval procedure reflects an attempt to decrease sensitivity. Simply put, reliability may be increased but validity with respect to the true nature of stuttering and speech may continue to be compromised. Needless to say, much of the profession has failed to implement these time procedures.

## Clinic Room Fluency: An Invalid Marker of Improvement

More than 60% of 162 efficacy reports only collected frequency counts of stuttering within a clinical setting, where fluency levels are generally at their highest after therapy. Most reports made little or no attempt to evaluate fluency beyond the clinic following completion of the therapeutic protocol (Bloodstein, 1995), possibly because many appeared to believe that short periods of clinic room fluency signified a long-term effective treatment (Perkins, 1983). However, numerous reasons exist as to why pre-post measures of within-clinic fluency levels do not accurately represent the efficacy of any therapeutic protocol.

### Habituation to Test Material and Setting

One factor that should be considered is the similarity of the post-test stimuli to the pre-test stimuli and therapy stimuli. For example, if the same reading material is used across testing situations, almost everyone is likely to show improvement due to familiarity with the material. Even if speech samples are taken during conversation as well as reading, care needs to be taken to ensure that different topics are discussed.

Generally, those receiving therapy for stuttering spend countless hours receiving treatment in the same environment. Yet stuttering is a dynamic pathology and the manifestation of its behaviors often varies from situation to situations (e.g., speaking in the clinic room with clinician versus answering the telephone). Environmental influences and speaking situations have been known to affect speaking situations (Boberg & Sawyer, 1977; Silverman, 1975) and speaking in a controlled, familiar, and comfortable environment may be the easiest situation possible. For any fluency gains made in the clinic to be considered evidence of true improvement, they must extend across a variety of speaking situations and audiences. Perhaps a better but still imperfect test of improved fluency may be to have patients use the telephone to call 20 to 30 businesses using assigned scripts to decrease the possibility of using covert strategies. The telephone provides access to a variety of conversational partners using a medium that those who stutter typically find difficult. These calls may be rated for fluency as well as other salient parameters, such as speech naturalness, ease of speech, and spontaneity. Such methods of testing might add a metric of generalization using "real" and challenging encounters over a short period of time, providing some evidence that gains extend across speaking situations and are not restricted to contrived and repeated test environments. Many patients may not even feel comfortable performing this task prior to therapy due to a previous history of failure. However, some evidence of therapeutic efficacy may be garnered if after therapy patients are able to confidently make these telephone calls and show evidence of improved speech across the parameters being measured.

The bottom line is that the dynamic and heterogeneous nature of stuttering creates clear problems when interpreting the efficacy of studies that employ pre-post fluency measures. To test every patient in every speaking situation is impossible. In other words, to determine the efficacy of a therapeutic protocol and determine any decreased impact of the pathology, information is required that assesses the "experiential" nature of the disorder. Those who stutter inherently know when speech is easy or more difficult, when they can relinquish the use of covert strategies, and when their speech approaches "normalcy" with regard to fluency, naturalness, and effort expended. For this reason, it is necessary to simply ask the person who stutters at all stages of therapy whether or not the designated intervention strategy is proving to be effective. However, in some cases frequency counts of overt stuttering can be the only viable measurement tool. Many children who stutter may have yet to develop the skills to verbalize the experiential nature of stuttering, especially those who are at incipient stages, and who may not yet have sufficient experience with the pathology to have developed a covert experiential repertoire of stuttering characteristics.

## Transference and Emotional Investment

Closely related to the habituation factors discussed above is the possibility of transference. Over time, following numerous hours of therapeutic intervention, good rapport is established and a clinical bond can develop between clinician and client. The clinical bond that develops between client and clinician often becomes strong and creates "transference" between client and clinician (Pearson, 2001). The therapeutic milieu is not an ordinary social interaction. An exchange of feelings can take place between clinician and patient. It may be especially easy for stuttering patients to place a high level of trust in their clinicians as, for many, it is often rare to find someone who will sit and listen unconditionally without judging them by their speech patterns. This transference can be confounding when measuring treatment efficacy as therapy recipients tend to perform at their highest levels when employing behavioral fluency techniques in the presence of their clinicians (Kalinowski et al., 2004). The author (JK) recalls a period of his life in which he was a young adult receiving stuttering therapy in a university setting. He describes how every semester he would show up at the therapy stuttering severely. Every semester he was paired with a student clinician with whom he was able to quickly establish rapport. During the clinical sessions, he was able to diligently incorporate all the therapy techniques taught to him from the clinician's "recipe" book, and reproduce them because he felt so comfortable in her presence and wanted her to succeed in her clinical practicum. He also reports, being able to get into a "therapeutic mode" and use therapy techniques optimally simply by smelling the clinician's perfume! This classically conditioned response is a clear example of how transference between clinician and client can have an impact on therapeutic results and why assessment measures need to go beyond clinic room fluency and tap into the experiential nature of the disorder. It should be noted that the apparent gains made by the author in therapy seldom carried over into the real world and never for extended periods. For that reason he continued to receive stuttering therapy throughout his undergraduate and masters programs.

Along similar lines, clinicians who subscribe to a particular method of treatment become emotionally invested in their protocols of choice (Kerr, 2002). Generally, these protocols are time-consuming and carry with them years of great personal commitment in their attendant thought and deliberation. This emotional investment can influence the perception of therapeutic outcomes. For example, clinicians who are highly invested in their protocols may fail to acknowledge certain stuttering symptoms that their therapeutic orientation does not cover. Their desire to see their patients succeed may also hinder testing in more difficult situations where the patient's tenuous therapeutic speech is more likely to fail. We have previously seen what appears to be evidence of emotional investment in therapisst treating children who stutter in the North Carolina school system. These therapists were asked to provide information pertaining to the number of children they treated that had fully recovered from stuttering. We were not surprised to find that the median recovery rate among clinicians was only 13.9%. However, an interesting trend was that longer practicing clinicians reported recovery rates that were almost twice as high as clinicians with less experience. As most clinicians used a similar battery of treatments, it seems evident that the higher proportion of reported recoveries by the more experienced therapists is most likely related to psychologic investment. Thus, it seems probable that when assessing the efficacy of their own treatment methods, a period of time must elapse before typical therapists can release themselves from their emotional and psychologic ties to particular therapies and be able to assess the results they have achieved with greater objectivity.

### Lack of Long-Term Measures

A common approach that many therapies have taken in the past is viewing the therapeutic process as short-term. Many "intensive" therapies are completed in 3 or 4 weeks during which all the skills thought to be necessary for producing fluent speech are learned and practiced. After that, the "maintenance" of fluent speech is essentially the responsibility of the client. A number of problems related to this approach are addressed in detail in the next chapter. However, for now it should be noted that stuttering continues to be an involuntary pathology throughout life, and no amount of training or practice makes it otherwise. For that reason, assessment of the therapeutic process should take place over the long term, as combating the impact of the involuntary neural block can be a lifelong process. Many studies only report pre- and post-therapy measures and do not consider how patients fare in the long term, even though a body of data exists to suggest that post-therapeutic relapse to stuttering is the common long-term outcome.

It should be noted that efficacy studies conducted more recently are beginning to provide more post-therapy measures of clinical efficacy (e.g., Boberg, 1976, 1981; Kalinowski et al., 2004; Kroll, 2003; Langevin & Kully, 2003; Ryan & Van Kirk, 1974). However, they continue to be limited. Oftentimes therapeutic gains will be reassessed one year post-therapy (Andrews & Tanner, 1982; Boberg, 1981; Howie, Tanner, & Andrews, 1981) and occasionally up to five years (Kuhr & Rustin, 1985; Prins, 1970; Ryan & Van Kirk, 1974). However, these long-term measures often make use of frequency counts that are generally taken in clinical settings and often by the same therapists who provided the therapy, again allowing for the possibility of the confounding effects noted above. We accept that long-term testing and retesting can be difficult, especially considering factors such as participant morbidity (i.e., losing contact with the clinic) and difficulties collecting frequency count data in different speaking situations. Again, however, we reiterate that the person who stutters is the one who knows best how well any intervention method is working and, thus, the best "efficacy" data is most likely collected from therapy recipients via self-reports that delve into the experiential nature of the disorder. This type of information can be continuously gathered over the long term (e.g., up to 10 years post-therapy) across large numbers of patients receiving therapy to determine the true therapeutic impact. Thus, collecting long-term frequency counts may not only be difficult, but also may provide misleading or incomplete measures of long-term efficacy.

### Clinic Room Fluency: Summary

Clearly, it appears that pre-post therapy stuttering frequency counts alone are lacking in validity when it comes to addressing the impact of therapy, and it is naïve to think otherwise. Thus, these counts of overt stuttering behaviors probably should not be used as the primary tool for reporting the efficacy of stuttering treatments. We propose that "experiential" data from the person who stutters provides a wealth of information from the only truly valid perspective—the person who stutters. When addressing the experiential nature of the disorder and the "qualities" associated with truly fluent speech, it is necessary to address not only the flow of speech (e.g., stuttered versus not stuttered), but also other factors that are clearly salient to the person who stutters during the "experience" of speaking.

# Naturalness and Ease of Effort of Speech: Smearing the Disorder

One objective of any stuttering treatment protocol should be to produce speech that as well as being free from overt stuttering is also immediate, spontaneous, effortless, and natural sounding— in other words, indistinguishable from the speech of persons who do not stutter (Dayalu & Kalinowski, 2002; Kalinowski & Dayalu, 2002). Normally fluent people speak automatically, using a minimal amount of effort, little vigilance, and have almost no cause to worry about potential pitfalls while speaking. In contrast, implementing therapeutic speech models requires constant monitoring and effort. The results of using therapeutic techniques is a ubiquitous unnatural "droned" quality (Dayalu & Kalinowski, 2002; Franken et al., 1992; Ingham et al., 1985; Kalinowski et al., 1994; Runyan & Adams, 1979; Runyan et al., 1990). In other words, post-therapeutic speech neither sounds nor feels like the truly fluent speech of the normally fluent speakers. Yet, pre-post assessments of stuttering rarely consider these factors which inevitably play crucial roles in determining the extent that the therapeutic speech patterns will continue to be used beyond the clinic room where they are continually reinforced by clinicians whose primary goal is to achieve decreases in frequency counts via the use of speech retraining techniques such as prolongation, gentle onsets, continuous phonation, light articulatory contacts, and so forth. Simply put, the therapeutic focus has placed such value in reducing counts of stuttered syllables over time that the very natural and effortless feel that characterizes the speech of most normal speakers is neglected in stuttering therapy. So are we really shocked when we see relapse rates that may exceed 70%?

The point that can be made is that speech naturalness is among the most important parameters to be measured when conducting assessment at any point during the therapeutic course. In clinical research, measures of speech naturalness ratings are often obtained by playing speech samples to naïve listeners. A naïve listener is someone who has little experience with stuttering from personal, social, or academic standpoints. Typically, they consist of undergraduate college students. Without being provided a definition of stuttering, these naïve listeners are asked to rate speech samples on a scale of 1 to 9, with 1 being highly natural and 9 being highly unnatural. This method and scale has been used since 1984 (Martin et al., 1984) and is an accepted procedure for acquiring measures of speech naturalness. Interestingly Kalinowski et al. (1994) used 64 naïve raters to assess pre- and post-therapeutic speech of both mild and severe stutterers who received intensive behavioral speech therapy using a motoric speech retraining protocol known as the Precision Fluency Shaping Program (PFSP). Not surprisingly, frequency counts indicated that after therapy most clients' speech was relatively free from overt stuttering. However, when naturalness measures were taken, the raters indicated that they found the post-therapeutic speech of both groups to sound less natural than their speech sound before therapy. In other words, though their pretherapeutic speech contained overt stuttering it still sounded better to the untrained ear than the posttherapeutic speech with its ubiquitously droned nature. Not surprisingly, using unnatural post-therapeutic speech can create social discomfort and embarrassment both in the person who stutters and in the listener, even more so than the production of overt stuttering events.

Thus, "motoric" manipulations to the speech subsystems via therapeutic techniques typically impede the natural manner of speech production (Armson & Kalinowski, 1994; McClean et al., 1990; Story et al., 1996) or make speech sound "funny" to the listener. How does it feel to the person producing it? The person who stutters may feel relatively little discomfort practicing novel speech patterns in a reinforcing clinical environment or even when alone in their home or car. However, while generalizing novel speech patterns beyond clinical settings, therapy recipients begin to face new challenges from untrained listeners. Inherently, those who stutter know that they are not producing speech in the same manner as everyone else. It simply feels as different as it sounds. After coming from the clinic, many may not be ready to feel the reactions and suffer the social penalties and discomfort of using artificial speech patterns in the real world, a factor which may put many on the path to relapse (Kalinowski & Dayalu, 2002, Saltuklaroglu & Kalinowski, 2002). In his class the author (JK) recalls how after receiving intensive stuttering therapy he ventured into a New York City night club.

Using his best therapeutic speech, he asked a young lady "Would you like to dance?" Rather than providing a verbal response, she removed a can of pepper spray from her purse and proceeded to spray the face producing the zombie-like speech.

A recent study by O'Brian et al. (2003) highlights the argument made above. They collected both objective (i.e., frequency counts) and self-reported data from adult stutterers who had completed a motoric speech retraining program. The self-reported data from the participants consisted of a number of subjective ratings, again made on a 9-point scale. The lower end of the scale represented positive ratings and the higher end represented negative ratings. According to their ratings, participants indicated that they found using therapeutic skills outside the clinic both relatively difficult and uncomfortable. That is, 80% of the participants rated 4 or above with respect to their comfort level and 60% rated 5 or above with respect to the ease of using "prolonged" speech beyond the confines of the clinic. Thus, these data suggest that after undergoing this therapy, from the perspective of the participants, the resultant speech neither felt natural nor was easily implemented. To us, this is a red flag that relapse may be forthcoming. Though some behaviorists may argue that the participants simply needed more time using the novel speech patterns for them to achieve higher levels of comfort, we believe that the ratings provided were simply indicators that the participants were being asked to do something difficult, that also made them sound and feel abnormal.

Thus, closely related to speech naturalness is the ease with which speech is produced, another measure that has received little or no attention in studies measuring clinical efficacy. Sheehan (1984) drew attention to this point by stating:

> A stutterer may feel miserable at the strain and vigilance required to keep an artificial pattern going. But the resulting monotone might dramatically lower the frequency count. Conversely, a stutterer might relax his suppressive vigilance to feel much freer and more open, even though the frequency count might be reported as higher by an objective observer (Sheehan, 1984, pp. 223).

Starkweather also drew attention to this notion when he defined fluent speech as "the ability to talk at normal levels of continuity, rate, and effort." In their treatise on pseudofluency, Kalinowski and Dayalu (2002) also described how post-therapeutic speech requires constant monitoring and vigilance in order to create the resultant speech patterns which cannot be considered true fluency. They further stated that such effort expenditure can be both a physically and emotionally exhausting daily endeavor. In addition, 17 out of 20 participants in the O'Brian et al. (2003) study rated 5 or above on the 9-point rating scale on a question addressing the amount of time spent "thinking" about controlling stuttering, which is an excellent parameter for addressing the ease with which post-therapeutic speech is produced. The ratings obtained appear to suggest that considerable mental effort is required to maintain the use of therapeutic techniques to avoid the production of overt stuttering behaviors. Thus, the continued use of post-therapeutic speech may be analogous to asking someone to walk continuously on tiptoes. It will get you from point A to point B, but it will require substantial monitoring and effort, take more time, feel clumsy, soon become uncomfortable, and attract a great deal of unwanted attention from those watching.

Simply put, persons who stutter expend much greater amounts of energy to produce speech than those who do not stutter. Overt stuttering acts are notorious for the amount of energy expended in relatively short bursts of time. These acoustic bursts of energy are probably used to release central neural blocks. The energy used to release a block is much more apparent when physical manifestations (head jerks, facial contortions, etc.) and acoustic aberrations (repetitions and prolongations) occur simultaneously. However, the constant expenditure of energy during the use of covert strategies such as avoidances and substitutions often escape detection, yet can be unremitting. All the chapters in this textbook adhere to this orientation of stuttering and our goal for those who stutter is to emulate the speech of those who do not stutter, not just from a visible standpoint, but also with respect to the amount of energy expended during speech and in dealing with the covert symptomatology. That is, we do not want to use constant monitoring, droning, or unnatural speech. We may require the use of these strategies on an intermittent basis, but to use them continually is a prognosis for failure. Therefore, one goal of therapeutic efficacy should really be an assessment of energy expenditure—both overt and covert. It is our hypothesis that one source of failure in past therapies is that most people can only maintain certain levels of high energy expenditure for short periods of times. Thus, another view of the high relapse rates associated with many therapies is the constant draining of energy sources. It may simply be easier to stutter. Hence, we need a therapeutic approach that gives the most stuttering relief with the least amount of energy expended.

We encourage speech-language pathologists to gather information about the patient's feelings with regard to speech naturalness and the ease with which speech is being produced at every stage of therapy, from the initial consultation to the final clinical encounter in every setting possible. The viewpoint of the clinician is tainted. Clinicians (especially those with behavioral training) typically look for a decrease in overt stuttering and the use of therapeutic techniques as a sign of success. Furthermore, clinicians are typically experiencing the disorder and, as such, they cannot properly assess speech naturalness or effort expended. Without gaining this "experiential" perspective from the client, it is unlikely that clinicians will provide the client with speech patterns that will carry over beyond the clinic room.

We also suggest that the most appropriate tool currently available for determining speech naturalness and ease is a self-report format. Although using the ratings of naïve listeners provides informative measures for research purposes, acquiring this type of data can be a time-consuming process and unnecessary for clinical purposes. People who stutter simply know when speech sounds and feels right. Remember that stuttering is an intermittent disorder and even the most severe stutterer has times when truly fluent without using any therapeutic techniques. Thus, those who stutter know how it feels to be fluent and how it feels to stutter. Chances are, they are familiar with every type of speech that falls between these ends of the spectrum (e.g., stuttering, fluency, or relative level of pseudofluency). Stuttering clients can tell us at almost any time whether or not their speech sounds and feels natural to them and how much effort they are expending to keep the overt disfluencies beneath the surface. Thus, self-report provides the best measurement tool for such purposes, especially considering clients can provide their "experiential" perspectives at any time and in any speaking situation.

## Self-Reports Are Primary Tools for Measuring the Efficacy of Stuttering Treatments

Acquiring subjective data from individuals who stutter is clearly an invaluable procedure for evaluating the efficacy of any therapeutic protocol. When the symptoms of a pathology are 80% invisible, as clinicians, we require the perspective of those who stutter to tell us how much we are helping them. In the past there have been charlatans that used unconventional methods to tell us we were cured. For example, in the 1840s, a certain Dr. Dieffenbach told people who stutter that their affliction was caused by an enlarged tongue. His "cure" was to remove a triangle-shaped wedge from the front of the tongue and sew the remaining portion back together. After much bleeding and pain (not much for anesthetics back then) he told the patients they were cured. Indeed, for a while their stuttering probably did not bother them as much, as the pain associated with the surgery was probably enough to induce careful articulation and unnatural speech patterns that inhibited the stuttering to some extent. However, stuttering inevitably returned, most likely after the tongue finally healed and their speech patterns returned to normal. In the early 1900s, Benjamin Bogue established a specialized school to "cure" stuttering. His "secret" cure could not be revealed until one actually attended, only to find out that it simply involved some finger tapping in conjunction with speech production, a condition that imposes a rhythmic nature on speech and is known to temporarily enhance fluency, though it is nearly impossible to maintain. In the history of our field, these characters live on in infamy. However, if someone had stopped to ask the person who stuttered if they felt different about their speech after being deceived by Dieffenbach or Bogue, if they had indeed been "cured," the true nature of these interventions may have been revealed earlier, rather than after many had suffered needlessly at their hands.

Self-reports are powerful measuring tools in evaluating the effectiveness and efficiency of the stuttering treatment programs. They allow the person who stutters to provide valuable information with respect to both their experiences with stuttering and its treatment. Simply put, information obtained about the person who stutters via self-report format should be primary for assessing the efficacy of any intervention technique.

Self-reports have certain advantages over overt measures. First, they tap into the covert aspects of the disorder that comprise the largest portion of the pathology that may be unremitting, even though notable changes are observed in frequency count measures. For example, a person may undergo therapy for an extended period and be able to produce stutter-free speech in the clinic. However, the covert "experiential" nature of the disorder may continue to factor largely into their communications in the outside world. Therapy recipients may continue to feel that their speech is tenuous, unstable, and likely to break down at any time. For this reason, outside the therapy room, they may continue to avoid many speaking situations, use substitutions and circumlocutions, and generally feel that speech is still "difficult" in most situations. In such cases, it would be difficult to claim therapeutic success based solely on frequency counts. However, with the use of well-constructed questionnaires, we can gather this information from the person who stutters and let him or her tell us directly about how well our vehicles of change are truly working in the real world, across a variety of speaking situations. The O'Brian et al. (2003) data highlight the value of self-reports in stuttering efficacy. The discrepancies in the data between the frequency counts and self-report measures suggest a certain frailty in post-therapeutic speech. Simply put, the post-therapeutic decrease in stuttered syllables obtained is inconsistent with the self-reports regarding comfort levels and ease of use, which to us is a red flag suggesting that the bulk of the stuttering syndrome continues to lie beneath the surface and continues to be expressed via covert behaviors. In another recent study, Riley et al. (2004) showed that the frequency counts of stuttered syllables were highly correlated with the patients self-report of stuttering severity ($r = .75$), but not with the avoidance behaviors. Thus, frequency counts of overt behaviors may provide a small window of the overall severity, but are not the best indicator of the extent that the pathology manifests covertly. Furthermore, it may also be that most clinicians use frequency counts as the primary measure for assigning severity.

The importance of self-report as a primary tool in the assessment of stuttering cannot be overstated. A person may be completely stutter-free for a period of time following intervention (the author [TS] remained stutter-free for a month after intensive behavioral therapy before relapsing), yet the degree of awareness and speech monitoring that is necessary to maintain the speech bespeaks a constant awareness of stuttering, a need to monitor speech, and the continued use of covert strategies. People who stutter are clearly aware of the effects of stuttering even when seemingly fluent to an outside observer. Even the speech of those appearing overtly mild can be filled with hesitations, avoidances, and even small blockages that are not detectable to the casual observer. We simply need to ask the person who stutters about the impact of all these behaviors. With the exception of a few rare therapy recipients, it appears unlikely that even those who show no overt signs of stuttering in the clinic would continue to report being free from all signs and symptoms of stuttering. However, the clear paucity of this "experiential" data should be considered a shortcoming in many available efficacy data sets.

A number of questionnaires are available to tap into the experiential nature of the disorder. Some, such as the Perceptions of Stuttering Inventory (PSI; Woolf, 1967), S-scale (Erickson, 1969), and the Children's Attitudes About Talking—Revised (CAT-R; DeNil & Brutten, 1991) make use of simple true/false statements. The person who stutters evaluates each statement and determines if it pertains to him or her. A total score is then determined for each questionnaire. Of the three questionnaires mentioned above, we tend to favor the use of the PSI. This questionnaire makes 60 statements, 20 of which are associated with avoidance of stuttering, 20 with expectancy to stutter, and 20 with the struggle associated with stuttering. The statements used are well-constructed and provide a wealth of knowledge into the covert nature of the pathology as measured by these three salient parameters. We recently conducted an efficacy study of the SpeechEasy™ fluency device (discussed in a later chapter) and used the PSI as a measure of effectiveness. With respect to interpreting our overt counts, this efficacy study may be subject to similar restrictions as found in others. However, we also measured speech naturalness and used pre-post measures of the PSI to gather information from the persons who stutter with respect to how well the SpeechEasy™ was helping them deal with the stuttering experience. We were encouraged to find that all participants reported decreases in avoidance, struggle, and expectancy behaviors associated with stuttering one year after beginning to use the SpeechEasy device (Stuart et al., in press).

Another format is the Likert scale. Persons who stutter rate themselves on a particular parameter associate with stuttering using a numeric scale (e.g., 1–5, 1–7, and 1–9) where the opposite ends of the scales represent strongest and weakest self-assessments of the parameter in question. The use of these types of scales can provide valuable information as they, unlike true/false statements, are continuous rather than categorical scales, a characteristic which may make them more sensitive to measuring therapeutic changes. Examples of these types of scales include the Perceptions of Self Semantic Differential Task (Kalinowski et al., 1987) and the Southern Illinois University Speech Situation Checklist (Hanson, Gronhovd, & Rice, 1981). Another scale that can provide valuable information is the Self-Efficacy Scale for Adult Stutterers (Ornstein & Manning, 1985). This 42-item questionnaire addresses the ability of a person who stutters to approach numerous easy and difficult speaking situations. Each situation is rated on a scale of 0 to 100 and an overall average across the items can be determined. This questionnaire also provides a window into particular types of speaking situations that a therapy recipient may find more difficult, and thus may be used as "real life" tests of fluency.

Because self-reports can provide information about speaking across a variety of situations and circumstances, we can use them for evaluating a therapeutic procedure. Simply put, self-reports can provide a global measure of stuttering amelioration with respect to day-to-day situations, not just those that are typically best (e.g., clinic-room fluency). For this reason, we believe that honest self-reports provide data that should carry considerably more weight than the overt measures of stuttering frequency, making them the true "acid test" of any form of stuttering intervention (Kalinowski et al., 2004). However, even when using self-reports, a few precautions should be taken. First, self-reports must be collected from samples of 30 or more individuals in order to obtain a representative sample that nullifies the statistical effects of any extreme values. Second, they should employ formats that are easy to administer and easily amenable to repeated administrations. Third, the questionnaire used needs to assess the full repertoire of experiential behaviors found at level 1 of our model. These may include assessments of word, sound, or situational avoidances, ease of speech, speech naturalness, compensation strategies, anticipatory strategies, and reactions to stuttering. It is for this reason that we have often favored the PSI. It uses a simple format and provides a relatively comprehensive examination of covert stuttering behaviors.

## Summary

Rather than truly measuring therapeutic efficacy, most studies that claim improvements may simply be providing evidence of a temporary state of "stuttering inhibition." As we delve a little deeper into what makes people who stutter more fluent, we begin to see that these transient states can be easily induced using sensory methods of speech input (e.g., listening to speech) or motor methods that make changes to the way that speech is produced. However, as evident by the stability in the epidemiology (e.g., incidence and prevalence) and relapse data, these short-term gains rarely translate into long-term remission. Therefore, it appears that for the most part, our assessment of stuttering has used a flawed metric. Using frequency counts alone is an inadequate measure of clinical efficacy, as they only assess the peripheral surface manifestations of the pathology. By only looking at decreases in overt stuttering moments, we see the pathology as being one-dimensional, rather than the multi-layered, dynamic, and complex syndrome that it really is. For this reason, we must continually examine speech naturalness, ease of speech production, and the impact that our therapy is having on the management of the stuttering experience.

Similar to depression, panic attacks, post-traumatic stress disorders, and so forth, stuttering needs to be associated with a central and an experiential sense of "loss of control" and only the person who stutters can provide information that can be used to assess the impact of the pathology and the treatment method.

Thus, without self-reports, overt measures alone are incomplete at best. We have used self-reports as secondary tools to validate overt measures but we suggest that a reversal in the relative levels of importance of the two procedures would help efficacy measures gain much needed credibility and validity. In other words, self-report should be the primary tool and overt measures need only be used to bolster the experiential data provided by people who stutter.

# References

Adams, M. R. (1985). The speech physiology of stutterers: Present status. *Seminars in Speech and Language, 6,* 177–197.

Adams, M. R., & Hayden, P. (1976). The ability of stutterers and non-stutterers to initiate and terminate phonation during production of an isolated vowel. *Journal of Speech and Hearing Research, 19,* 290–296.

Adams, M. R., & Ramig, P. (1980). Vocal characteristics of normal speakers and stutterers during choral reading. *Journal of Speech and Hearing Research, 23,* 457–469.

Agnello, J. G. (1975). Voice onset and voice termination features of stutterers. In L. M. Webster & L. C. Furst (Eds.), *Vocal tract dynamics and dysfluency* (pp. 40–70). New York: Speech-Language-Hearing Association.

Alfonso, P. J. (1990). Definition and subject-selection criteria for stuttering research in adult subjects. In J. A. Cooper (Ed.), *Research needs in stuttering: Roadblocks and future directions* (Asha Report No. 18, pp. 15–24). Rockville, MD: American Speech-Language-Hearing Association.

Andrews, G., & Tanner, S. (1982). Stuttering: The results of 5 days treatment with an airflow technique. *Journal of Speech and Hearing Disorders, 47,* 427–429.

Armson, J. & Kalinowski, J. (1994). Interpreting results of the fluent speech paradigm in stuttering research: Difficulties in separating cause from effect. *Journal of Speech and Hearing Research, 37,* 69–82.

Bloodstein, O. (1995). *A handbook on stuttering* (5th ed.). San Diego, CA: Singular Publishing Group, Inc.

Boberg, E. (1976). Intensive group therapy program for stutterers. *Human Communication, 1,* 29–42.

Boberg, E. (1981). Maintenance of fluency: An experimental program. In E. Boberg (Ed.), *Maintenance of fluency: Proceedings of the Banff Conference.* New York: Elsevier.

Boberg, E., & Sawyer, L. (1977). Maintenance of fluency following intensive therapy. *Human Communication, 2,* 21–28.

Borden, G. J. (1983). Initiation versus execution time during manual and oral counting by stutterers. *Journal of Speech and Hearing Research, 26,* 389–396.

Borden, G. J., Baer, T., & Kenney, M. K. (1985). Onset of voicing in stuttered and fluent utterances. *Journal of Speech and Hearing Research, 28,* 363–372.

Bothe, A. K. (Ed.). (2003). *Evidence-based treatment of stuttering: Empirical bases, clinical applications, and remaining needs.* Mahwah, NJ: Lawrence Erlbaum.

Braun, A. R., Varga, M., Stager, S., Schulz, G., Selbie, S., Maisog, J. M., Carson, R. E., & Ludlow, C. L. (1997). Altered patterns of cerebral activity during speech and language production in developmental stuttering. An H2(15)O positron emission tomography study. *Brain, 120*(pt 5), 761–784.

Caruso, A. J., Abbs, J. H., & Gracco, V. L. (1988). Kinematic analysis of multiple movement coordination during speech in stutterers. *Brain, 111*(pt 2), 439–456.

Cohen, J. (1960), A coefficient of agreement for nominal scales. *Educational and Psychological Measurement, 20,* 37–46

Colcord, R. D., & Adams, M. R. (1979). Voicing duration and vocal SPL changes associated with stuttering reduction during singing. *Journal of Speech and Hearing Research, 22,* 468–479.

Conture, E. G., Colton, R. H., & Gleason, J. R. (1988). Selected temporal aspects of coordination during fluent speech of young stutterers. *Journal of Speech and Hearing Research, 31,* 640–653.

Conture, E. G., Rothenberg, M., & Molitor, R. (1986). Electroglottographic observations of young children's fluency. *Journal of Speech and Hearing Research, 29,* 384–393.

Cordes, A., & Ingham, R. (1995). Stuttering includes both within-word and between-word disfluencies. *Journal of Speech and Hearing Research, 38,* 382–386.

Costello, J. M. & Ingham, R. J. (1984). Assessment strategies for stuttering. In R. F Curlee. & W. H. Perkins (Eds.). *Nature and treatment of stuttering: New directions* (pp. 303–333). San Diego, CA: College-Hill Press.

Cross, D., & Luper, H. (1979). Voice reaction time of stuttering and nonstuttering children and adults. *Journal of Fluency Disorders, 4,* 59–77.

Cross, D., & Luper, H. (1983). Relation between finger reaction time and voice reaction time in stuttering and nonstuttering children and adults. *Journal of Speech and Hearing Research, 26,* 356–361.

Cullinan, W. L., & Springer, M. T. (1980). Voice initiation and termination times in stuttering and nonstuttering children. *Journal of Speech and Hearing Research, 23,* 344–360.

Dayalu, V. N., & Kalinowski, J. (2002). Pseudofluency in adults who stutter: The illusory outcome of therapy. *Perceptual Motor Skills, 94,* 87–96.

De Nil, L. F. & Brutten, G. J. (1991). Speech associated attitudes of stuttering and nonstuttering children. *Journal of Speech and Hearing Research, 34,* 60–66.

De Nil, L. F., Kroll, R. M., Kapur, S., & Houle, S. (2000). A positron emission tomography study of silent and oral single word reading in stuttering and nonstuttering adults. *Journal of Speech, Language, and Hearing Research, 43,* 1038–1053.

Di Simoni, F. C. (1974). Preliminary study of certain timing relationships in the speech of stutterers. *Journal of the Acoustical Society of America, 56,* 695–696.

Dworzynski, K., & Howell, P. (2004). Predicting stuttering from phonetic complexity in German. *Journal of Fluency Disorders, 29,* 149–173.

Erickson, R. L. (1969). Assessing communication attitudes among stutterers. *Journal of Speech and Hearing Research, 12,* 711–724.

Few, L. R., & Lingwall, J. B. (1972). A further analysis of fluency within stuttered speech. *Journal of Speech and Hearing Research, 15,* 356–363.

Finn, P. (2003). Self change from stuttering during adolescence and adulthood. In A. Bothe (Ed.), *Evidence-based treatment of stuttering: Empirical bases and clinical applications* (pp. 117–138). Mahwah, NJ: Lawrence Erlbaum Associates, Publishers

Foundas, A. L., Bollich, A. M., Corey, D. M., Hurley, M., & Heilman, K. M. (2001). Anomalous anatomy of speech-language areas in adults with persistent developmental stuttering. *Neurology, 24,* 207–215.

Foundas, A. L., Bollich, A. M., Feldman, J., Corey, D. M., Hurley, M., Lemen, L. C., & Heilman, K. M. (2004). Aberrant auditory processing and atypical planum temporale in developmental stuttering. *Neurology, 63,* 1640–1646

Foundas, A. L, Corey, D. M, Angeles, V., Bollich, A. M., Crabtree-Hartman, E., & Heilman, K. M. (2003). Atypical cerebral laterality in adults with persistent developmental stuttering. *Neurology, 25,* 1378–1385.

Fox, P. T., Ingham, R. J., Ingham, J. C., Hirsch, T. B., Downs, J.H., Martin, C., Jerabek, P., Glass, T., & Lancaster, J. L. (1996). A PET study of the neural systems of stuttering. *Nature, 11,* 158–161.

Franken, M. C. (1987). Perceptual and acoustic evaluation of stuttering therapy. In H. F. M. Peters & W. Hultstijn (Eds.), *Speech motor dynamics in stuttering* (pp. 285–294). New York: Springer-Verlag.

Franken, M. C., Boves, L., Peters, H. F. M., & Webster, R. (1992). Perceptual evaluation of the speech before and after fluency shaping therapy. *Journal of Fluency Disorders, 17*, 223–242.

Freeman, F. J. (1984). Laryngeal muscle activity of stutterers. In R. F. Curlee & W. H. Perkins (Eds.), *Nature and treatment of stuttering: New directions* (pp. 104–116). San Diego, CA: College-Hill Press.

Freeman, F. J., & Ushijama, T. (1978). Laryngeal muscle activity during stuttering. *Journal of Speech and Hearing Research, 21*, 538–562.

Goldsmith, H. (1983). Some comments on "articulatory dynamics of fluent utterances of stutterers and nonstutterers." *Journal of Speech and Hearing Research, 26*, 319–320.

Gronohovd, K. D. (1977). A comparison of the fluent oral reading rates of stutterers and nonstutterers. *Journal of Fluency Disorders, 2*, 247–252.

Guntupalli, V. K., Kalinowski, J., & Saltuklaroglu, T. (in press). The need for self-report data in the assessment of stuttering therapy efficacy: Repetitions and prolongations of speech ≠ the stuttering syndrome. *International Journal of Language and Communication Disorders.*

Ham, R. E. (1989). What are we measuring? *Journal of Fluency Disorders, 14*, 231–243.

Hanson, B. R., Gronhovd, K. D., & Rice, K. L. (1981). A shortened version of the Southern Illinois University Speech Situation Checklist for the identification of speech-related anxiety. *Journal of Fluency Disorders, 6*, 351–360.

Healey, E. C., & Adams, M. R. (1981). Speech timing skills of normally fluent and stuttering children and adults. *Journal of Fluency Disorders, 6*, 233–246.

Healey, E. C., & Gutkin, B. (1984). Analysis of stutterers' voice onset times and fundamental frequency contours during fluency. *Journal of Speech and Hearing Research, 27*, 219–225.

Hillman, R. E., & Gilbert, H. R. (1977). Voice onset time for voiceless stop consonants in the fluent reading of stutterers and nonstutterers. *Journal of Acoustical Society of America, 61*, 610–611.

Howie, P. M., Tanner, S., & Andrews, G. (1981). Short- and long-term outcome in an intensive treatment program for adult stutterers. *Journal of Speech and Hearing Disorders, 46*, 104–109.

Ingham, R. J. (2002, November). *An er-fMRI study of stuttering and simulated stuttering (128).* Paper presented at the American Speech-Language-Hearing Association, Atlanta, GA.

Ingham, R. J. (2003). Emerging controversies, findings, and directions in neuroimaging and developmental stuttering: In A. Bothe (Ed.), *Evidence-based treatment of stuttering: Empirical bases and clinical applications* (pp. 27–64). Mahwah, NJ: Lawrence Erlbaum Associates, Publishers.

Ingham, R. J., Cordes, A. K., & Finn, P. (1993b). Time-interval measurement of stuttering: Systematic replication of Ingham, Cordes, and Gow (1993). *Journal of Speech and Hearing Research, 36,* 1168–1176.

Ingham, R. J., Cordes, A. K., & Gow, M. L. (1993a). Time-interval measurement of stuttering: Modifying interjudge agreement. *Journal of Speech and Hearing Research, 36,* 503–515.

Ingham, R. J., Fox, P. T., Costello, D., Ingham, J., & Zamarripa, F. (2000). Is overt stuttered speech a prerequisite for the neural activations associated with chronic developmental stuttering? *Brain and Language, 75,* 163–194.

Ingham, R. J., Martin, R. R., Haroldson, S. K., Onslow, M., & Leney, M. (1985). Modification of listener judged naturalness in the speech of stutterers. *Journal of Speech and Hearing Research, 28,* 495–504.

Jancke, L., Hanggi, J., & Steinmetz, H. (2004). Morphological brain differences between adult stutterers and non-stutterers. *BioMed Central (BMC) Neurology, 4,* 23.

Johnson, W. (1942). A study of the onset and development of stuttering. *Journal of Speech Disorders, 7,* 251–257.

Kalinowski, A. G., Kalinowski, J., Stuart, A., & Rastatter, M. P. (1998). A latent trait approach to the development of persistent stuttering. *Perceptual Motor Skills, 87,* 1331–1358.

Kalinowski, J, & Dayalu, V. N. (2002). A common element in the immediate inducement of effortless, natural-sounding, fluent speech in people who stutter: "The second speech signal." *Medical Hypotheses, 58,* 61–66.

Kalinowski, J., Guntupalli, V. K., Stuart, A., & Saltuklaroglu, T. (2004). Self-reported efficacy of an ear-level prosthetic device that delivers altered auditory feedback for the management of stuttering. *International Journal of Rehabilitation Research, 27,* 167–170.

Kalinowski, J., Lerman, J. W., & Watt, J. (1987). A preliminary examination of the perceptions of self and others in stutterers and nonstutterers. *Journal of Fluency Disorders, 12,* 317–331.

Kalinowski, J., Noble, S., Armson, J., & Stuart, A. (1994). Naturalness ratings of the pretreatment and post-treatment speech of adults with mild and severe stuttering. *American Journal of Speech Language Pathology, 3,* 61–66.

Kerr, A. G. (2002). Emotional investment in surgical decision making. *Journal of Laryngology and Otolaryngology, 116,* 575–579.

Knox, J. A. (1975). *Acoustic analysis of stuttering behavior within the context of fluent speech.* Unpublished doctoral dissertation, University of Iowa, Iowa City.

Kroll, R. M. (2003). Importance of treatment efficacy research in the area of stuttering. *Logopedics, Phoniatriacs, Vocology, 28,* 92–93.

Kuhr, A., & Rustin, L. (1985). The maintenance of fluency after intensive in-patient therapy: Long-term follow-up. *Journal of Fluency Disorders, 10,* 229–236.

Kully, D., & Boberg, E. (1988). An investigation of interclinic agreement in the identification of fluent and stuttered syllables. *Journal of Fluency Disorders, 13,* 309–318.

Langevin, M., & Hagler, P. (2003). Development of a scale to measure peer attitudes toward children who stutter. In A. Bothe (Ed.), *Evidence-based treatment of stuttering: Empirical bases and clinical applications* (pp. 139–172). Mahweh, NJ: Lawrence Erlbaum Associates, Publishers.

Langevin, M., & Kully, D. (2003). Evidence-based treatment of stuttering: III. Evidence-based practice in a clinical setting. *Journal of Fluency Disorders, 28,* 219–235.

Lebrun, Y. & Bayle, M. (1973). Surgery in the treatment of stuttering. In Y. Lebrun & R. Hoops (Eds), *Neurolinguistic approaches to stuttering* (pp. 82–89). The Hague: Mouton.

Liberman, A. M., & Mattingly, I. G. (1985). The motor theory of speech perception revised. *Cognition, 21,* 1–36.

Love, L. R., & Jeffress, L. A. (1971). Identification of brief pauses in the fluent speech of stutterers and nonstutterers. *Journal of Speech and Hearing Research, 14,* 229–240.

Mallard, A. R., & Kelly, J. S. (1982). The precision fluency shaping program: Replication and evaluation. *Journal of Fluency Disorders, 7,* 287–294.

Mallard, R. R., & Westbrook, J. B. (1985). Vowel duration in stutterers participating in precision fluency shaping. *Journal of Fluency Disorders, 10,* 221–228.

Martin, R. R., Haroldson, S. K., & Triden, K. A. (1984). Stuttering and speech naturalness. *Journal of Speech and Hearing Disorders, 49,* 53–58.

McClean, M. D., Kroll, R. M., & Loftus, N. S. (1990). Kinematic analysis of lip closure in stutterers' fluent speech. *Journal of Speech and Hearing Research, 33,* 755–760.

McClean, M. D., & Tasko, S. M. (2004). Correlation of orofacial speeds with voice acoustic measures in the fluent speech of persons who stutter. *Experimental Brain Research, 159,* 310–318.

McClean, M. D., Tasko, S. M., & Runyan, C. M. (2004). Orofacial movements associated with fluent speech in persons who stutter. *Journal of Speech, Language, and Hearing Research, 47,* 294–303.

McKnight, R. C., & Cullinan, W. L. (1987). Subgroups of stuttering children: Speech and voice reaction times, segmental durations, and naming latencies. *Journal of Fluency Disorders, 12,* 217–233.

Melnick, K. S., Conture, E. G., & Ohde, R. N. (2003). Phonological priming in picture naming of young children who stutter. *Journal of Speech, Language, and Hearing Research, 46,* 1428–1443.

Metz, D. E., Onufrak, J. A., & Ogburn, R. S. (1979). An acoustic analysis of stutterers' fluent speech prior to and at the termination of speech therapy. *Journal of Fluency Disorders, 4,* 249–254.

Metz, D. E., Samar, V. J., & Sacco, P. R. (1983). Acoustic analysis of stutterers' fluent speech before and after therapy. *Journal of Speech and Hearing Research, 26,* 531–536.

Murphy, M., & Baumgartner, J. (1981). Voice initiation and termination time in stuttering and nonstuttering children. *Journal of Fluency Disorders, 6,* 257–264.

Natke, U., Sandrieser, P., van Ark, M., Pietrowsky, R., & Kalveram, K. T. (2004). Linguistic stress, within-word position, and grammatical class in relation to early childhood stuttering. *Journal of Fluency Disorders, 29,* 109–122.

Nippold, M. A. (2004). Phonological and language disorders in children who stutter: Impact on treatment recommendations. *Clinical Linguistics and Phonetics, 18,* 145–159.

Neumann, K., Euler, H. A., von Gudenberg, A. W., Giraud, A. L., Lanfermann, H., Gall, V., & Preibisch, C. (2003). The nature and treatment of stuttering as revealed by fMRI: A within- and between-group comparison. *Journal of Fluency Disorders, 28,* 381–409.

O'Brian, S., Packman, A., Onslow, M., & O'Brian, N. (2003). Generalizability theory II: Application to perceptual scaling of speech naturalness in adults who stutter. *Journal of Speech, Language, and Hearing Research, 46,* 718–723.

Onufrak, J. A. (1980, November). *A follow-up analysis of stutterers' speech after successful speech therapy.* Paper presented at the annual convention of the American Speech-Language-Hearing Association, Detroit, MI.

Ornstein, A. F., & Manning, W. H. (1985). Self-efficacy scaling by adult stutterers. *Journal of Communication Disorders, 18,* 313–320.

Pearson L. (2001). The clinician-patient experience: Understanding transference and countertransference. *Nurse Practitioner, 26*(6), 8–11.

Perkins, W. H. (1971). *Speech pathology: An applied science.* St. Louis, MO: Mosby.

Perkins, W. H. (1975). Articulatory rate in the evaluation of stuttering treatments. *Journal of Speech and Hearing Disorders, 40,* 277–278.

Perkins, W. H. (1981). Measurements and maintenance of fluency. In B., Borger (Ed.), *Maintenance of fluency* (pp. 37–82). New York: Elsevier.

Perkins, W. H. (1983). Learning from negative outcomes in stuttering therapy: II. An epiphany of failures. *Journal of Fluency Disorders, 8,* 155–160.

Pindzola, R. H. (1986). Acoustic evidence of aberrant velocities in stutterers' fluent speech. *Perceptual Motor Skills, 62,* 399–405.

Preibisch, C., Neumann, K., Raab, P., Euler, H. A., von Gudenberg, A. W., Lanfermann, H., & Giraud, A. L. (2003). Evidence for compensation for stuttering by the right frontal operculum. *Neuroimage, 20,* 1356–1364.

Prins, D. (1970). Improvement and regression in stutterers following short-term intensive therapy. *Journal of Speech and Hearing Disorders, 35,* 123–135.

Ramig, P. R. (1984). Rate changes in the speech of stutterers after therapy. *Journal of Fluency Disorders, 9,* 285–294.

Ramig, P. R., Krieger, S. M., & Adams, M. R. (1982). Vocal changes in stutterers and nonstutterers when speaking to children. *Journal of Fluency Disorders, 7,* 369–384.

Riley, G. D. (1994). *Stuttering severity instrument for children and adults* (3rd ed.). Austin, TX: Pro-Ed.

Riley, J., Riley, G., & Maguire, G. (2004). Subjective screening of stuttering severity, locus of control and avoidance: Research edition. *Journal of Fluency Disorders, 29,* 51–62.

Robb, M. P., Lybolt, J. T., & Prince, H. A. (1985). Acoustic measures of stutterers speech following an intensive therapy program. *Journal of Fluency Disorders, 10,* 269–279.

Runyan, C., & Adams, M. R. (1979). Unsophisticated judges' perceptual evaluations of the speech of "successfully treated" stutterers. *Journal of Fluency Disorders, 4,* 29–48.

Runyan, C. M., Bell, J. N., & Prosek, R. A. (1990). Speech naturalness ratings of treated stutterers. *Journal of Speech and Hearing Disorders, 55,* 434–438.

Ryan, B. P., & Van Kirk, B. (1974). The establishment, transfer, and maintenance of fluent speech in 50 stutterers using delayed auditory feedback and operant procedures. *Journal of Speech and Hearing Disorders, 39,* 3–10.

Salmelin, R., Schnitzler, A., Schmitz, F., & Freund, H. (2000). Single word reading in developmental stutterers and fluent speakers. *Brain, 123,* 1184–1202.

Saltuklaroglu, T., & Kalinowski, J. (2002). The end-product of behavioural stuttering therapy: Three decades of denaturing the disorder. *Disability Rehabilitation, 15,* 786–789.

Samar, V. J., Metz, D. E., & Sacco, P. R. (1986). Changes in aerodynamic characteristics associated with therapy. *Journal of Speech and Hearing Research, 29,* 106–113.

Sheehan, J. G. (1970). *Stuttering: Research and therapy.* New York: Harper & Row.

Sheehan, J. G. (1984). Problems in the evaluation of progress and outcome. In W. H. Perkins (Ed.), *Stuttering disorders* (pp. 223–239). New York: Thieme-Stratton.

Shenker, R. C., & Finn, P. (1985). An evaluation of effects of supplemental "fluency" training during maintenance. *Journal of Fluency Disorders, 10,* 257–267.

Silverman, F. H. (1975). How "typical" is a stutterer's stuttering in a clinical environment? *Perceptual Motor Skills, 40,* 458.

Smith, A., Denny, M., Shaffer, L. A., Kelly, E. M., & Hirano, M. (1996). Activity of intrinsic laryngeal muscles in fluent and disfluent speech. *Journal of Speech and Hearing Research, 39,* 329–348.

Smith, A., Luschei, E., Denny, M., Wood, J., Hirano, M., & Badylak, S. (1993). Spectral analyses of activity of laryngeal and orofacial muscles in stutterers. *Journal of Neurology, Neurosurgery, and Psychiatry, 56,* 1303–1311.

Starkweather, C. W., Hirschman, P., & Tannenbaum, R. S. (1976). Latency of vocalization onset: Stutterers versus nonstutterers. *Journal of Speech and Hearing Research, 19,* 481–492.

Starkweather, C. W., & Meyers, M. (1979). Duration of subsegments within the inter-vocalic interval in stutterers and nonstutterers. *Journal of Fluency Disorders, 4,* 205–214.

Story, R. S. (1990). *A pre- and post-therapy comparison of articulatory, laryngeal, and respiratory kinematics of stutterers' fluent speech.* Unpublished doctoral dissertation, University of Connecticut, Storrs.

Story, R. S., Alfonso, P. J., & Harris, K. S. (1996). Pre- and post-treatment comparison of the kinematics of the fluent speech of persons who stutter. *Journal of Speech and Hearing Research, 39,* 991–1005.

Stromsta, C. (1986). *Elements of stuttering.* Oshtemo, MI: Atmorts Publishing.

Till, J. A., Reich, A., Dickey, S., & Seiber, J. (1983). Phonatory and manual reaction times of stuttering and nonstuttering children. *Journal of Speech and Hearing Research, 26,* 171–180.

Travis, L. E. (1931). *Speech pathology: A dynamic neurological treatment of normal speech and speech deviations.* New York: D. Appleton Co.

Van Riper, C. (1982). *The nature of stuttering* (2nd ed.). Englewood Cliffs, N.J.: Prentice-Hall.

Vishwanath, N. S. (1989). Global and local-temporal effects of a stuttering event in the context of a clausal utterance. *Journal of Fluency Disorders, 14,* 245–269.

Watkins, R. V., & Johnson, B. W. (2004). Language abilities in children who stutter: Toward improved research and clinical applications. *Language, Speech and Hearing Services in School, 35,* 82–89.

Watson, B. C., & Alfonso, P. J. (1987). Physiological bases of acoustic LRT in nonstutterers, mild stutterers, and severe stutterers. *Journal of Speech and Hearing Research, 30,* 434–447.

Weiss, A. L. (2000). What child language research may contribute to the understanding and treatment of stuttering. *Language, Speech and Hearing Services in School, 35*, 90–92.

Wingate, M. E. (1969). Sound and pattern in "artificial" fluency. *Journal of Speech Language and Hearing Research, 12*, 677-686.

Winkler, L., & Ramig, P. R. (1986). Temporal characteristics in the fluent speech of child stutterers and nonstutterers. *Journal of Fluency Disorders, 11*, 217–229.

Woolf, G. (1967). The assessment of stuttering as struggle, avoidance, and expectancy. *The British Journal of Disorders of Communication, 2*, 158–171.

Wu, J. C., Maguire, G., Riley, G., Fallon, J., LaCasse, L., Chin, S., Klein, E., Tang, C., Cadwell, S., & Lottenberg, S. (1995). A positron emission tomography [18F]deoxyglucose study of developmental stuttering. *Neuroreport, 15*, 501–505.

Wu, J. C., Maguire, G., Riley, G., Lee, A., Keator, D., Tang, C., Fallon, J., & Najafi, A. (1997). Increased dopamine activity associated with stuttering. *Neuroreport, 10*, 767–770.

Zebrowski, P. M. (1991). Duration of the speech disfluencies of beginning stutterers. *Journal of Speech and Hearing Research, 34*, 483–491.

Zebrowski, P. M., Conture, E. G., & Cudahy, E. A. (1985). Acoustic analysis of young stutterers' fluency: Preliminary observations. *Journal of Fluency Disorders, 10*, 173–192.

Zimmermann, G. (1980). Articulatory dynamics of fluent utterances of stutterers and nonstutterers. *Journal of Speech and Hearing Research, 23*, 95–107.

# 4

# Contemporary Methods of Treating Stuttering

> *"An expert is a man who has made all the mistakes which can be made in a very narrow field."*
>
> —*Niels Bohr (1885–1962)*

Most students enter the field of communication disorders with intentions of becoming skilled clinicians who can help others manage their communicative impairments. Thus, it is often with eager anticipation that these students approach the "treatment" section of courses in this field. After all the arguments among academicians about theoretical orientations have been said and done, what matters most to clinically oriented students is acquiring efficient and effective treatment methods. If a treatment works, students and patients care less about the theoretical orientation that made it sound. However, theoretical orientations that become popular also yield treatment methods that become popular and, in turn, any evidence of clinical efficacy from a treatment can help to further popularize a theoretical approach. Hence, when dealing with a pathologic condition, arguments regarding theoretical orientations must continue to arise with the hope of providing increasingly better options for treatment. Such is the case in the field of stuttering.

In the previous chapter we presented our theoretical orientation toward stuttering and how all symptomatology cascades outward from a neural hitch or block in the central nervous system. Based upon this model, we discussed what we believe to be the best assessment procedure for measuring therapeutic efficacy. The next obvious step is to provide students with the most effective therapy procedures from our perspective. Our theoretical orientation is simply one of stuttering "inhibition"—whereby the involuntary block responsible for all stuttering symptoms is suppressed or inhibited, allowing fluent speech patterns to predominate without interference from the neural hitch. However, our model does not dismiss past therapeutic methods. Though it is clear to us that many past approaches suffer from shortcomings such as high relapse rates, unnatural droned speech, difficulty in implementation, and extensive therapeutic intervention periods, we also recognize that many of these intervention methods, especially those in which the peripheral speech system is mechanically manipulated, provide powerful sources of stuttering inhibition. For this reason, we do not dismiss behavioral motor speech retraining techniques. We simply wish to find more effective means of integrating them into therapeutic procedures so as to quickly and easily inhibit stuttering while decreasing the possibilities of the shortcomings listed above. Therefore, before providing our orientation to the treatment of stuttering, in this chapter it is necessary for us to dissect some past treatment approaches with respect to understanding how they operate in adults and children who stutter, how they provide some levels of short-term remission, and why they may fail in providing long-term amelioration. In the next chapter, before providing our ideas regarding therapy, we provide a unifying conceptual framework that accounts for most powerful phenomena that reduce stuttering or "inhibit" the central involuntary block.

When treating stuttering, we may ask whether we wish to help people who stutter remove all aberrant behaviors from their speech, simply learn to accept themselves as stutterers, or some combination thereof. That is, do we attempt to remove all stuttering behaviors, an idealistic although a somewhat naive goal, or do we attempt to "heal" the person who stutters, so as to provide sufficient self-acceptance to function adequately in this world of generally fluent speakers? Or, do we attempt to provide some combination of these two ideals? We explore three general contemporary therapeutic approaches that have been widely used over the last half-century with varying degrees of success. First, we explore behavioral fluency-shaping approaches, which teach skills that were thought to be standard "recipes" for fluency. These therapies assumed that speaking behaviors could be brought under continuous voluntary control with the correct training of proper speech behaviors (whatever they may be). They also operated under the notion that by targeting and removing all overt stuttering behaviors, covert behaviors would also be removed and full "healing" would follow. Next, we examine the methods of the incomparable Charles Van Riper. Along with advocating motoric changes to speech production, he also sought to allow persons who stutter to accept, confront, and become desensitized to their pathology, often by stuttering in a fluentlike manner—a notion that may seem paradoxic at first. By doing this, patients were allowed to gain some semblance of control over the pathology in order to deal with it in a realistic manner. Finally, we explore cognitive coping strategies. These methods of "talk therapy" do not attempt to directly remove stuttering behaviors, but rather they attempt to "rationalize" the pathology or view the pathology with an appropriate sense of perspective. These cognitive approaches attempt to point to the self and, thus, provide those who stutter with coping and support systems designed to lessen the impact of stuttering on everyday life.

## Fluency-Shaping Approaches

These are primarily mechanistic techniques methods that are taught in a systematic behavioral hierarchy and are thought to instate "normal speech production." These mechanistic methods usually reduce or eliminate overt repetitious stuttering disruptions, at least for the short term. Whether stuttering was seen as a bad habit under learning theory or as an organic deficit under the speech motor paradigm, behavioral permutations of these procedures have been implemented to help ingrain fluent speech patterns. The idea is that after the initial "learning' phase, continuous maintenance and diligence will allow fluency skills to transfer and become superimposed upon stuttered speech, making then eventually automatic.

The basic "technique" that is taught to people who stutter upon entering most behavioral therapies is the extension or "prolongation" of vowels and voiced continuant sounds. The primary intended purpose of this technique is to reduce the rate of speech (Goldberg, 1981; Goldiamond, 1965; Ingham, 1984). The impetus behind using prolonged speech has often been twofold. First, it was thought that by slowing down, new and supposedly more appropriate speech patterns could be ingrained into the speech motor system and older more inappropriate habits (i.e., stuttering) could be supplanted. That is, it was assumed that speech motor programs that are most conducive to producing fluent speech are most easily learned and ingrained at slow speech rates that reduce the demands placed on the speech motor system (Bloodstein, 1995). Second, and perhaps more importantly, the slowing down was thought to be necessary because of the strong belief that those who stutter do not have the same speech temporal capacities for speech execution as normally fluent speakers. The slowing down was thought to allow a "flawed" system to produce a forward flowing speech that is not typically normal sounding, but free from repetitions.

Therapies can be administered either intensively or on an extended schedule. Intensive therapies often consist of 100 or more therapy hours packed into a three or four-week period, with or without follow-up. In contrast, therapy recipients on an extended schedule can receive weekly or biweekly sessions for months or even years. The type of schedule prescribed is often dependent on the availability of time and services, severity of stuttering, financial resources, and individual preferences. However, it may be fair to state that intensive therapies (see the Stuttering Foundation of America Web-site: http://www.stutteringhelp .org/reflists/ref_icl.htm for a list of such programs across the USA and Canada) require effort as well as time and financial commitment, but also often carry with them "promise" of alleviation of some of the burdens of stuttering. However, we again note that relapse in 3 to 6 months is a major problem after the fluency derived from almost all intensive programs wears off. The number of these intensive camps has waned in the last decade or so, as has the amount of time required to complete programs in these camps. They perhaps help a few hundred people per year, or a couple of thousand in a decade or so. Thus, this degree of help is relatively small compared to the large numbers of people who stutter in North America and around the world.

Regardless of the intervention schedule, during the first few days of therapy, speech rates are usually reduced drastically—even as slow as a syllable every two seconds (Webster, 1974; 1979). This prolongation rate can be up to 10 or more times slower than normal speech rates, which have commonly been found to be around 4 to 5 syllables per second (Netsell, 1981; Pickett, 1980). However, it should be noted that at this extremely slow rate of speech it is almost impossible to stutter. However, we have argued that this type of speech can even be called one long stutterlike prolongation (Dayalu & Kalinowski, 2002), which is why we say that these therapies are good at eliminating repetitions. Yet, even in the most severe cases of stuttering, the imposition of these extremely unnatural speech patterns almost eliminates all other overt signs of overtly disrupted speech. Every prolonged syllable is an extended droned production—which may not be unlike the involuntary prolongations that can characterize stuttering. From this basic foundation, a series of secondary "fluency skills" can be added that are thought to be compatible with fluent speech. These fluency skills are designed to target the speech subsystems (e.g., respiratory, laryngeal, and articulatory) individually and reduce the possibility of stuttering behaviors manifesting in these sites. For example, if stuttering is characterized by excessive laryngeal tension or difficulty initiating speech then the use of "gentle onsets" (Webster, 1980) or an "airflow control" (Schwartz, 1977) technique may be deemed appropriate to combat manifestations in the larynx. These techniques are designed to keep air flowing smoothly through the vocal folds and keep speech moving in a forward direction. Gentle onsets are thought to help in initiation as the vocal folds can be adducted slowly during speech initiation using a breathy vocal attack.

Although these secondary fluency skills attempt to target speech subsystems individually, it should be noted that the speech motor system is not compartmentalized. That is, changes that are effected in one speech subsystem will have influences on the others. The entire peripheral speech mechanism (i.e., from the lungs, through the larynx and vocal tract, and up to the pharyngeal and oral articulators) are bound together in a unified and coordinated structure (Browman & Goldstein, 1992). Any alteration in one system is likely to affect the others and alter the final speech product. It may be naïve of us to think that we can really focus upon making changes to one speech subsystem at a time. The use of prolonged speech in itself serves to slow down the speech periphery. In doing so, speech output is altered. That is, speech takes on a droned quality, which has become a "therapeutic signature" in stuttering therapy. When we begin to layer additional secondary "techniques" on top of the already slowed prolonged forms, speech becomes even slower and the droned quality becomes even more "different" from normal production. Thus, the implementation of prolonged speech with contributions from the secondary techniques such as gentle onsets, continuous phonation, airflow, and light articulatory contacts slows down the dynamics of speech production and creates gross changes in the overall perceptual quality of the speech end product that are best described as "droning." These behaviors are supposedly prophylactic in nature but are used at a cost. They are socially conspicuous; they often sound highly unnatural and need constant monitoring. In their favor, if one uses them long enough and diligently enough, they will remove most secondary behaviors. Oftentimes the need to use such exaggerated behaviors diminishes in some people, showing the power of stuttering inhibitions via mechanistic techniques.

In chapter 3, we outlined some of the differences in the perceptually fluent speech of those who stutter relative to those who do not. Recall that one factor that may have contributed to such differences was a history of therapy. Considering the droned "therapeutic signature" that often characterizes post-therapeutic speech, these differences are not surprising and have been demonstrated empirically. Following therapy, stutterers have been found to acoustically demonstrate longer voice onset times and vowel durations and an increased proportion of voiced segments (Metz, Onufrak, & Ogburn, 1979; Metz, Samar, & Sacco, 1983; Metz, Schiavetti, & Sacco, 1990; Samar, Metz, &

Sacco, 1986; Shenker & Finn, 1985). Kinematic studies of perceptually fluent post-therapeutic speech of stutterers have also shown greater inspiratory volumes and expiratory flows, as well as reduced amplitude for lip and jaw movements on consonantal sounds relative to normally fluent control subjects (Story, Alfonso, & Harris, 1996). Stutterers who received treatment have also demonstrated longer duration of jaw movement and time to peak velocity in the upper lip, lower lip, and jaw, as well as sequencing reversals of these articulators on perceptually fluent productions of the word "sapapple" (McClean, Kroll, & Loftus, 1990). Simply put, after therapy stutterers are producing speech differently and it is reflected in both acoustic and kinematic measures. In other words, the use of prolonged speech in conjunction with other fluency-shaping techniques cumulatively produces interdependent modulations in speech production that are perceived as a globally conspicuous and unnatural prosodic quality or droning. Table 4–1 outlines various "fluency skills" with respect to how they have been perceived to impact speech production in stutterers and what we suspect they may be doing to speech production with respect to contributing to the droned therapeutic signature. However, though it lacks functionality, sometimes droning is not a bad thing, as the droned quality seems to inhibit stuttering.

## Droning Inhibits Stuttering

Immediately upon imposing extensively droned speech, stuttering is almost invariably eliminated. Most therapy recipients are rendered nearly "invulnerable" to stuttering when their rate of speech is decreased to a syllable every two seconds and the entire dynamic of their speech system has been radically altered to produce droned speech. That is, the chances of stuttering at this rate are extremely low and the person receiving therapy can inherently feel this "invulnerability." The therapeutic course could be considered successful at this point, as most therapies only use the criterion of the elimination or reduction of discrete stuttering behaviors as a measure of success. However, at this impossibly slow rate, this droned therapeutic speech may be almost unintelligible, and is completely nonfunctional, especially at two seconds per syllable. Yet, naturalness and communicative

**Table 4–1.** The Intuitive Rationale Behind Some Commonly Used Therapeutic Techniques and Our Proposed Explanations for Their Ameliorative Effects

| Therapeutic Technique | Behavioral Therapeutic Purpose | Intended Subsystems of Modulation | Proposed Ameliorative Effect |
|---|---|---|---|
| Gentle (easy) onsets | Measure amplitude slope of laryngeal onset to reduce tension. | Phonatory | Slows speech and contributes to droned quality. |
| Prolonged speech | Reduces the demands on the speech motor system by reducing speed of articulatory movements. | Phonatory Articulatory Respiratory | Contributes to droned quality by increasing lengths of vowels and hence the articulatory dynamics of the vocal tract. |
| Airflow techniques | Initiate airflow at the beginning of utterances to avoid a "locking of the vocal folds." | Laryngeal Respiratory | Contributes to halting quality imposing air stream management in appropriate places in speech flow. |
| Continuous phonation | Reduces the demands on the system by increasing the relative amount of voiced content. | Phonatory | Contributes to droned quality by increasing relative amount of voiced content. |
| Light articulatory contacts | Reduce excessive tension in the articulators to avoid blocking on consonantal sounds. | Articulatory | Contributes to droned quality by turning consonants into vowel-like sounds. |

functionality have rarely been considered when stuttering is treated under the tenets of behavioral therapy (Bloodstein, 1995; Kalinowski et al., 1994; Onslow, Costa, Andrews, Harrison, & Packman, 1996), and as long as the speech is forward flowing and free from overt stuttering, the success criterion is met. However, when speech naturalness in stuttering therapy began to be examined in the mid 1980s (Martin, Haroldson, & Triden. 1984), it became a thorn in the side of those seeking only to eliminate overt stuttering manifestations; it seems that unnaturalness and stuttering are inversely related, or stuttering increases with increased naturalness. Since then a series of studies has shown that naturalness of speech is a very important factor to consider when opting for the use of any therapeutic technique (Kalinowski, Noble, et al., 1994; Franken, Van Bezooijen, & Boves, 1997). Simply put, if the resultant speech product does not sound and feel natural, no matter how free from overt stuttering it may be, relapse is likely to follow.

In Figure 4–1 we have outlined the typical course of a fluency-shaping program with respect to the amount of "droning" involved, speech naturalness, functionality, stability of the speech product, and the use of covert strategies for reducing stuttering. It is highly unlikely that at any point after the initial period of the therapeutic course (i.e., the "Drone Zone") will the speech of the therapy recipient be less susceptible to stuttering. Furthermore, while in the "Drone Zone," covert compensatory strategies such as substituting words, avoiding difficult words sounds or situations, and using circumlocutions around difficult words seem to be virtually eliminated. These strategies, skillfully employed for years in order to speak without displaying overt stuttering behaviors, appear to serve no purpose when a person is feeling an invulnerability to stuttering.

Once fluency techniques are mastered at the slowest of speech rates where it is virtually impossible to stutter, speech rates are gradually increased and the techniques are retaught and synchronized with each newly imposed rate. Every incremental increase in speech rate represents an attempt to make therapeutic speech more natural sounding and functional. Simply put, it is an attempt to gradually exit the Drone Zone (see Figure 4–1). With gradual increases in speech rate, more complex

DRONING

| PreTherapy | Initial phase of Therapy | Middle phase of Therapy | End of Therapy | One Month Post Therapy |
|---|---|---|---|---|
| Predroning | Maximum Droning "The Drone Zone" | Decreased droning | Minimal Droning | Intermittent droning (at best) |
|  |  | Pseudodroning | | |
| Stutter-filled speech VERY UNSTABLE | Completely stutter-free speech VERY STABLE | Stutter-free speech for most but signs of stuttering appear in severe cases LESS STABLE | Stutter-free speech for "top" students but frequent signs of stuttering in most others UNSTABLE | Stuttering-free speech when droned or for short periods thereafter VERY UNSTABLE |
| Natural sounding speech | Unnatural and nonfunctional speech | Still unnatural sounding but better functionality | Continues to lack in naturalness for many | Naturalness fluctuates with amount of droning imposed |
| Avoidances, substitutions, and circumlocutions permeate speech | Speech is completely free from avoidances, substitutions, and circumlocutions | Avoidances, substitutions, and circumlocutions begin to reappear | Avoidances, substitutions, and circumlocutions are salient for many | Avoidances, substitutions, and circumlocutions permeate speech |

RELAPSE

**Figure 4–1.** Continuum of possible speech productions in those who stutter, from pretherapeutic to one month post-therapeutic, illustrating the incompatibility between speech naturalness and the absence of overt stuttering behaviors, and the simultaneous use of avoidances, substitutions, and circumlocutions.

and functional activities are often introduced into the therapeutic regime with the intention of generalizing the use of the newly learned speech patterns. That is, targeted increases in speech rates progress from being used in simple to complex forms, from being produced with lots of clinical cues to being produced independently, and from being produced in clinical settings to being produced in natural settings. However, it is also upon increasing speech rates and attempting to make speech sound more natural by removing the droned quality, that the breakdown in the forward flow of speech often begins and stuttering begins to resurface, especially in the more severe stutterers. This instability in the forward flow of speech is also marked by the return of ingrained covert substitutions, avoidances, and circumlocutions, sometimes to a greater extent than at pretherapeutic levels, as the impetus for producing forward flowing speech may be greater in therapeutic settings. Dayalu and Kalinowski (2002) offered the term "pseudofluency" to describe such speech. It remains unnatural sounding, requires constant monitoring and effort to produce, and is subject to breakdown. We suggest that the term "pseudofluency" is synonymous with "pseudodroning." While the droned quality is not as salient as at the initial stage of therapy, it continues to resonate throughout speech. As such, pseudodroning is less stable and more subject to breakdown than speech that is completely droned. The underlying assumption is that any breakdown in fluency is because the "correct" motor speech patterns have not yet been ingrained into the motor speech program of the person who stutters. Thus, when overt stuttering begins to reappear at faster rates of speech, the prescribed remedy is a regression to a slower rate in which the droned quality is again most salient.

By the end of the therapeutic course, which is often 3 to 5 weeks after the starting date, following countless hours of rate control and skill practicing, some therapy recipients appear to be successful, in that they are able to produce forward flowing, stutter-free speech at relatively high speech rates and in a variety of contexts. However, others (usually the more severe cases) do not seem to be able to produce stutter-free speech unless they continue to add a salient droned quality, moving from pseudodroning back to the Drone Zone, sounding highly unnatural, and even then, only in the simplest of speaking situations (Saltuklaroglu, Kalinowski, & Guntupalli, 2004). Upon leaving the nurturing and reinforcing therapeutic cocoon, all therapy recipients are instructed to keep practicing their "techniques" and imposing slower speech rates with a higher droned quality as necessary in order to further ingrain their newly "repro-grammed" speech patterns. There is no social penalty for droned speech in the therapeutic cocoon. In fact, it is reinforced to the hilt, so that it can be instated "forever"—or so the theory goes. It is supposed to follow the same manner of speech acquisition and typical motor learning in newborn infants—but it seems something is wrong with this line of thinking and it never achieves this sort of automaticity or naturalness. For some, the future may look promising, as evident by their ability to produce pseudodroned stutter-free speech at speech rates that seem com-municatively functional. However, others return to the outside world with pseudodroned speech that is tenuous at best, unable to produce stutter-free speech without regressing to the Drone Zone. For them, the fear of stuttering is often as real as ever and they may revert to the use of avoidances, substitutions, and cir-cumlocutions in order to hide both overt stuttering behaviors and their unnatural post-therapeutic speech. These therapy recipients are often the first to question what went wrong and why they have seemingly failed to reprogram their speech motor system. They have been told that using the techniques and stuttering are mutually exclusive, and if they are stuttering they are simply not using the techniques appropriately. This is simply untrue. There is no scientific evidence to suggest that stuttering and the use of any behavioral technique cannot coexist. We do know that cer-tain behavioral techniques inhibit stuttering but there is no evi-dence to suggest that stuttering cannot exist with "proper" use of technique (whatever that may be). That is, stuttering can exist at any speech rate, using gentle onset or full diaphragmatic breaths, and there is no one to blame. We suppose that this knowledge might relieve a lot of those who stutter from the guilt and shame of not using techniques or having techniques fail them in the fight against this insidious involuntary disorder.

We suggest that it is the mechanically imposed droning itself that inhibits the neural stuttering block. The global devia-tions from perceptually natural speech that are found in droned speech supply the inhibitory power over stuttering. In the next chapters we argue that droning provides a form of mechanically induced "gestural redundancy," a quality in speech that reflects imitative processes and has inhibitory power over stuttering.

Furthermore, droning seems to possess an inherent inhibitory effect over stuttering for a short period of time after it is removed as well as when it is continually implemented. That is, some people who stutter seem susceptible to "carryover fluency" as evident by their relatively effortless dance through therapy following the initial stage of extensive droning, and their ability to produce stutter-free speech for short periods of time post-therapy in a variety of contexts and situations, regardless of whether or not fluency skills appear to be implemented. The "carryover" inhibitory effect of droning on stuttering has been demonstrated empirically. Stutterers who were asked to say a continuous /a/, which may be somewhat analogous to droning without the dynamic articulatory modulations, showed a 30% decrease in stuttering in the ensuing speech as compared to a control condition. However, when a 4-second silence was inserted between the production of the steady vowel and the intended utterance, no reduction in stuttering frequency was observed (Dayalu, Saltuklaroglu, Kalinowski, Stuart, & Rastatter, 2001), demonstrating that when using the production of a single sustained vowel as the source of inhibition, though some carryover occurs, it is relatively short-lived.

It should be noted that producing natural-sounding stutter-free speech without the use of fluency skills is sometimes frowned upon by those espousing behavioral fluency shaping techniques. These clinicians have been trained to monitor the use of specific target behaviors (i.e., techniques) thought to induce fluency, and witnessing fluency in the absence of these behaviors does fit with the designated therapeutic protocol. Thus, these clinicians may continue to remind therapy recipients of the constant need to use their "skills" and may claim that this carryover or "lucky fluency" that they are experiencing is fleeting and unstable. We suggest that "lucky" fluency is simply a form of fluent speech that is generated from extended droning that allows stuttering inhibition that may last for weeks or months. This inhibition can be sustained with more droning and that is why clinicians frown on "natural speech." They may know that the period of inhibition needs to be supported via droning or the use of other inhibitory methods. However, if stuttering can be adequately inhibited using a particular strategy or set of techniques and the inhibition remains for a period of time, then why not take advantage of this true natural-sounding fluent speech until it is time to inhibit again? When we discuss our therapeutic approach we will again consider this question.

Others, however, do not seem to be as amenable to the inhibitory carryover from droned speech, and seem to continually need to revert back to the Drone Zone in order for speech to proceed without stuttering. For these therapy recipients, the management of stuttering is nearly always more difficult. The more deviance from natural speech, the more effort and energy that is expended to achieve the inhibited state, and the more likely it is that the new speech forms will not be continually implemented.

## The Relapse Spiral

Initially, there is something magical about removing the aberrant energy expenditure used to overcome repetitions, struggle behavior, head jerks, arm movement, and eye blinking, from a person with a moderate-to-severe stutter. The relative normalcy is often awe-inspiring. To see a person wrapped up in a cumulative boa constrictor, released via a simple droning technique is amazing and gratifying to any clinician who has taught the technique being used. Yet, the release from stuttering and the newfound stutter-free speech comes with a couple of uninvited riders. The first rider is the unnaturalness of post-therapeutic speech relative to pretherapeutic speech and the speech of non-stuttering speakers (Saltuklaroglu, Kalinowski, & Guntupalli, 2004). In other words, it is characterized by the "droned" therapeutic signature. The other rider is the continuous monitoring that is required to continuously impart these techniques, as for most they rarely achieve promised levels of "automaticity." This continuous monitoring and guarding against breakdown requires a great deal of energy expenditure. Thus, for many, these two riders spell relapse. The question is why these two riders are not acknowledged as soon as we hear the speech after therapy. It is all a matter of relativism. After the "boa constrictor" stage of stuttering, simply being able to use a droned speech form is a new freedom relative to the struggle and degree of aberrance that previously existed. However, like most humans, those who stutter seek to be like those without a disorder. As stuttering is intermittent even in the most severe cases, there are often times when those who stutter may be indistinguishable from those without the pathology. However, as soon as droning is implemented, it permeates all speech utterances, and the red flag of a communicative impairment is immediately raised. Thus, even though the new speech may be relatively struggle-free and forward flowing, the global changes make it sound far from normal. Thus, we see a "Catch-22" in stuttering therapy. Do I stutter and sound natural some of the time or do I remove most overt stuttering and sound unnatural all the time? Just about everyone who undergoes traditional therapies must answer this question and attempt to strike a balance. It can be confusing and lead to relapse. What seems apparent is that fluent speech without controls is fine when it works for an individual, but typically droning and some degree of control is needed at some point to inhibit stuttering.

Relapse rates following behavioral therapies are at least 70% (Craig & Calver, 1991; Craig & Hancock, 1995). For many who never seemed to quite adjust to continuous pseudodroning and who had to continually revert back to the Drone Zone in order to produce forward-flowing speech, relapse does not seem surprising. After all, droning requires a concerted effort and its continuous imposition on every syllable is more conspicuous and unnatural sounding than the previous discrete stuttering behaviors that were intermittent at best. A drastic compromise in speech naturalness is the price to pay for forward-flowing speech, a price that is often too high and results in the abandonment of therapy techniques and a return to stuttering. For others who seemed to master pseudodroning during therapy and exit the program with high levels of forward-flowing and relatively natural-sounding speech, the relapse course may not be as direct. Without the continued implementation of droning, the inhibitory effects wane and overt stuttering begins to resurface. It is only when droning is reinstated that stuttering once again disappears. However, by doing so, naturalness is again compromised. Hence, upon re-entry to the "real world" pseudodroning includes intermittently juggling between sounding natural and maintaining stutter-free speech. The two simply do not appear to be  compatible. It follows that all speech produced by people who stutter may fall on a continuum ranging from stuttered and natural sounding to stutter-free and unnatural sounding (see Figure 4–1). Though this account of relapse may seem pessimistic, from our interactions with hundreds of those who stutter it is relatively accurate. What it does provide is a clue that fluent speech is not a learned behavior. Other motor skills (e.g., walking, skating, bicycle riding, and writing) are usually learned during a single learning stage and rarely show relapse after thousands of hours of practice or therapy, especially for automatic processes like speech. It seems strange that a constant governor must be applied to speech production when it is such an automatic process. This is analogous to driving a car with the brakes constantly applied while having a foot on the gas. You may wonder why you still lose control of the car. The trick may be to learn when to slow the car down and use the brake to minimize the effect of loss of control. In stuttering this means learning how best to implement certain techniques that help maintain forward and natural speech flow while still inhibiting the otherwise omnipresent possibility of an involuntary neural block.

Obviously for a therapy to have the best chance of working, we need to guard against relapse. We discussed achieving the balance between stutter-free and natural-sounding speech. If droning inhibits stuttering, then it seem paradoxic to believe that those who stutter can sound natural and produce stutter-free speech with the use of motoric therapy techniques. Thus, our methods of intervening describe how best to engage a fluency-enhancing mechanism to inhibit stuttering while making only minimal changes in motor speech output so as to maximize speech naturalness and reduce the chances of relapse. By analyzing patterns of stuttered speech with respect to the types, durations, and loci of overt moments of stuttering, therapists can play a key role in selecting appropriate methods of inhibition to achieve this balance.

## Peripheral or Central Inhibition

Attributing the ameliorative effects of stuttering therapy to the reprogramming of the peripheral speech subsystem by subsystem (see Table 4–1) now seems highly suspect considering the fact that the motor speech mechanism functions as a unified system and the subsystems cannot be independently modulated. Rather, we suggest that prolonged speech and the other fluency techniques inhibit stuttering at a central level by deriving the droned prosodic quality that is globally imparted upon speech. The combinations of prolonged speech with other speech modulations such as "gentle onsets," "airflow," "continuous phonation," and "light articulatory contacts" seem to make interactive contributions to the droned quality, thus altering motor to sensory feedback and creating a central inhibitory effect on stuttering (see Table 4–1). Therefore, it is not the precise coordinated motoric movements of the techniques per se that are responsible for decreased levels of stuttering, but rather the cumulative, interactive, and interdependent manner in which the combinations of motoric machinations modulate the peripheral speech motor system and impose the droned quality upon speech that inhibits stuttering.

Stuttering should not be considered a disorder of the peripheral motor speech system and attempting to compartmentally reprogram a highly complex, unified system that has never proven to be compromised seems illogical (Armson & Kalinowski, 1994). If "correct" speech patterns could be learned in the same way as any other motor routine, fluent speakers could be trained in the same manner as athletes or musicians. The high relapse rates following behavioral speech retraining seem indicative that the origin of the pathology is not peripheral in nature. Rather, the overt stuttering manifestations at the level of the lungs, larynx, and articulators are simply symptoms of a central neurologic pathology (Kalinowski, Dayalu, Stuart, Rastatter, & Rami, 2000). This pathology seems to be effectively inhibited by the person who stutters by generating salient alterations in motor to sensory feedback from speech. As such, the implementation of prolongation and other fluency skills are not correcting a peripheral flaw in speech production. Instead, they induce salient prosodic changes that create "gestural redundancy" in the brain. This term is explained fully in the next chapter. What it implies is that when gross detectable changes are made to the manner of speaking, our brains pick up more speech information per unit time, a scenario that is conducive for engaging the central mechanism for inhibiting stuttering.

## Behavioral Therapies for Children

Since the days of Wendell Johnson, notions regarding the provision
of therapy to children who stutter have changed dramatically.
Recall, that Johnson (1942) believed that stuttering developed
from normal nonfluency because overly perfectionistic parents
drew negative attention to the mild disfluencies produced by
their children. Thus, therapy was targeted toward parents and
caregivers, teaching them to ignore stuttering in their child.
Recall also, that this approach yielded an approximately 80%
recovery rate—most likely thanks to natural spontaneous recovery. These seemingly positive results allowed the Johnsonian
approach to influence the treatment of stuttering children until
the 1980s, long after therapy for adults had become more behaviorally oriented.

In the 1980s, the studies finding significant kinematic and
acoustic differences (greater durations, differing temporal patterns
of lip and jaw movement) in the speech in those who stutter relative to normally fluent speakers brought the speech motor paradigm to the forefront. Rather than being viewed as just a bad
habit, it began to be suspected that stuttering was associated
with organic deficits that caused reduced temporal motor capacities for correctly executing and coordinating speech (Caruso
et al., 1988). For the adult stuttering population, this change
in orientation was not about to bring many great changes in the
administration of therapy. Under both learning theory and the
speech motor paradigm, the use of prolonged speech remained
the primary method of intervention for adults. However, in children, the notion of an organic compromise brought with it
radical changes in the implementation of therapy. No longer
was stuttering to be ignored under the pretense that it did not
exist until parents made it exist. Now, it was thought that a
true tangible culprit existed for manifestations of stuttering and
that these aberrant speech behaviors should be brought to the
attention of all concerned and dealt with directly. Suddenly,
identifying early stuttering behaviors became the right thing to
do. In addition, parents could no longer be directly blamed for
inducing stuttering in their children. Early intervention made
sense and became the right thing to do. It was logically assumed
that if "correct" speech patterns were to be overlaid upon

stuttering, it would occur most easily if attempted during its most incipient stages.

Not surprisingly, stuttering children started to be treated by direct behavioral therapy, namely, using simplified variations of prolonged speech. Therapists provided strong models of prolonged speech forms with names such as "easy speech" and "turtle talk." Children were simply asked to replicate these speech patterns moving from simple to more complex forms, with increasingly less cueing, and moving from clinical settings to more naturalistic environments. Children are generally adept imitators, a characteristic that is discussed in detail in the next chapter. As such, replicating prolonged speech forms in clinical settings is often accomplished quite easily. Furthermore, patterns of childhood stuttering can be less severe than those of adults, and often do not carry the attendant covert baggage. These characteristics give the illusion of high therapeutic success in a relatively short time within a clinical setting.

As the direct approach to childhood stuttering therapy became popular, a new model for explaining childhood stuttering began to emerge. This was known as the "demands and capacities model" (Starkweather, 2002; Starkweather, Gottwald, & Halfond, 1990). This model simply states that children begin to exhibit disfluencies when the demands placed upon their speech system outweigh the motor speech system's natural speech and language capacities. If the demands placed upon the system continue to grossly outweigh their corresponding capacities, stuttering may become ingrained. The demands on the system may stem from various sources that may be either internal (i.e., within the child) or external (i.e, environmental factors). Internal demands may include muscular coordination; a range of linguistic skills including semantics, grammatic abilities, syntax, and pragmatic skills such as turn-taking, conversation initiation, and conversation maintenance; articulation and phonology; anxiety levels; and general cognitive abilities. External demands may include the speech and language characteristics of others such as their natural rate and prosody, expectations of others related to producing accurate linguistic forms, stress, teasing, or just about any other external factor that increases the communicative pressures on a child. Thus, children develop at different rates and show differential capacities of coping with the gamut of internal and external demands on the speech mechanism. Under this model, stuttering is simply thought to develop in children whose capacities fall behind their demands. Thus, in addition to promoting direct therapy, the next generation of childhood stuttering clinicians also continued to advocate reducing the demands on children's speech systems so as to allow their natural capacities to "catch up" and reduce the chances of stuttering continuing to permeate and becoming engrained in the motor speech system.

Although this direct approach appeared to be quite different from the previous Johnsonian approach, the wide acceptance of the demands and capacities model continued to show a strong influence of Johnsonian dogma on the therapeutic approaches to childhood stuttering. After all, Johnson's "monster study" could be described under the "demands and capacities model" as an attempt to exert sufficient external demands on the speech system to induce stuttering. Thus, even after direct intervention became consistently advocated, parents were still told to positively reinforce speaking and not associate stuttering with any form of punishment. They were told to model "easy" slowed speech patterns and reduce the levels of communicative pressures in the child's speaking environment. Use of this model provided an explanation that parents could understand easily. The speech motor and language system of their child just did not seem to be keeping up with the natural demands placed upon him or her. Direct intervention could help impose fluency via speech retraining. Johnsonian ideas were also retained as it was thought that parents could also help indirectly by providing a nurturing and reinforcing speaking environment that was not conducive to stuttering. Parental modeling of slow, easy speech patterns was thought to be especially appropriate for very young children who are not yet capable of participating in structured, direct therapy sessions. In addition, parents could reduce the overall rates of exchanges during communication by using appropriate pauses during turn-taking. One problem with this approach is that similar to the Johnsonian approach, parents steeped in the demands and capacities model may continue to blame themselves when their children fail to recover from stuttering. They may believe that they could not provide speaking environments that met the natural capacities of their child. In addition, children who received direct therapy and failed to recover from stuttering may blame themselves for failure, especially when they see other children recovering, as is the case 80% of the time due to natural recovery. Children who engage in turtle talk, easy speech, and other therapeutic techniques presented in the clinic and still fail to recover may have a sense of failure and blame themselves for this failure. Feeling the responsibility for this failure, for a pathology that is truly involuntary and can be beyond volitional control may be analogous to children who blame themselves for their parents divorcing.

Direct intervention in children appeared to be a step in the right direction after the Johnsonian notions of ignoring the pathology. Compared to adults, children seemed to be relatively easy to treat. In many children, stuttering was not fully ingrained and the possibility of full recovery (even without intervention) still existed. In addition, children generally (though by no means always) tend to exhibit milder forms of the pathology that appear to be more amenable to change, and carry with them fewer covert behaviors. However, possibly the most important factor for helping children to become fluent via direct intervention in a therapeutic setting is their ability to imitate. Children are adept imitators of others. Imitation is an ability that is refined in humans and is crucial to the initial phases of language development and motor skills. Think how you learn athletic skills or how to play a musical instrument. The first step is to watch others who do the skill proficiently and try to imitate them. As we grow older we tend to imitate less unless we decide to learn new skills. What is important here is that imitation is an act that is generally done fluently among all human populations, including infants, adults, those with developmental delays and other pathologic populations. This "fluent" characteristic of imitation is of exceptional importance and is discussed in detail in the next chapter as we begin to understand the mechanism of stuttering inhibition. For now, it is sufficient to say that direct therapy for stuttering children may exploit their ability to fluently imitate the speech patterns of others. Therapy for children involves a great deal of modeling by the clinician and direct imitation by the children receiving therapy. Many clinicians marvel at the abilities of these stuttering children to fluently reproduce their patterns of "turtle talk" or "slow easy" speech. As soon as the child hears the model in the clinical room, most often, they are able to easily replicate it. Thus, measuring the fluency of stuttering children in clinical settings can produce data that appear very compelling, a factor that, along with natural spontaneous recovery, possibly explains the optimistic data reported in efficacy studies on direct behavioral interventions for stuttering children (Kalinowski, Dayalu, & Saltuklaroglu, 2002).

However, from our experience, many children who stutter and their parents report that the children have little difficulty producing the designated behavioral speech targets within the nurturing and reinforcing confines of the clinic room or therapy at home. As with adults, possibly the most difficult aspect of motoric speech retraining in children is extending the derived improvements beyond the clinic and the structured home therapy. Many times, children will simply abandon the imitated speech patterns as soon as they leave the therapy session. Many school-age children state that they just cannot or do not want to use their therapeutic speech in the classroom or when talking to friends—stating they would rather stutter. Many claim they simply forget to use their therapy techniques, which is not surprising, considering the amount of monitoring and attention that is required to continually impose them. Forgetting to use the techniques is also a claim from many adults. Thus, for those children who do not experience spontaneous recovery, direct intervention may teach children some methods of stuttering inhibition, but the relief seems to be temporary. Stable prevalence rates of stuttering suggest that similar to Johnsonian therapy, this direct therapy does little to boost recovery rates from stuttering. However, it may help promote recovery in some children who teeter on the edge. For others, learning to use motoric speech manipulations to inhibit stuttering may provide varying levels of relief from the burdens of stuttering and may help decrease overall severity levels.

In an effort to promote early intervention and generalization of speaking skills beyond the clinic, Onslow's Lidcombe program (see chapter 2) attempts to train parents to provide direct therapy to their incipiently stuttering children. Interestingly, one of the most frequently used techniques that parents are taught to use involves asking children to repeat their stuttered utterances using slow, easy forms of speech that are modeled by the parents. Thus, this therapy also seems to capitalize on children's natural propensity for imitating. While we do not question the logic behind early intervention and using the parents as therapists to aid in generalization, we are still yet to be convinced that this approach produces rates of recovery that can be proven to exceed those of natural spontaneous processes. To be convincing, empirical data from Lidcombe studies would need to indicate *eradication* of stuttering within the groups tested that significantly exceeds spontaneous recovery rates. Simply put, if the group data still show stuttering during testing, we can be sure that a proportion of children did not fully recover even in the test environments. The test environments are so amenable to fluency enhancement that even the control subjects, those who do not receive therapy, often exhibit 50 to 75% decreases in stuttering over time in the same environments. Most of the improvement is observed between the first session and the second session for both the treated and the nontreated participants in most longitudinal, repeated measures studies. In addition, we would like to see a less stringent selection criteria for children accepted into the program, so as to be sure that all parents and children have an equal chance of being accepted into the therapeutic program.

We conclude this section by restating the difficulty in ascertaining the efficacy of any therapy for childhood stuttering. Before any therapy can be considered effective, it needs to be weighed against the epidemiologic data. For the past decade or so, Yairi's research group has been involved in longitudinal studies investigating the progression of stuttering in about 150 preschool children. They have continued to find recovery rates of about 76%, with most of the recoveries occurring within 48 months of onset. Therefore, though early intervention makes logical sense, any time full recovery occurs during the initial phase of stuttering, it is impossible to rule out the contributions of spontaneous recovery. Yet we still continue to treat young children who stutter. It is our ethical obligation and we may be accelerating the recovery path as well as providing effective techniques for continued stuttering inhibition.

# Van Riperian Therapy—Stuttering Modification

Many therapies have focused on confrontation and acceptance of stuttering. The most accepted and used of these therapies were the methods of Charles Van Riper. In the final chapter of his seminal text *The Nature of Stuttering*, Van Riper provides his ideas on how the disorder originates. He saw stuttering occurring as a result of disordered "timing" during speech execution. One of the main ideas that Van Riper attributed to be a source of disordered timing was disrupted feedback loops during speech production. According to the zeitgeist, "servotheory" was popular for explaining speech production. Servotheory like cybernetics simply employs the notion that a mechanism can adjust itself based on the feedback it is receiving. For example, if any of you have taken the graduate record examination (GRE) on the computer, you may have found that if you answer some questions correctly, the questions that follow become more difficult. If you produce one or two wrong answers, the subsequent questions become easier. The computer program employs a "servomechanism" to adjust its output based on the answers being fed into it. Another example of a servomechanism, which Bloodstein (1995) uses, is a digital thermostat that is set a certain temperature. If the temperature deviates two or three degrees above or below the set temperature the heater or the air conditioning unit will be activated to make the adjustment to the desired setting. Again, the "servomechanism," here the digital thermostat, adjusts its output based on the input it is receiving. Speech was thought to operate in a similar manner. As we receive acoustic and proprioceptive (knowing the relative positions of our articulators) feedback during speech, we can make motor adjustments to speech production to ensure that what we intend to say is produced without errors. Although Van Riper explored a number of sources for the proposed "timing" deficit, he seemed to favor the notion that the servosystem used in speech production may be somehow compromised in those who stutter. Learning theory was also popular in psychology during Van Riper's clinical days and, thus, it is not surprising that his therapy meshed servotheory (e.g., cybernetics) and learning theory.

As a lifelong "stutterer" and long-time clinician, Van Riper was aware of the day-to-day battles with stuttering. He understood that effectively managing stuttering often required a great deal more than the simple ability to replace conspicuous stuttering behaviors with altered speech patterns, which were often more awkward and conspicuous than the ones they were replacing. He also understood that stuttering was a complex syndrome that manifested slightly differently in everyone it afflicted. As such, before attempting to change moments of stuttering, Van Riper's therapy aimed at teaching stutterers to identify with their disorder and confront it in such a way so as to lower its impact on their communication and lifestyle. Therefore, unlike fluency-shaping therapy, Van Riperian therapy did not follow a standard recipe. Instead, it was tailored by a clinician trained in a Van Riperian school to meet the needs of each client individually. This approach certainly took a certain amount of vigor, acceptance, and dedication from the client. It required stutterers to confront many aspects of their disorder, including their own negative emotions and the hostile attitudes of others. For those who covet "fluency" and will do almost anything to hide their disorder, denial is most often a very powerful defense mechanism. Thus, this type of open confrontation with stuttering can be emotionally taxing and can lead one to drop out from therapy. Van Riper's program required mental toughness and resiliency in its initiation, continuation, completion, and follow-up. Not surprisingly, it seemed to have a high mortality rate or drop-out rate. However, at the same time, his methods also produced some excellent examples of successful therapeutic intervention and continue to influence stuttering therapies across the world. Van Riper, Johnson, and Sheehan dominated the therapy world until the influence of systematic behaviorism would eventually cause them to lose favor to behavioral fluency-shaping methods that were more standardized, easier to administer, did not require the same amount of confrontation with the disorder, and therefore did not subject its therapy recipients to the same levels of emotional upheaval. We will examine the four stages of Van Riper's therapy.

## Identification

The first stage of therapy focuses on the identification of behaviors that make up the stuttering syndrome. In this part of therapy, the person who stutters is asked to identify and describe moments of stuttering with respect to stuttering type, duration, and severity of behaviors; the use of covert strategies for avoiding certain words or sounds; emotions before, during, and after the moment of stuttering; physiologic reactions such as changes in heart rate, breathing, and temperature; and ancillary nonspeech behaviors (e.g., eye movements, head jerks, facial contortions, lip quivers, nasal flairs, fist pounding, etc.). In other words, the clinician helps the therapy recipient identify with every aspect of stuttering. This can be a daunting task for even the most prepared. Most who stutter typically never attempt to highlight their compensatory strategies. It may not be unusual for the stutterer to perceive himself or herself to be stuttering more than normal during this stage. Perhaps this is because, maybe for the first time, he or she is being made to confront every aspect of the disorder and not just the "larger" stuttering events that do the most to hinder communication. In other words, regardless of how severe or innocuous a stuttering behavior may seem, the therapy recipient is required to identify and describe it. The notion behind identification was that one could not change inappropriate behavior until it was known exactly what was inappropriate.

During the identification stage, therapy recipients may be simply asked to talk with the clinician or read out loud, during which the therapist may stop the conversation at any time to discuss the types of stuttering behaviors being displayed. At this stage the person who stutters learns about the speech production mechanism and all the perturbations that he or she does to maneuver this mechanism in manners that create stuttered speech streams. Most of this is videotaped so that behaviors can be highlighted, analyzed, and dissected into their component parts. It is this microanalysis that is believed to start breaking the cycle of self-reinforcement of maladaptive behaviors that are manifest in stuttering.

Another strategy may be to send the client out into the real world and record a number of conversations. Again, these recordings can be replayed in the clinic room while both client and clinician listen and pick apart the stuttering events taking place. It should be noted that during this phase, though the clinician may produce examples of easier forms of stuttering, no attempt is made to actually modify the client's behaviors. However, the simple task of identification prepares clients for the next stage, which focuses on becoming desensitized to stuttering. That is, by continually identifying and confronting aspects of stuttering, many therapy recipients begin to desensitize themselves to the impact of the disorder. Thus, identification is often a form of "passive desensitization" that opens the door to the next phase of therapy.

## Desensitization

Van Riper moved from identification to desensitization. While identification was really "passive desensitization," the desensitization phase is actually both active desensitization and the beginning of stuttering modification via pseudostuttering. Whereas the identification stage sought primarily to identify behaviors and feelings associated with stuttering, the desensitization phase attempts to separate the behaviors from the feelings. In other words, it attempts to remove the negative emotions from the act of stuttering—a goal that may be quite difficult considering that negative emotions have often been entrenched in the psyches of those who stutter for years. It should be noted that a great deal of desensitization is already accomplished in the identification stage by the continuous examination of the act of stuttering. However, during this second stage, the goal is for clients to become immune to the emotional effects of stuttering. In other words, this is a form of counterconditioning. Throughout life, the stutterer has usually come to associate moments of stuttering with negative feelings in themselves and the negative attitudes of others. Considering the penalties associated with overt stuttering, this pairing of negative emotion to the overt stuttering behaviors is expected. Thus, in order to become desensitized to stuttering during this therapeutic period, the therapist must help the client tear away the negativity associated with stuttering and replace it with a positive or, at least a neutral emotional state.

One of the main therapeutic strategies used during this stage is "pseudo" or artificial stuttering. A systematic hierarchy is often implemented whereby clinicians replicate models of the client's stuttering and then clients are asked to voluntarily reproduce their own stuttering patterns. It was believed that by voluntarily reproducing these moments of stuttering, clients could begin to shed the feelings of lost control. If stuttering behaviors could be reproduced in a controlled setting and no aspect of it was involuntary, then it was believed the stutterer may begin to feel more in control of the moment. Furthermore, if the social penalties for stuttering were removed under conditions of voluntary stuttering, then the dissociation of true stuttering from negative emotions could begin. As such, pseudostuttering has proven to be a valuable therapeutic tool that was thought to help one become desensitized to stuttering. As it turns out, it may be easier to speak after pseudostuttering as some forms of pseudostuttering have been found to be truly inhibitory to true stuttering. For example, early studies showed reductions in stuttering of up to 80% in intended utterances when the utterances were preceded by the voluntary production of syllabic repetitions (Fishman, 1937; Meissner, 1946). In one of our studies, prior to producing a different target utterance, participants produced 1 to 3 different pseudostuttered (i.e., volitionally repeated three times) words. Stuttering frequency in the target utterances was reduced by 40% (Saltuklaroglu, Kalinowski, Dayalu, Stuart, & Rastatter, 2004). Perhaps more interestingly, the same levels of stuttering reduction were achieved when the same syllabic stimuli were only passively presented to participants before they produced the target utterance, supporting a link between speech perception and production that is further explored in the next chapter. This study provided interesting possibilities for stuttering inhibition via "active" and "passive" pseudostuttering; we followed it up with a similar experiment that examined solely the use of syllabic repetitions as objects of perception and production for stuttering inhibition. In a recent study, we found that producing almost any combination of syllabic repetitions prior to speaking could effectively inhibit stuttering in subsequent utterances by about 70% (similar to what was found in the early studies by Fishman and Meissner). However, when these syllabic forms were presented passively, the highest levels of stuttering inhibition (~65%) were only found when the syllables presented matched the first syllable in the intended utterance. These studies again highlights the inhibitory value of pseudostuttering, the relationship between speech perception and production, and possibly the role of syllabic repetitions in the spontaneous recovery that occurs in up to 80% of children, especially those displaying these easy repetitive behaviors.

Desensitization to stuttering readies a stutterer for the modification stage. One of the difficulties with fluency-shaping therapies is that fluency skills are expected to be used in situations that are historically fear evoking. This can be a self-fulfilling prophecy for breakdown. For example, if using the telephone has been a situation that historically has always resulted in anticipatory fears, overt stuttering, and negative reactions, then simply learning to use prolongation and gentle onsets most likely will not reduce this fear. As such, upon approaching this situation a stutterer may tense up with the anticipation of stuttering, fail to implement the necessary techniques, and suffer the consequences of stuttering. Repeated episodes like this can lead to a quick relapse. However, Van Riper's desensitization attempts to minimize this possibility. In essence, it attempts to emancipate the stutterer from stuttering. Simply put, if the fear of stuttering and the reactions to stuttering no longer exist, then the chances of successfully implementing any technique of speech modification would appear to be considerably higher. By gaining control over emotional states, it was thought that speech could be more easily manipulated.

## Modification Phase

After learning to stand up to and openly face stuttering, it was time to establish better speech speaking patterns, or in Van Riper's view, establish correct timing for speech production. The emotional turmoil that often resulted from the first two stages of therapy was now to be rewarded by learning methods of stuttering more fluently. During this stage, Van Riperians taught essentially three techniques for modifying hard disruptive patterns of stuttering into patterns that they hoped were less disruptive and did little to hinder communication. These three techniques were "cancellation" (after), "pull-outs" (during) and "preparatory sets" (before). Each of them is used to integrate a more fluent way of stuttering into the speech production pattern of the person who stutters. The main difference between the three techniques lies in when they are implemented relative to the moment of stuttering. Cancellations are produced after a stuttering episode has been completed. They operate on the basic learning theory that inappropriate behaviors need to be canceled and not reinforced, as they would be if the stutterer were allowed to continue and finish his or her utterance. After going through the episode, a stutterer is taught to stop and then repeat or cancel the stuttered word using a more easily produced form such as a slight prolongation. Stuttering usually diminishes on the second attempt or abates, thus seemingly removing the self-reinforcement from the stuttering. According to basic learning therapy it is important to make sure that this reinforcement is extinguished and a new more appropriate behavior is integrated.

Pullouts are produced during the moment of stuttering. That is, having been taught to identify moments of stuttering and not react negatively to them, therapy recipients should now be able to catch themselves during a stuttering episode and "ease" out of it, rather than continuing along with excessive struggle and tension. Pullouts simply alter the natural resolution of the stuttering moment, allowing the stutterer to take an active role in manipulating the outcome of a stuttering moment so that it does not resolve involuntarily on its own. The premise here is that stuttering will occur but that the person who stutters can determine, at least in part, the type and duration of the stuttering moment. It is by manipulating the post-onset moment that some amount of control is garnered. At the beginning of the modification stage, pullouts can be quite nebulous, only altering the final portion of the block by replacing it with an easy prolongation. Thus, the use of pullouts tries to show that although stuttering remains an involuntary pathology, individual moments of stuttering can be manipulated. With continued therapy and further establishment of control, pullouts often become shorter in length.

Finally, preparatory sets are analogous to the use of fluency-shaping skills. Rather than enter a speaking situation that is likely to be stuttered unprepared, the use of a prepared "motor plan" for execution may pre-empt the possibility of stuttering occurring within an intended utterance. Preparatory sets may include some prolongation or "gliding" into sounds with light articulation and increased phonation, so as to reduce the possibility of stuttering before it occurs. Essentially this is analogous to adopting some altered or novel speech pattern that the stutterer knows may not sound or feel completely natural, but will, at least during the intended utterance, allow speech to be produced without significant disruption. Some might say you are mildly stuttering on the word in which you anticipate stuttering.

The modification stage of therapy is analogous to learning inhibitory techniques under a fluency-shaping umbrella. However, there is one main difference. Stuttering modification techniques are directly implemented out of a standard recipe book and they are not used continually through the speech production. For them to be efficiently implemented, the stage needs to be set beforehand via the two previous therapy stages. In contrast, fluency-shaping procedures dive straight into speech modification, implementing methods of prolongation from the first day of therapy.

## Stabilization Phase

The fourth and final stage in Van Riperian therapy is stabilization. At this point the stutterer should have acquired a sufficient arsenal of strategies for coping with all aspects of the stuttering syndrome, as well as effective strategies for dealing with moments of stuttering, bringing them under some control and producing overt stuttering patterns that do not severely hinder communication, draw negative attention, or induce negative emotions. In other words, therapy recipients should now be "fluent stutterers." The goal now, and for the rest of their lives perhaps, is to remain that way. As such, the stabilization phase prepares the stutterer to face the challenges of stuttering in everyday life.

Even after extensive therapy, the newfound concept of a fluent stutterer is often not fully ingrained and the use of modification techniques is not automatic. In many cases, the old behaviors and negative emotions can be looming just beneath the surface. For this reason, it is important to implement a plan for stabilizing the therapeutic gains and helping them achieve some degree of automaticity. This final stage of therapy is of utmost importance as the responsibility for implementing this plan now falls on the shoulders of the therapy recipient. During this phase the clinician may work with the client on accepting his or her self-concept as a stutterer and applying fluent stuttering to everyday speaking situations. In other words, clients are expected to be able to apply their awareness of stuttering and their new fluent stuttering techniques in the real world, seeking out increasingly more difficult speaking situations. In addition, they are expected to maintain their attitudinal gains with respect to positive emotional states and continue to separate the behaviors and feelings associated with stuttering.

One of the clinician's important roles during the stabilization stage is to outline a functional and realistic plan that the therapy recipient can put to work every day. In addition to facilitating the use of modification techniques (e.g., cancellations, pull-outs, and preparatory sets), the clinician may help the new fluent stutterer achieve speech patterns that sound more natural by increasing speech rates and applying natural prosody while using inhibition techniques to help bridge the gaps between speech segments. Finally, the clinician may continue to advocate the use of pseudostuttering in everyday interaction. This can be employed as a method of keeping the stutterer "honest," making them understand that they are still a stutterer but now have methods of controlling stuttering as well as continuing to reinforce the notion that overt stuttering does not evoke negative reactions. Again, the use of pseudostuttering may also be inhibitory to true stuttering, thereby providing the therapy recipient with another avenue for producing fluent speech.

## Van Riper's Approach to Treating Children Who Stutter

In discussing the treatment of children who stutter, Van Riper (1973) distinguishes between treatment for the "beginning" stutterer and treatment for the "confirmed" stutterer. If these two classes of stutterers were described under Bloodstein's phases, the beginning stutterers would be those in phase I or II. However, Van Riper targets his therapy for confirmed stutterers to children between the ages of 7 and 14. His justification for this is that stuttering past the age of 14 can be considered to be adult-like and can be treated as such. Depending on their age and degree of stuttering, children below the age of 7 may require some combination of treatments as beginning and confirmed stutterers.

For the beginning stutterer, Van Riper (1973) outlines a basic program that involves direct therapy with the child, though it does not directly target speech production. There are seven basic steps in this program which are: making speech pleasant, providing models of fluency for the child to imitate, designing activities that are conducive to fluent speech (e.g., low-stress activities that can involve the use of known fluency-enhancing devices such as shadowing or speaking in rhythm), providing ample reinforcement for fluent speech, desensitizing the child to stuttering, counterconditioning negative emotions with more positive ones, and preventing negative stimuli from precipitating covert stuttering behaviors such as avoidances. In short, this is a considerably simpler form of therapy than what is targeted toward parents. It involves significant amounts of counseling and is generally designed as a means of prevention. That is, it is intended to halt the progress of incipient stuttering and prevent the child from becoming a "confirmed" stutterer. It is done under the assumption that the child is experiencing bouts with disfluency that have not yet been ingrained into the speech mechanism and following such a procedure will prevent this from occurring.

In dealing with the child who is a confirmed stutterer, the approach Van Riper took is closely structured to the four stages of therapy he used with adults with a few variations. These variations are based on some notable differences between children and adults who stutter that create both advantages and disadvantage during the therapeutic process. The main difference between adults and children that can be advantageous to therapy is that the pathology is newer to the child and therefore not as ingrained; unpleasant experiences may not be as reinforced or etched into the child's psyche. Any fears or negative reactions should be generally less severe than in adults who have spent years in the stuttering shackles. Thus, although some children quickly develop "full-blown" cases of stuttering, generally speaking, children have "less" of the whole pathology than adults, and, hence, it should be easier to remove. However, a number of factors also make the treatment of stuttering children more difficult. Children rarely ask to be in therapy. Instead, it is often a parent or teacher who refers them. Because of this, and the fact that they have not suffered to the same extent as adults, it may be difficult to keep a child motivated to attend therapy. The implementation of the first two stages of therapy can also be difficult with children. They may not be willing to endure the rehashing of negative emotions because of a promise that at a later stage they will be provided with tools to combat stuttering. Along these same lines, in severe cases, children may be in the throes of pain associated with stuttering, yet lack the desire, maturity, or even the linguistic abilities to be able to express their feelings verbally. When approaching the treatment of children who stutter under this approach, all these factors need to be considered.

In consideration of the above, Van Riper promotes the notion of a strong clinical bond between child and therapist, perhaps even stronger than that between the adult stutterer and therapist . He suggests that this bond is imperative as children, especially severely stuttering children, are unlikely to want to subject themselves to therapeutic intervention unless they have trust in the therapist and understand that they will not be judged or seen in negative light for their stuttering.

From this point, the therapeutic course may be structured similarly to the adult, with progression through the four stages. However, each therapeutic stage may be simplified. For example, in the identification phase, there may be less direct confrontation with overt and secondary behaviors. Instead, the child and clinician may simply talk innocuously about the general range of overt and covert stuttering behaviors that the child displays. Similarly, during the desensitization stage, the main goal of the clinician is to help reduce penalties such as the unpleasantness, frustration, and stigma associated with stuttering. Much like fluency-shaping approaches, the modification stage of Van 'Riperian therapy takes advantage of the child's capacity to imitate. Rather than telling the child how to stutter more fluently, the clinician models easy forms of stuttering with reduced tension and less communicative penalty, with the intent of having the child replicate these behaviors and assimilate them into their forms of stuttering.

In discussing the stabilization stage of therapy with children who stutter, Van Riper appears to paint an overly optimistic picture. He suggests that children require little stabilization and states that "Often the whole disorder melts away when the child begins to stutter easily" (Van Riper, 1973, p. 445). As such, in his discussion of stabilization for children, he simply advocates implementing conditions to remove stressors from environments such as home and school, where the child spends most of his or her time. These methods have obvious Johnsonian roots and sound remarkably similar to treatments provided under a "demands and capacities" umbrella. Much like other childhood therapies for stuttering, Van Riper's optimistic views of recovery tend to suggest that spontaneous recovery may have played a large role in the recoveries that were possibly attributed to his therapeutic methods. It may not be surprising that forms of stuttering become less severe as the recovery process begins, or that stabilization is an easy process in children who are recovering spontaneously. As such, much like other forms of therapy for children, we suggest that Van Riperian therapy may have accelerated the recovery course for many children who were already destined to recover, or even helped a few children recover who were on the "edge." However, we doubt that this therapy or any other therapy for children has directly provided the "curative" agent for recovery from childhood stuttering.

## Cognitive "Talk" Therapies

The third type of therapy that we examine in this chapter does not directly target moments of stuttering. Instead of attempting to remove or modify overt moments of stuttering, these "talk therapies" simply attempt to bring the stutterer to rationalize and cope with the everyday battles that those who stutter almost invariably face. In dealing with stuttering on a day-to-day basis, it is possible for those who stutter to begin to obtain neurotic or irrational views and see the world from a distorted perspective. By talking about the disorder and meeting with others who have shared similar experiences, people who stutter may be able to gain acceptance from others and while doing so, learn to see themselves in a more positive light. Stuttering carries a disproportionate weight of importance to many who stutter, and by talking about it with others, the disorder may be brought into perspective and assigned an appropriate level of importance. Talk therapies can be implemented in lieu of behavioral protocols or simultaneously with behavioral protocols.

One way that this type of approach is implemented is via support groups. Stuttering support groups now exist in almost every major city and numerous smaller centers across the United States. Many of these support groups are chapters of the National Stuttering Associations (NSA). The NSA is an association made for and by people who stutter to inform others about the disorder. It publishes a newsletter to help keep its members connected and has a Web site where relevant information can be found (www.nsastutter.org). Aside from the various chapter meetings that may occur two or three times a month, the NSA hosts an annual convention. Attending this convention can be a very powerful experience for a person who stutters, especially the first time one attends. Just the sense of not being alone and being able to share similar experiences with more than a thousand people who have come together for the same reason can be an empowering experience for anyone who stutters. It can be a gratifying experience and an event that is looked forward to every year by many people who stutter. The NSA is supportive of all people who stutter and tends to take a neutral stance toward other therapy approaches and scientific endeavors. It recognizes that all stutterers are a heterogeneous group and what may be helpful to one person may not be the best approach for others. Thus, support groups allow people who stutter to come together to talk about their experiences, share success stories, failures, embarrassments, and any other aspect of life that is affected by their stuttering. Much like other support groups, stuttering support groups attempt to provide a sense of belonging and non-judgmental support to members of the group. People may choose to use therapy skills, but overt stuttering is quite accepted and never penalized within the group confines.

The Stuttering Foundation of America (SFA; www.stuttersfa.org) is another group providing services, support, and resources for those who stutter. The Web site offers numerous links providing a wide range of information about stuttering as well as the availability of therapy in centers around the world. The SFA also publishes books, brochures, and videotapes on stuttering. The SFA was started in 1947 by Malcolm Fraser and is now the oldest nonprofit association for stuttering in the world. Over the years, leaders in the field such as Dean Williams, Charles Van Riper, Joseph Sheehan, and Wendell Johnson have attended and presented at its meetings. The current president of the SFA is Jane Fraser, who is Malcolm Fraser's daughter. Thus, perhaps because of its association with the pioneers in therapy, the SFA tends to provide helpful advice, yet takes a more conservative view toward treatment.

Another resource for people who stutter is the American Speech-Language and Hearing Association's (ASHA) special division on fluency (www.asha.org/about/membership-certification/divs/div_4.htm). Consistent with ASHA's emphasis on clinical intervention, one goal of this division is to provide speech-language pathologists with the tools and knowledge to best help the stutterers they treat. However, this special division group also supports scientific endeavors and are advocates for people who stutter.

## Conclusions

Although scientists, academics, clinicians, and even people who stutter may continue to argue regarding the optimal treatment approach, it should be clear that no method of treatment works for everyone who stutters. Everyone who stutters is different and without understanding of the underlying cause of the central block, we have no means of permanently removing it. Thus, attempting to provide a standard method of symptom management for everyone who stutters is probably naïve as stuttering symptoms manifest in so many different ways and have a diverse range of effects across people. One thing that becomes apparent is that with the amount of effort we have put into producing therapies and the relatively limited success we have seen in reducing the impact of stuttering across the population as a whole, our understanding of stuttering and the development of effective long-term symptom management may still be in its infancy. What we hope this section has provided is not a choice of three approaches that clinicians can adhere to when selecting a therapy technique, but a number of techniques that clinicians may add to their individual repertories of tools so that they may be able to use their best judgments when tailoring therapies to an individual, so as to produce the best combinations of stuttering "inhibition" and coping strategies.

Because no single approach stands out as being superior to the others, it is imperative that clinicians become skillful in being able to identify methods of treatment that work for a given individual. This ability often comes with experience, knowledge of an individual's patterns of stuttering, and sometimes, repeated failures. However, in order to better select therapeutic techniques, it may also be necessary for clinicians to understand how the methods they are using to inhibit stuttering are operating, which is the theme of the next chapter, and how they may be best combined, which is addressed in subsequent chapters.

# References

Armson, J. & Kalinowski, J. (1994). Interpreting results of the fluent speech paradigm in stuttering research: Difficulties in separating cause from effect. *Journal of Speech and Hearing Research, 37,* 69–82.

Bloodstein, O. (1995). *A handbook on stuttering* (5th ed.). San Diego, CA: Singular Publishing Group.

Browman, C. P., & Goldstein, L. (1992). Articulatory phonology: An overview. *Phonetica, 49,* 155–180.

Caruso, A. J., Abbs, J. H., & Gracco, V. L. (1988). Kinematic analysis of multiple movement coordination during speech in stutterers. *Brain, 111,* 439–456.

Craig, A. R., & Calver, P. (1991). Following up on treated stutterers: Studies of perceptions of fluency and job status. *Journal of Speech and Hearing Research, 34,* 274–289.

Craig, A. R., & Hancock, K. (1995). Self-reported factors related to relapse following treatment for stuttering. *Australian Journal of Human Communication Disorders, 23,* 48–60.

Dayalu, V. N., & Kalinowski, J. (2002). Pseudofluency in adults who stutter: The illusory outcome of therapy. *Perceptual and Motor Skills, 94,* 87–96.

Dayalu, V. N., Saltuklaroglu, T., Kalinowski, J., Stuart, A., & Rastatter, M. P. (2001). Producing the vowel /a/ prior to speaking inhibits stuttering in adults in the English language. *Neuroscience Letters, 22,* 111–115.

Fishman, H. C. (1937). A study of the efficacy of negative practice as a corrective for stammering. *Journal of Speech Disorders, 2,* 67–72.

Franken, M., Van Bezooijen, R., & Boves, L. (1997). Stuttering and communicative suitability of speech. *Journal of Speech, Language, and Hearing Research, 40,* 83–94.

Goldberg, S. A. (1981). *Behavioral cognitive stuttering therapy (BCST): The rapid development of fluent speech.* San Francisco: Intelligroup.

Goldiamond, I. (1965). Stuttering and fluency as manipulatable operant response classes. In L. Krasner., & P. L. Ullmann (Eds.), *Research in behavior modification*. New York: Holt, Rinehart & Winston.

Ingham, R. J. (1984). *Stuttering and behavior therapy*. San Diego, CA: College-Hill Press.

Johnson, W. (1942). A study of the onset and development of stuttering. *Journal of Speech and Hearing Disorders, 7*, 251–257.

Kalinowski, J., Dayalu, V. N., & Saltuklaroglu, T. (2002). Cautionary notes on interpreting the efficacy of treatment programs for children who stutter. *International Journal of Language and Communication Disorders, 37*, 359–361.

Kalinowski, J., Dayalu, V. N., Stuart, A., Rastatter, M., & Rami, M. K. (2000). Stutter-free and stutter-filled speech signals and their role in stuttering amelioration for English speaking adults. *Neuroscience Letters, 27*, 115–118.

Kalinowski, J., Noble, S., Armson, J., & Stuart, A. (1994). Naturalness ratings of the pretreatment and post-treatment speech of adults with mild and severe stuttering. *American Journal of Speech Language Pathology, 3*, 61–66.

Martin, R. R., Haroldson, S. K., & Triden, K. A. (1984). Stuttering and speech naturalness. *Journal of Speech and Hearing Disorders, 49*, 53–58.

McClean, M., Kroll, R., & Loftus, N. (1990). Kinematic analysis of lip closure in stutterers' fluent speech. *Journal of Speech and Hearing Research, 33*, 755–760.

Meisner, J. H. (1946). Relation between voluntary non-fluency and the frequency of stuttering in oral reading. *Journal of Speech Disorders, 11*, 13–18.

Metz, D. E., Onufrak, J. A., & Ogburn, R. S. (1979). An acoustic analysis of stutterers' fluent speech prior to and at the termination of speech therapy. *Journal of Fluency Disorders, 4*, 249–254.

Metz, D. E., Samar, V. J., & Sacco, P. R. (1983). Acoustic analysis of stutterers' fluent speech before and after therapy. *Journal of Speech and Hearing Research, 26*, 531–536.

Metz, D. E., Schiavetti, N., & Sacco, P. R. (1990). Acoustic and psychophysical dimensions of the perceived speech naturalness of nonstutterers and posttreatment stutterers. *Journal of Speech and Hearing Disorders, 55*, 516–525.

Netsell, R. (1981). The acquisition of speech motor control: A perspective with directions for research. In R. Stark (Ed.), *Language behavior in infancy and early childhood* (pp. 127–153). Amsterdam: Elsevier-North Holland.

Onslow M., Costa L., Andrews C., Harrison E., & Packman A. (1996). Speech outcomes of a prolonged-speech treatment for stuttering. *Journal of Speech and Hearing Research, 4*, 734–749.

Pickett, J. M. (1980). *The sounds of speech communication: A primer of acoustic phonetics and speech perception.* Baltimore: University Park Press.

Saltuklaroglu, T., Kalinowski, J., Dayalu, V. N., Stuart, A., & Rastatter, M. P. (2004). Voluntary stuttering suppresses true stuttering: A window on the speech perception-production link. *Perception and Psychophysics, 66,* 249–254.

Saltuklaroglu, T., Kalinowski, J., & Guntupalli, V. K. (2004). Towards a common neural substrate in the immediate and effective inhibition of stuttering. *International Journal of Neuroscience, 114,* 435–450.

Samar, V. J., Metz, D. E., & Sacco, P. R. (1986). Changes in aerodynamic characteristics of stutterers' fluent speech associated with therapy. *Journal of Speech and Hearing Research, 29,* 106–113.

Schwartz, M. F. (1977). *Stuttering solved* (5th ed.). New York: JB Lippincott.

Shenker, R. C., & Finn, P. (1985). An evaluation of effects of supplemental "fluency" training during maintenance. *Journal of Fluency Disorders, 10,* 257–267.

Starkweather, C. W. (2002). The epigenesis of stuttering. *Journal of Fluency Disorders, 27,* 269–287.

Starkweather, C. W., Gottwald, S., & Halfond, M. (1990). *Stuttering prevention: A clinical method.* Englewood Cliffs, NJ: Prentice-Hall.

Story, R. S., Alfonso, P. J., & Harris, K. S. (1996). Pre- and posttreatment comparison of the kinematics of the fluent speech of persons who stutter. *Journal of Speech and Hearing Research, 39,* 991–1005.

Van Riper, C. (1971). *The nature of stuttering.* Englewood Cliffs, NJ: Prentice-Hall.

Webster, R. L. (1974). A behavioral analysis of stuttering: Treatment and theory. In K. S. Calhoun, H. E. Adams, & K. M. Mitchell (Eds.), *Innovative treatment methods in psychopathology.* New York: Wiley.

Webster, R. L. (1979). Empirical considerations regarding stuttering therapy. In H. H. Gregory (Ed.), *Controversies about stuttering therapy.* Baltimore: University Park Press.

Webster, R. L. (1980). Evolution of a target based behavioral therapy for stuttering. *Journal of Fluency Disorders, 5,* 303–320.

# 5

# Stuttering Inhibition via Mirror Neurons and the Perception-Production Link

> *"You do not really understand something unless you can explain it to your grandmother."*
> —*Albert Einstein*

According to the model we proposed, all stuttering phenomena originate from central involuntary block that occurs intermittently in the brain. These blocks create a cessation of speech flow that sets in motion a self-releasing, biological regulatory mechanism that uses acoustic gestures (we will explain "gestures" shortly) or repetitions. The use of gestural oscillations to facilitate the release of a block is quite successful for the most part; often two, three or four repetitions are all that is needed for the block to be released and for forward flowing of speech to resume. Simply put, these easy oscillations are quite effective for releasing the central neural block, especially in the incipient stage of the disorder during which 70 to 80% of those who stutter use these repetitive gestural behaviors to spontaneously remit from the disorder (Yairi & Ambrose, 1999). Clearly, this biological regulatory gestural mechanism is both apt at creating forward-flowing speech and self-remitting the stuttering pathology.

The biological regulatory mechanism fails in remitting about 20% of incipient stutterers and the relative severity of stuttering in these individuals, or the relative "amount" of the pathology that the individual may come to possess, becomes associated with both the frequency and intensity of his or her neural stuttering blocks. However, numerous conditions exist that can reduce the relative frequency and intensity of these blocks within an individual. Under these conditions, we typically observe increased levels of fluency, and from our paradigmatic standpoint we say that the central stuttering neural block is "inhibited." In the previous chapter we discussed a number of fluency shaping and stuttering modification techniques that are often used to inhibit or release the neural block. For example, while those coming from a speech motor dynamics paradigm may claim that the use of prolongation serves to correct a temporal motor production deficit; from our standpoint, we say that prolongation and other mechanistic techniques are simply examples of motorically derived "stuttering inhibition." The use of droned speech or consciously prolonged speech is simply a way to keep the neural speech "pipeline" open via continuous sound production. This is analogous to keeping the water on at low drip so that the water pipes do not freeze in the wintertime. The dripping water is bothersome but compared to frozen pipes it can be tolerated for short-periods of time until the plumber can fix the problem. Here the problem will not be fixed and the use of droned speech can prevent or "inhibit" the freezing of the pipes, at least on an intermittent basis.

At least during the incipient stages, what we observe is a simple oscillatory problem in which a neural hitch is overcome or bypassed by simple peripheral repetitions via the speech production system. Syllabic repetitions that are composed primarily of vocalic nuclei (e.g., ba, ba, ba) are transmitted to the CNS. These rapid oscillatory acoustic gestural bursts provide the harmonic or "gestural" tuning necessary to supplant most blocks or release the system back into forward-flowing speech. Thus, most natural recovery from childhood stuttering occurs this way without intervention. This is nature's own recovery mechanism. However, there are numerous other phenomena that are also inhibitory in nature and can serve to release the neural block.

Although the concept of stuttering inhibition is relatively simple (i.e., the suppression of the involuntary neural block), we have not yet explained how the process of inhibition works. Stated otherwise, what is it that keeps the water flowing through the neural pipes of people who stutter? The objective of this chapter is to explain the inhibition of the block or how we keep the flow going through the pipes. First, as the block occurs at a central level, the final suppression or inhibition of the block must also occur at this level. Hence, the inhibition of stuttering must be neural in nature. To begin to understand this neural process, it is best to begin by examining the most potent of all stuttering inhibitors.

## Choral Speech

By far, the most compelling phenomenon that we, and possibly many others, have observed with regard to the stuttering pathology is the ease with which all its symptoms can be suppressed when a person who stutters speaks in unison with another speaker (Andrews, Howie, Dozsa, & Guitar, 1982; Cherry, & Sayers, 1956; Kalinowski, Stuart, Rastatter, Snyder, & Dayalu, 2000). This is the "choral speech" effect. If you were to ask a person who stutters moderately to severely to read a passage to an audience, the request may be met with avoidance, fear, anger, pain, and any number of other negative emotions from past experiences of failure, no matter how small the audience. However, if you were to make the same request, with the stipulation that the person who stutters would not be reading alone, it is doubtful that any negative emotion would arise. There would be no risk involved and no potential penalty. It is a win-win situation for speaker and listener. The listener hears natural, free-flowing reading and the speaker (with the assistance of a second speaker) produces relatively natural, free-flowing speech, without fear of failure. For a person who stutters, eliminating the risk of speech failure is part of the idealized notion of becoming indistinguishable from the person who does not stutter. Normally, every speaking situation is met automatically with an ongoing and exhausting risk analysis that would leave any mathematician, economist, military defense stagiest, even perhaps Game Theorist John Nash, astounded. Under choral speech conditions, the risk is eliminated, leaving the person who stutters with a "feeling of invulnerability" to any speech breakdown (Kalinowski & Saltuklaroglu, 2003a; 2003b; Kalinowski, Saltuklaroglu, Guntupalli, & Stuart, 2004). This invulnerability is reasserted in the almost complete elimination of stuttering and the experiential sense of freedom.

People who have stuttered for a long time often know about the power of choral speech. They often report learning of this neurologic phenomena in childhood when reading with others in groups, saying the "Pledge of Allegiance" in a group, or praying in unison. In these situations they will be almost invariably fluent, and feel comfortable speaking. Conversely, stuttering returns when the second speaker is removed and the stutterer is left to speak alone. In this sense, stuttering is a unique pathology. To the best of our knowledge, it is the only involuntary neurologic pathology whose symptoms can be immediately eliminated via the simple presence of another person's speech.

Records of stuttering in civilizations exist since at least the times of the Egyptians who had a hieroglyph to denote it. Similarly, we suspect that the "magic" of the choral speech effect has been known for just as long. Throughout history those who stutter may have participated in religious ceremonies or rituals, possibly expecting their speech to fail when their time came to speak, but then finding that it was produced fluently during unison speech with the religious leader. People who stutter acquire a sense of when they will be more fluent and when they will stutter more and there is something extremely powerful and comforting about beginning to speak in unison with another speaker. Those who stutter simply know that while the second speaker is present, their own speech will continue to flow smoothly and stuttering will not factor into the utterance. This is the sense of "invulnerability" that comes from the choral speech effect and seems to remove all the anguish and anticipation about speaking that normally comes with stuttering. In other words, this sense of invulnerability diametrically counteracts all the ingrained covert effects of stuttering and endows those who stutter with a sense of complete freedom of speech (Kalinowski & Saltuklaroglu, 2003a; 2003b). As such, with the almost complete removal of all stuttering symptoms, it is not surprising that choral speech is considered the gold standard for fluency enhancement and stuttering amelioration.

Considering that the truly desired speech objectives of nearly everyone who stutters is to sound "normal" and feel like they are producing speech in the same effortless and stable manner as those who do not stutter, choral speech accomplishes this better than any other fluency-enhancing strategy available. This "normalization" of speech patterns and the subsequent removal of all secondary stuttering behaviors is also the obvious goal for most contemporary types of stuttering therapy. For 75 years stuttering has been predominantly treated by behavioral therapy aimed toward systematic retraining of the articulatory, laryngeal, and respiratory systems (Saltuklaroglu & Kalinowski, 2002). However, the choral speech hallmark of invulnerability sets a lofty standard that is rarely met by any therapeutic intervention. Before examining how choral speech operates, we provide a detailed description of the parameters of stuttering that choral speech operates upon to set this gold standard.

## 1. Overt Stuttering

Perhaps the most obvious change in speech production under choral speech, and the one that is most easily documented, is the removal of nearly all (e.g., 90–100%) overt stuttering behaviors (Andrews et al., 1982; Cherry & Sayers, 1956; Kalinowski et al., 2004). Aberrant speech patterns that are normally filled with repetitions, prolongations, silent postural fixations, and an array of secondary struggle behaviors are almost immediately and magically transformed into a smooth flowing stream of speech that is nearly indistinguishable from the speech of those who do not stutter. The "magic" is that the only thing required for this to occur is that the person who stutters perceives a "second speech signal" and simply joins in, speaking in a normal manner. This signal may be acoustic or visual (watching movements of the lips) in nature but it must contain information about the "gestural status of the vocal tract" (Kalinowski, Dayalu, Stuart, Rastatter, & Rami, 2000; Kalinowski et al., 2000; Saltuklaroglu, Dayalu, Kalinowski, Stuart, & Rastatter, 2004). It works optimally when the linguistic information being produced by the two speakers is synchronized (i.e., the two speakers speak the same material). These acoustic and visual second speech signals, can completely "turn off" this involuntary and debilitating pathology that is otherwise highly resistant to therapeutic intervention. Figure 5–1 shows how a choral signal can inhibit the pathology by bypassing the central block.

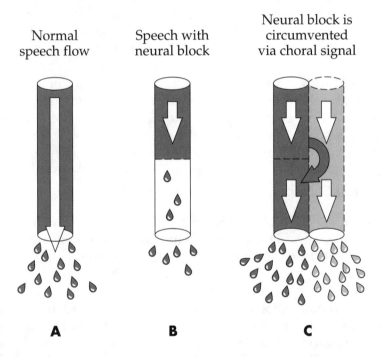

**Figure 5–1.** Speech flow through the neural pipeline. **A.** Normal speech flow. **B.** Speech impeded by a central involuntary block. **C.** The use of a choral second speech signal to bypass the involuntary block and allow speech to proceed normally.

When second speech signals are removed from the most severe stutterers, the pathology almost immediately returns. Stuttering is "turned back on" when the accompanying speaker is removed. In less severe cases, there may be some "carryover" fluency before the speaker hits the first block which may last for a few seconds or even minutes after removal of the second speaker. In other words, if choral speech is thought to keep the flow through the pipes moving, once choral speech is removed, it is likely that it takes time for another blockage to occur and it may not be as severe. We are also finding signs of a long-term carry-over effect in some people, a phenomenon that we are continuing to investigate. Hence, the magic of choral speech lies in the fact that it is passive, exogenous, and constant (Saltuklaroglu, Dayalu, & Kalinowski, 2002; Saltuklaroglu, Kalinowski, Dayalu, Guntupalli, Stuart, & Rastatter, 2003). It can maintain the *"patency"* of the neural channel or network and temporarily instate a relatively normalized speech system.

## 2. Ease of Attainment and Implementation

Another part of the so-called "magic" of choral speech is that, in stark contrast to the long and drawn out therapeutic protocols that have been used to inhibit stuttering, the inhibition of stuttering via choral speech is achieved almost immediately and requires no training or motor manipulation of the peripheral speech mechanism (Guntupalli, Kalinowski, Saltuklaroglu, & Nanjundeswaran, 2005; Kalinowski et al., 2004; Kalinowski & Saltuklaroglu, 2003a; 2003b). Behavioral speech therapy takes weeks and often months or even years to complete. In contrast, choral speech like the use of all "second speech signals" is relatively passive. The person who stutters has only to listen to or look at the second speech signal to achieve a dramatic inhibition of the stuttering block.

Many speech therapy clinics continue to treat returning clients with the assumption that this involuntary disorder can be brought under volitional control with continued practice and more therapy. Unfortunately, stuttering is involuntary by nature and definition and, therefore, the novel speech patterns taught by behavioral therapists never seem to be fully internalized to overcome stuttering, often resulting in a sense of failure and vulnerability on the part of the therapy recipient. In contrast, under choral conditions, fluency is "reflexively" achieved. That is, it is usually immediate and nearly always stable. It is almost unfailing under even the most traditionally difficult of speaking conditions (e.g., speaking in front of an audience). Because of its immediate nature and the lack of motor manipulation, it seems logical that the perception of the second speaker by people who stutter is directly impacting the speech production centers of the brain and somehow immediately engaging a neural mechanism that is capable of overriding the central involuntary neural block.

We will argue that all conditions that override the central stuttering block (e.g., choral speech, droned speech, and even the production of overt stuttering behaviors) all operate on the central nervous system to inhibit the central block. (Saltuklaroglu, Kalinowski, & Guntupalli, 2004). However, ease of use and implementation clearly differentiates the functional capacities of stuttering inhibitors. Van Riperian therapies and behavioral methods of prolongation are both intended to increase the functionality of the inhibitors. They try to make them easier to use and implement as well as more presentable to the listener than overt stuttering—which is not always achieved when speech naturalness is compromised. The point here is that choral speech exceeds any of the other methods with respect to the ease with which the central block is inhibited.

## 3. Rate of Speech

The behavioral concept of retraining the speech motor system follows the assumption that stuttering is a peripheral rather than central disorder and that people who stutter suffer from a compromised speech motor system that can be unlearned or compensated for via peripheral machinations (Packman & Onslow, 2002).

It follows that speech retraining (via prolongation and any of the other fluency techniques) involves decreasing the rate of speech, creating slow and deliberate articulatory patterns in an attempt to control the speech periphery. In contrast, under choral conditions that induce "reflexive" fluency, speech rate is not a factor per se. Under choral conditions, people who stutter can speak fluently at any speech rate. This has been empirically demonstrated in a series of studies using altered auditory feedback, which we will come to recognize as a permutation or variation of choral speech. Altered auditory feedback is discussed in detail in the next chapter. However, for now it is sufficient to say that it involves hearing one's own voice differently so as to create the illusion of a second speaker speaking in unison. When speaking at both slow and fast rates under altered feedback, participants have been shown to speak approximately 80% more fluently (Kalinowski, Armson, Roland-Mieszkowski, Stuart, & Gracco, 1993; Kalinowski, Armson, & Stuart, 1995; Kalinowski, Stuart, Sark, & Armson,1996), showing that as the block is inhibited via choral speech, the motor speech periphery of those who stutter is free to perform its job at any rate of speech, in a similar manner to how it operates in normally fluent people. When keeping the neural channel open, the central involuntary block is inhibited and the person who stutters is usually empowered to speak as rapidly or slowly as desired. As a slow rate of speech is not necessary to inhibit stuttering under choral conditions, we again see evidence that stuttering does not occur as a result of a temporal motor deficit. Like the slow but constant water flow, running in pipes to prevent the freeze-up that we mentioned earlier, one can imagine keeping a car running all the time to keep it form stalling. Though the car may not stall, it is an inefficient means of accomplishing this task, much like the use of droned speech for stuttering. Over time, the compensations are more costly and wasteful than the initial problem itself. Hence, when attempting to control stuttering by treating the peripheral speech motor system, we merely attack the more proximal (i.e., near) symptoms rather than the distal (i.e., far) source of the pathology, which can be a relatively less efficient and effective vehicle for treatment.

## 4. Naturalness of Speech

Choral speech generally operates without the need to impose behavioral strategies of motoric speech retraining. Without any changes in speech production, the natural quality of one's own speech is retained throughout any utterance. A normal rate is maintained as well as the natural prosody and inflexion patterns that make each person's speech unique. In contrast, the decreased rates of speech associated with behavioral speech retraining usually come with the aforementioned vulnerability associated with droned, robotic, zombie-like speech patterns that often draw more attention than the stuttering behaviors they attempt to replace (Dayalu & Kalinowski, 2002; Saltuklaroglu et al., 2003).

## 5. Stability of the End Product

The invulnerability to stuttering that characterizes choral conditions is made evident in the spontaneous, natural sounding, fluent speech that is relatively impervious to breakdown regardless of linguistic material, rate of speech, speaking situation, and even audience size. To the best of our knowledge, when using true choral speech (i.e., derived from a second speaker speaking in unison), the choral speech effect has never been shown to diminish (Kalinowski & Dayalu, 2002; Saltuklaroglu et al., 2002). In other words, stuttering inhibition via choral speech appears always to be possible, suggesting that choral speech is the one fluency enhancer that remains truly stable; perhaps our therapy techniques should seek to replicate this effect as much as possible. In contrast, claiming that post-therapeutic speech is "unstable" may be understated. The countless hours spent attempting to ingrain and use the novel speech patterns, along with the droning, unnatural productions add up to an end product that is usually highly volatile (Dayalu & Kalinowski, 2001; Dayalu & Kalinowski, 2002; Kalinowski & Dayalu, 2002; Kalinowski, Noble, Armson, & Stuart, 1994; Saltuklaroglu & Kalinowsli, 2002; Saltuklaroglu et al., 2004; Stuart & Kalinowski, 2004). Speech production continues to be similar to walking a tightrope—one slip and the speaker tumbles back into the realm of stuttering. With the fear of breakdown and sounding unnatural comes the return of covert stuttering behaviors, such as word and sound avoidances, substitutions, and circumlocutions. Not surprisingly this vulnerability also becomes evident in the high relapse rates following behavioral therapy (Craig & Hancock, 1995).

## 6. Covert Stuttering Behaviors

Under choral conditions, there is simply no risk of speech failure. Speech is produced relatively easily, almost eliminating the need for word and sound avoidances, substitutions, and circumlocutions. Additionally, when speaking in unison, traditionally difficult situations such as speaking to an audience or using the telephone lose their fear-evoking capacities. Simply put, under choral speech conditions all the fears and apprehensions about speaking that we normally associate with stuttering are removed. This is the true sense of invulnerability and the truly magical characteristic of choral speech that separates it from any other form of stuttering inhibition technique. When covert fears are removed and the possibility of stuttering ceases to factor into speech production, the person who stutters achieves a level of speech normalcy that is seldom achieved elsewhere.

## Fluency Versus Pseudofluency

The above descriptions highlight the differences in end product resulting from spontaneous choral speech and arduous behavioral speech retraining. The vulnerability to stuttering that seems to permeate all aspects of post-therapeutic speech is simply antithetical to the use of choral speech. The shortcomings of forward flowing post-therapeutic speech has prompted the moniker "Pseudofluency" (Dayalu & Kalinowski, 2001, 2002). As made evident by the above comparisons, pseudofluency is all that true fluency is not. pseudofluency is laborious, tenuous, and filled with a chronic sense of impending speech failure or vulnerability to stuttering. In other words, when stuttering is treated by simply masking its peripheral symptoms, the pathology may still be thought to be present, albeit in a "denatured form" (i.e., replaced by continuous prolongations) (Satukalroglu & Kalinowski, 2002). In contrast, under choral speech conditions, almost all evidence of the pathology is removed.

However, as with most naturally occurring phenomena, rather than being a categorical distinction, fluency and pseudofluency are simply two ends of a continuum. While it may be clear that true choral speech represents the truly fluent end of the continuum and slow (e.g., 2 seconds per syllable), droned speech represents the truly pseudofluent end of the continuum, most speech achieved by people who stutter in therapy or via permutations of choral speech falls somewhere between these two poles. Thus, for us, the goal of any therapeutic intervention for stuttering is to derive speech that approaches the truly fluent end of the continuum to the greatest extent possible.

## Choral Speech in the Therapeutic Milieu

At this point you may be starting to ask about the clinical applications of choral speech. Its powerful and universal effects do indeed appear magical, yet they may seem to lack some practicality. After all, it would be impossible for someone who stutters to continually speak in unison with another speaker. So what are the applications of choral speech? In the past, choral speech has been used by therapists to demonstrate the stutterer's inherent capacity to speak fluently. Before beginning fluency-shaping or Van Riperian therapies, a clinician may speak in unison with the therapy recipient to show the optimal outcome of their therapy. Of course, the post-therapeutic speech never achieves the degree of true fluency that is attained during the choral speech demonstration and the blame may be cast upon the therapy recipient for not adequately adhering to the therapeutic protocol. It seem ironic to us that such a powerful tool has served only as a demonstration of fluent speech and has not been better implemented into therapeutic protocols.

One reason that choral speech has not been adequately exploited for therapeutic purposes is because its effects have lacked adequate explanation, though a number have been offered. These have included the reduction in communicative responsibility (Eisenson & Wells, 1942), the inducement of novel patterns of vocalization (Wingate, 1976), and the provision of an external timing mechanism (Johnson & Rosen, 1937), reflecting the influence of various paradigmatic approaches to stuttering. Yet attempts to confirm any of these postulated explanations have been unfulfilled and the choral speech phenomenon has remained an enigma. If we take a Kuhnian stance, we may say that regardless of the adopted paradigm, choral speech has remained an unexplained anomaly and a large thorn in the side of those espousing the need for control over the speech periphery. In fact, it may even be fair to say that failing to adequately explain the choral speech phenomenon has led to a crisis in the field of stuttering that has led to the inception of our theoretical approach. Our approach to stuttering inhibition provides a compelling and parsimonious explanation for choral speech and explains other powerful fluency-enhancing conditions in terms of being derivations of their effect. Hence, we now explain the neural mechanism that we believe is responsible for the powerful fluency-enhancing effects of choral speech. However, before the description of "mirror neurons" will make sense, it is necessary for us to make a slight departure from the realm of stuttering and explain some of the nature of normal speech perception and production using a contemporary model developed by scientists at Haskins Laboratories.

## Gestural Models of Speech Perception and Speech Production

To fully communicate using speech, humans need the abilities of both production and perception. What exactly do we mean by production and perception? Speech production is often discussed in terms of its motor execution, with reference again to the peripheral speech mechanism (i.e., the lungs, larynx, and articulators). However, we must not forget that all the programming and planning required for this execution, as well as the linguistic knowledge required for meaningful speech, begins in the brain. Similarly, speech perception does not refer to "hearing" or "seeing" speech per se. Speech perception refers to the neurophysiologic processeses in the brain that allow us to interpret and process incoming sensory stimuli as speech information. Therefore, both speech perception and production have strong neural components. To better understand the inhibition of stuttering it is necessary to understand how the two processes of perception and production may be intricately tied together at a neural level and how this connection may be exploited by those who stutter to inhibit the central involuntary block.

Let us start by asking a seemingly simple question. What is both necessary and sufficient to perceive speech? Asked in another way, what does it take for our brains to recognize a sensory stimulus as speech? We are not the first to ask this question. Speech scientists have been exploring the nature of speech perception and production for years and once thought that the answer should be fairly straightforward. After all, we are all quite adept at recognizing speech immediately. Most of us can also produce speech relatively easily, a skill that is acquired during early childhood and without any formal training. However, even after 60 years of research in the area, we have yet to understand the true nature of speech and why it remains for most people on this planet, the most efficient and effective modality of linguistic communication. What we are implying is that speech is "special" and we are by no means the first to see speech in this way. It appears to be a specialized human process and one that elevates us above other species in our communicative capabilities. It is fair to state that human beings are biologically predisposed or "hardwired" for communication. But what is speech and what is it that makes it special?

## Speech Perception

Let us begin our examination of the speech processes by looking first at perception. When we think about speech, the first thing that we probably think of is the way it sounds or its acoustics. It was once thought that speech was no more than an "acoustic alphabet," with each sound being mapped individually and sequentially into the brain to spell out the different words that form our languages. Using this perspective, in 1944 Alvin Liberman and Frank Cooper, two optimistic and naïve (by their own admission) scientists attempted to build an "optical character reader" that could translate written words into a series of meaningful acoustic speech signals so that blinded veterans returning from World War II might be able read newspapers (Liberman, 1993). They created various sets of acoustic nonspeech signals that were intended to be representative of individual letters in the English language. They expected to be able to train people to "read" using this system at about 50 words per minute. This estimate was quite ambitious. After 90 hours of practice, their best trainee was only able to read at 4 words per minute. Thus, converting letters to a nonspeech acoustic alphabet has not proven to be any more efficient than using Morse code, which reconstructs letters as a series of dots and dashes. Though it now may seem almost intuitive, this finding provided a compelling clue that speech is a great deal more complex than a simple acoustic alphabet that strings sounds together. Though text-to-speech capabilities are now a reality, it has taken a great deal of technologic advances in computing and speech synthesis to make them possible. Even now, text to speech features are based on accepted acoustic combinations of sounds moving sequentially from one letter to the next, and if the computer (which is the general medium for speech synthesis) does not recognize a letter combination, it may be unable to produce the desired speech output.

Other evidence also exists to indicate that speech may not be a simple acoustic entity. As Liberman, and Ignatius Mattingly began to develop their "motor theory" of speech perception (Liberman & Mattingly, 1985), they became aware that if speech perception was solely dependent on the integrity of our auditory system for receiving acoustic information we would never be able to communicate with the rapid-fire efficiency with which we are accustomed. Though most normal speech rates are in the range of 4 to 5 syllables per second (Netsell, 1981; Pickett, 1980), it has been found that speech can be followed even at rates of about 400 words per minute (Orr, Friedman, & Williams, 1965), which may equate to about 12 syllables per second or 30 phonemes per second (Liberman, Cooper, Shankweiler, & Studdert-Kennedy, 1967). Even at half this rate, it would be simply overwhelming for our auditory system if it were required to individually perceive and interpret each sound coming in sequentially. It has even been shown that humans have difficulty correctly sequencing a stream of nonspeech sounds when they are presented at 4 sounds per second (Warren, Obusek, Farmer, & Warren, 1969; Warren, 1976). Thus, there must be something special about the nature of speech that allows us to process it so efficiently with the limitations imposed upon us by our auditory systems.

Another question is: If speech is an acoustic alphabet, why is that we can understand each other so easily when we speak the same language? Everyone has a different voice and has slightly different pronunciations of words, even before we consider the numerous accent and dialectal differences within languages; yet only in the most extreme cases do these differences impede our ability to communicate effortlessly with others who share our same linguistic code. If speech were an acoustic alphabet, would not all the acoustic differences present serious problems when it comes to understanding each other? Furthermore, if speech were simply an acoustic alphabet, would we not be able to train computers to recognize our speech in a similar manner?

Progress has been made in this area and many computer systems are now endowed with intricate voice recognition features. We can talk to computers on the telephone when we ask for directory assistance or check airline arrivals and departure times. However, try artificially stuttering, using a foreign accent or a different voice form, omitting or adding a speech sound, or applying background noise when talking to these computers. You will be immediately referred to a human operator who is much more adept at deciphering your spoken message. For computers to recognize human speech, the message needs to be delivered nearly perfectly. Computers are only programmed to recognize specific combinations of acoustic features, and when some variation is presented, their recognition capabilities are severely diminished. However, if a common language is shared, humans can immediately and effortlessly decipher almost anything that another speaker says, regardless of accent, fluency, articulatory disorders, or prosodic anomalies. The point is that although computers are now capable of recognizing and producing speech to some extent, they are not nearly as talented as humans at doing so, as the process is so specialized that we have not yet been able to figure out exactly how it occurs in our brains, so as to program computers to do it in a similar fashion. Even after all these years of research, we have yet to truly understand the mechanism that allows us to innately encode and decode speech, yet it appears that the answer does not lie solely within the acoustic speech signal.

Many hearing-impaired individuals are adept lip readers. During lip reading speech is being "perceived" and understood in the absence of an auditory signal. Try watching television with the volume turned down. Though you may not be able to understand everything that is being said, the lip movements being made by the actors or newscasters are clearly perceived to be speech movements and at least part of the message is often communicated. We also conducted an experiment whereby stuttering was substantially inhibited, by simply watching another person silently mouth the same words as the speaker. This silent visual analog of choral speech inhibited stuttering by approximately 80% (Kalinowski et al., 2000), which provided us with a vital piece of the puzzle for understanding the choral speech effect, namely, the second speaker need not be heard if he can be seen. For speech perception to occur, audition may be sufficient, but not necessary. The auditory channel is obviously a powerful conduit for receiving speech. We primarily use audition to receive the speech of others and even visual speech appears to be processed in what is traditionally considered to be the auditory cortex (Calvert et al., 1999; Campbell, 1998; Campbell et al., 2001; Nishimura, Hashikawa, Doi, Iwaki, & Watanabe, 1999; Sams, Aulanko, Hamalainen, Hari, Lounasmaa, & Lu, 1991; Sams, Mottonen, & Sihvonen, 2005; Tuomainen, Andersen, Tiippana, & Sams, 2005).

However, although numerous features can be sufficient, no single feature or cue has ever been found in an acoustic speech signal that is necessary for speech perception. Researchers at Haskins Laboratories have even found that they could create speech perception by using sine wave analogs of speech. These sine wave analogs contain no formants, glottal pulsing, or many of the other traditional cues that we normally associate with speech. They are simply composed of three or four rapidly changing pure tones that attempt to replicate the frequency and amplitude modulations of the formants throughout an utterance (Remez, Rubin, Pisoni, & Carrell, 1981). Yet, when one listens to these sine wave renditions, without any of the traditional speech cues, it is not difficult to hear meaningful sentences. This is not the same as listening to recordings of songs played backward, where one struggles to find some meaning in the convoluted acoustics of reversed speech. With the sine wave speech, most people are able to hear the same sentence and the words jump out almost immediately. For a demonstration of this phenomenon, it is worth visiting the Haskins Web site (www.haskins.yale. edu). So what is it that is being perceived when we hear or see speech? What is the common element that allows us to identify speech sounds and movements and effortlessly reproduce them?

## Speech Production

Our ability to speak to each other and understand one another is truly one of nature's marvels. Think about the muscular coordination required to produce meaningful streams of speech. Not only can we do this effortlessly, but we can alter our speech patterns, speak with a mouthful of food, or speak with an injury to the speech musculature, and still be understood. How did we acquire such precision and such flexibility in this task? Furthermore, who taught us how to do this? No one. We simply needed to be around others who were speaking during our infancy and, for most of us, the rest came easily and naturally. Does it not indeed seem as if we are specialized in some way for developing this system of oral communication? Where does it come from and what makes it possible? We answer those questions in the next section.

We can again gain some appreciation for our ability to produce speech when we compare it to what we have been able to accomplish in this area using computers. Even now, text-to-speech features are based on accepted combinations of sounds and if the computer (which is the general medium for speech synthesis) does not recognize a sound combination, it is often unable to produce the desired speech. Furthermore, synthesized speech has yet to match the meaning that is found in the prosodic features of natural speech. Have you ever heard a computer tell a joke? The timing and intonation patterns that are crucial to the delivery and make the joke humorous are simply absent. Though computers can be taught to produce a vast array of recognizable sound combinations, they have yet to capture contextual variability, spontaneity, prosody, and all other subtle nuances that make speech innately human. Thus, the speech synthesis available today seems to be a product of increased computing power, capable of assembling a vast array of algorithms for acoustic sound combinations, rather than an understanding of the "speech code," which due to its innately human nature offers a seemingly infinite number of acoustic combinations (Liberman et al., 1967).

### The Invariants in Speech Perception and Production

In chapter 3 we discussed the search for the "invariant" in stuttering or what is deemed necessary and sufficient to account for all aspects of the disorder. Similarly, the work at Haskins Labs beginning with the optical readers represented some of the initial research in the search for the invariants in speech perception and production. If scientists could discover exactly what quality it was that gave a particular sound its characteristic percept, then helping the communicatively impaired and developing technology for speech synthesis and speech recognition would become a more feasible task. However, though it appeared relatively simple at its onset (i.e., an acoustic alphabet), this endeavor turned out to be a Herculean task. With continued research that goes well beyond the scope of this text, speech scientists have amassed considerable evidence to show that the invariants of speech are not to be found in acoustic signals, visual signals, or even the kinematic muscular movements of the articulators during speech production. As with stuttering, the invariants of speech perception and production are thought to exist in the brain. The most basic unit or invariant in both speech perception and production is described as the speech "gesture" (Liberman & Mattingly, 1985).

## Gestures for Perception and Production

A stream of speech is best described as a series of "coarticulated speech gestures." Coarticulation refers to the blending of one sound with another in continuous speech (Emerick & Haynes, 1986; Liberman, 1993). When we speak, we do not produce speech sounds in isolation; rather we hear speech sounds combined in a continuous flow. Every sound in the sequence has some influence on its surrounding sounds, such that it is impossible to say where one sound ends and another begins. For example, put your hand in front of your mouth and say the word "pat." You should feel a slight puff of air as you release the plosive /p/ and coarticulate with the vowel /a/. Now do the same thing with the word "apple." You will not feel the puff of air after the /p/ this time. The /a/ following the /p/ generates aspiration on the /p/ such that the /p/ sound in "pat" is slightly different from that in "apple." In phonetics, these slight variations in the way a phoneme is produced because of contextual influences are known as "allophones." Now try alternating between the saying the words "sit" and "soot." Notice the difference in your lip postures before you even begin to say the /s/. This is due to the influence of the upcoming vowel. You can already anticipate the coarticulation between the /s/ and either the /i/ or /u/ vowel. It is these coarticulatory or contextual differences that result in the lack of an invariant speech feature both necessary and sufficient for perception. The acoustics, articulatory movements and allophonic variations in any sound, are a product of the other sounds with which they achieve coarticulatory dynamics. Add to this mixture prosodic and dialect variances and innumerable laryngeal and vocal tract differences among individuals and it becomes clearer why we have never been able to place our proverbial finger on an acoustic or kinematic invariant for speech production and perceptions. What we are left with, and what is important, is that in both cases described above we know that it is the /p/ or an /s/ sound being perceived and produced at the beginning of the word.

The seemingly simple task to find invariant speech cues, much like the task of finding the invariance in stuttering, progressed from proximal to distal, beginning with the acoustic signal, progressing to the kinematics of articulatory movements, and finally to the level of the brain. After we remove all these seemingly unnecessary "cues" that at some stage of the game may have been candidates for invariance, all we are left with is how our brains interpret the incoming stimuli. These are the percepts that we call speech "gestures." A speech gesture is simply the brain's representation of what is occurring in the vocal tract during speech. As we speak, our vocal tracts take on a variety of different shapes with an almost infinite number of articulatory configurations. Coarticulation is simply the movement from one vocal tract configuration to another. Therefore, as we perceive the speech of someone else, our brains simply understand the movements of their vocal tract. These movements make sense to us, as we can produce them ourselves in our own vocal tracts to convey the same message. Though each of our vocal tracts is different and produces different acoustic signals, and each of us may produce slightly different articulatory movements, we are still able to understand the speech of others and reproduce it in a similar manner as we share the same gestural code. This seems to be the best explanation for coarticulation. Coarticulation and contextual differences introduce an almost infinite number of combinations to the acoustics and kinematics of any phoneme production. However, if we understand that speech perception is not directly related to the acoustics, it makes more sense. If we understand that our brains perceive a gestural sequence of vocal tract events and we share this same code with others, we can begin to understand how this works. Our brains seem to have "categorical" perception for speech gestures (Liberman et al., 1967). Though the vocal tract is a continuous and dynamic system, our brains seem to know when we have shifted the dynamic configuration of the vocal tract from one gesture to another.

So what is the role of the acoustic speech signal and how can we explain the perception of silent, lipped speech? Both acoustic and visual speech signals provide cues as to the intended gestures. However, the acoustic signal simply provides a richer source of gestural information. If we examine a spectrogram, we can see voicing bars, vowel formants, formant transitions, high-frequency noise, stop gaps, and so forth. We hear all of this information and it is perceived by our brains as sets of unified speech gestures. Visual speech signals (i.e., lip movements) also provide cues to the intended gestures but they do not contain nearly the wealth of gestural information that is found in acoustic speech signals as lipped speech only provides information with regard to what is happening at the very front of the vocal tract at the level of the lips. Visual speech does not provide cues as to what is occurring deeper in the vocal tract or at the level of the larynx. It is probably for this reason that even the best lip readers rarely exceed about 30 to 40% accuracy (Spehar, Tye-Murray, & Sommers, 2004). Thus, speech gestures are made available to us by a wealth of redundant cues. None of these cues is necessary for perception by itself, but certain cues or combinations thereof appear to be sufficient. However, the sine wave speech shows us that we can even remove all of what speech scientists consider to be "traditional" speech cues and still be able to perceive speech as the changing sinusoidal waves provide a context for perceiving speech gestures and our brains appear to be able to "fill in the blanks."

Thus, speech gestures contain a redundancy of cues. Many gestures also share cues. For example, vowel sounds and voiced consonants all contain the voicing cue (which can be seen on a spectrogram as glottal pulsing). When we talk on the telephone we receive only acoustic cues. However, as stated, acoustic speech signals are rich in cues and we are able to easily understand one another over the telephone. During face-to-face conversation we benefit from increased redundancy due to the presence of auditory and visual cues, watching and listening to our conversational partners. These cues are generally synchronized as the lips are conveying cues that are consistent with the cues being generated deeper in the vocal tract. But what happens when these cues are not synchronized? One of the most famous phenomena in speech perception occurs when we provide inconsistent auditory and visual cues. When a person hears the syllable /ba/ while seeing the lip movements of someone producing /ga/. If we close our eyes and listen, we hear /ba/. If we turn off the volume and watch the speaker, we see /ga/. However, if we watch and listen together, we perceive /da/. This is known as the McGurk effect (McGurk & McDonald, 1976) and a demonstration can also be found on the Haskins Web site. This "illusion" is a demonstration of how our brains integrate speech cues to produce unified gestures. The two syllables share a great deal of gestural information such as manner of articulation (both are plosive sounds) and voicing. However, the place of articulation is different for both. So when hearing and listening to the two productions, the brain does its best to integrate the cues and form a unified gesture. In doing so, it "splits the difference" between the two places of articulation (lips for the /ba/ and palate for the /ga/) and create a unified gestural percept of /da/, which is generally associated with production on the alveolar ridge. If speech were simply an acoustic phenomenon, this effect would not be possible.

## The "Special" Nature of Speech

One of the reasons that we are able to communicate so efficiently at such a fast rate is because speech gestures are perceived and produced in "parallel." Rather than speech taking on the nature of an acoustic alphabet, where each sound is perceived and produced serially (one after another), speech gestures arise from rapidly changing vocal tract configurations. There is no way to tell when one gesture ends and another one starts because they overlap each other. Gestures are simply layered onto each other and the brain perceives them in parallel or at the same time

(Kalinowski et al., 2004; Liberman et al., 1967). This parallel processing makes speech perception a highly efficient process. Our brains have the ability to make complete sense of a rapidly incoming stream of gestures and we do not even need to think about processing it. The processing occurs automatically. Think about how you can listen to someone else speaking and be fully aware of what they are saying, while you are driving, reading a book, listening to music, or attending to any number of other tasks. How is it that we can absorb or produce such a vast amount of linguistic information in such a short period of time when we are not even attending these complex processes? If we look at the speech production, which may really be considered the flipside of perception (Liberman & Mattingly, 1985), how is it that we can execute such precise streams of gestural speech information without any formal coaching? Just about any other complex activity that requires precise muscular coordination (such as playing a musical instrument) takes substantial training to learn and is rarely mastered except by a few rare individuals whom we praise and marvel at their abilities. Yet few of us marvel at the ability to speak. It is just simply accepted as the primary means of human communication and a gift that seems to be magically bestowed upon most humans.

According to Liberman and Mattingly's (1985) revised motor theory, part of what makes speech perception and production so efficient and effective is that they both employ the same fundamental unit. Speech gestures are the invariants for both perception and production. In other words, if we can perceive it as speech, we can produce it as speech. The two processes are therefore inseparable at the neural level. Thus, during a conversational exchange, human beings simply trade commonly shared gestures. One person produces and the other perceives and then vice versa. The exchange works because gestures that hold meaning for the sender of information also hold meaning for the receiver of information. Therefore, during communication a link is created between sender and receiver (Liberman, 1998). Figure 5–2 shows this relationship between sender and receiver during spoken communication, showing the invariant neural objects of perception and production to be gestures in the vocal tract.

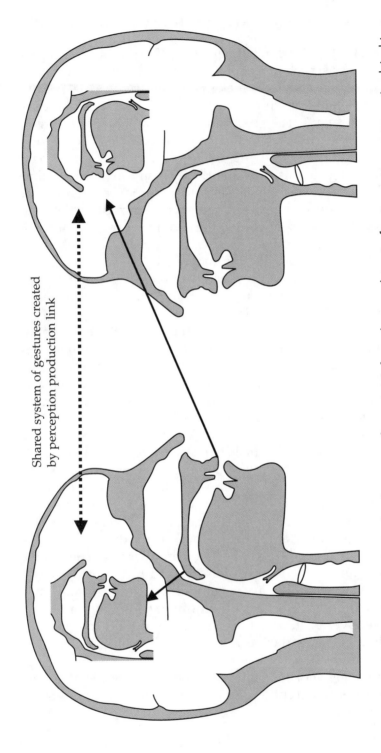

Shared system of gestures created by perception production link

**Figure 5–2.** Gestures (dynamic vocal tract configurations) from the vocal tract of one person are perceived in his or her own brain and that of the other person (via audition and vision). The same system of gestures is shared which allows for communication.

Although this is a truly condensed explanation of the motor theory of speech perception (Liberman & Mattingly, 1985) and does not do justice to the body of research that went into its formulation, we hope it will be sufficient to demonstrate the "special" nature of speech. The perception and production of unified speech gestures is a gift that is specialized and innate to humans. To us, motor theory provides the most complete and parsimonious framework for all phenomena we have described associated with speech, and all the inhibitory phenomena that we describe in the next chapter associated with stuttering. Motor theorists proposed that the specialization for speech processing is made possible by a "phonetic module" in the brain that processes speech gestures in parallel and easily transposes between percept and product. One of the shortcomings of this theory is that, no neuroanatomic or physiologic process has ever been identified that could verify this modularity, and to this date, it remains a point of contention within the theory. However, the recent discovery of mirror systems has provided compelling neurophysiologic support for this proposed modularity and, as such, supports the underlying tenets of the motor theory (Rizzolatti & Arbib, 1998). Thus, we now begin to examine how gestural communication evolved over the course of human evolution; how it develops as children acquire language; the mirror neuron mechanism thought to make it possible and account for the proposed phonetic modularity; and, how this may be tied to the inhibition of stuttering.

## Mirror Neuronal Systems

The human brain may be considered the "final frontier" for many scientists. Understanding the intricate cortical and subcortical workings about what makes us human will probably continue to challenge scientists for a long time. Having said that, we must acknowledge the progress that has been made in the area of neuroscience. If you have studied some neuroanatomy, you may recall describing neurons as being sensory or motor in nature. Sensory neurons send sensory information to the brain so we can sense or feel it and motor neurons send information from the brain to our body to regulate our body functions and allow us to move our muscles. Aside from neurons that connect sensory and motor processes (i.e., interneurons), this division was fairly straightforward until fairly recently. An Italian research group was the first to observe a set of neurons in part of a monkey's brain known as the rostral inferior premotor cortex (area F5) that fired both upon the observation and the execution of specific goal-directed actions, generally related to the hands. That is, they were activated not only when the monkey performed a goal-directed action (such as grasping, holding, or tearing), but also when the monkey observed another agent performing the same action. Neurons that were normally associated with motor processes fired when they received appropriate sensory stimuli. These neurons became known as "mirror neurons" (DiPellegrino, Fadiga, Fogassi, Gallese, & Rizzolatti, 1992; Gallese, Fadiga, Fogassi, & Rizzolatti, 1996; Rizzolatti & Craighero, 2004; Rizzolatti, Fadiga, Gallese, & Fogassi, 1996) and they seemed to be associated with recognizing and executing actions (Rizzolatti & Arbib, 1998). Figure 5–3 shows some examples of mirror neuron firing patterns.

Interestingly, the F5 cortical region in the monkey is considered to be the homolog or equivalent of Broca's motor speech area in humans. Relatively speaking, the F5 area of the monkey and Broca's area in humans share similar architecture in the frontal lobe. However, because electrodes cannot be inserted into humans, scientists still have not been able to achieve a direct measure of human mirror neuron activity. However, there has been strong evidence to support the existence of mirror neurons: behaviorally (Wohlschlager & Bekkering, 2002), using whole head magnetoencephalography (MEG; Avikainen, Forss, & Hari, 2002; Nishitani & Hari, 2000, 2002), transcranial magnetic stimulation (TMS; Fadiga, Criaghero, Buccino, & Rizzolatti, 2002; Meister et al.; 2003), and functional magnetic resonance imaging (fMRI; Grezes, Armony, Rowe, & Passingham, 2003). At this point you may be asking, "so what?" Why is finding motor neurons that fire upon receiving appropriate sensory input a big deal?

The discovery of "mirror neurons" in monkeys is evidence of a link between action and observation. As this link was found first in monkeys, these neurons have been given the name "monkey see, monkey do" neurons (Gallese, Keysers, & Rizzolatti, 2004).

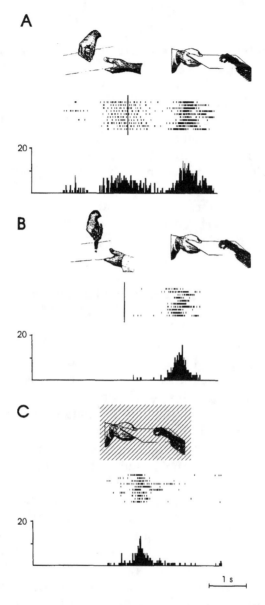

**Figure 5–3.** Firing patterns of monkey mirror neurons. **A.** Observation of and performance of food grasping actions elicits mirror neuron firing. **B.** Observation of an experimenter grasping with a tool does not elicit mirror neuronal firing, but firing occur when monkey grasps food. **C.** Grasping of the food by the monkey even in the dark elicts mirror neuronal firing. (This figure is reprinted from Rizzolattii, G., Fadiga, L., Gallesse, V., & Fogassi, L. (1996). Premotor cortex and the recognition of motor actions. *Cognitive Brain Research, 3*, 131–141, with permission from Elsevier Publishing.)

Their discovery has been heralded as one of the greatest scientific advances in the last decade. Noted neuroscientist V. S. Ramachandran states that he predicts that mirror neurons " . . . will do for psychology what DNA did for biology . . . " (http://www.edge.org/3rd_culture/ramachandran/ramachandran_p1.html). Before we explain how their discovery has borne fruit in our specific understanding of stuttering, we wish to provide a broad overview of this system as it relates to communication. Some understanding of the mirror system may provide an added perspective in understanding a number of communicative pathologies and, therefore, may be useful for prospective speech and language pathologists.

## Mirror Neurons and the Evolution of Language

After reading thousands of research articles, we (both authors of this textbook) agree that perhaps the most compelling article was entitled "Language within our grasp" (Rizzolatti & Arbib, 1998). We now make this article an assigned reading in our classes. It provides a convincing explanation for how language evolved from the primitive system of communication found in our predecessors to the complex system of vocal gestures that we use today, and how the presence of mirror neurons aided in this landmark evolutionary process.

At the most basic level, possessing a neural mechanism that is engaged during both the perception and production of goal-directed gestures provided our early ancestors with a neural mechanism for action recognition. In the evolutionary scheme of things, it is likely that the presence of the "monkey see, monkey do" mirror system led to our ability to imitate, later to the development of primitive communication, and finally language and speech as we know it today. However, it should be noted that, although the presence of the mirror system may have been a necessary contributor to these remarkable developments, by itself it was by no means sufficient. A number of other contributing factors were also necessary, including, the concurrent anatomic, neurophysiologic, and cognitive development of our species. If we accept Darwin's notions of evolution, we must acknowledge that this series of changes had adaptive value, naturally driven to ensure the survival of our species.

Imitation is considered to be a relatively advanced cognitive ability that requires the dissection and parsing (putting together) of numerous motor sequences (Arbib, 2001; Rizzolatti, Fogassi, & Gallesse, 2001). Although its definition is subject to some debate (see Heyes, 2001 for discussion), most agree that humans are the only species in which imitative abilities are truly developed. That is, although other species are able to emulate movements seen in others, humans appear to be the only species that can effectively internalize and generalize their meanings, so as to be spontaneously produced in other environments (Arbib, 2000, 2001; Heiser, Iacoboni, Maeda, Marcus, & Mazziotta, 2003). We humans learn by most skills, including language, via imitation and, therefore, it is not surprising that the ability is so highly developed in our species (Mataric & Pomplun, 1998).

If we dissect the simple process of imitation, an individual is required to recognize an action and then faithfully reproduce it. In other words, for imitation to successfully occur, it seems imperative that there be a link between observation and execution. Therefore, it is not surprising that mirror systems have been strongly implicated in the imitative mechanisms (Decety, Chaminade, Grezes, & Meltzoff, 2002; Heiser, Iacobini, Maeda, Marcus, & Mazziotta, 2003; Heyes, 2001; Iacoboni et al., 2001). However, though mirror systems are seen in monkeys, monkeys are unable to imitate with the same proficiency as humans. Therefore, the ability to imitate probably reflects some evolutionary capitalization of mirror systems combined with advances in other cognitive abilities (Arbib 2001; Heyes et al., 2001).

Skoyles (1998) made an astute observation regarding our ability to imitate, namely, that imitation is a skill that is performed fluently. In humans, fluent imitation may be observed regardless of linguistic knowledge or cognitive development. It is found in communicatively disabled populations such as those with mental retardation, suggesting that the ability to immediately imitate sequences of goal-directed gestures is not dependent on higher cognitive functions, assuming that the sequence in question can be represented accurately within the individual's gestural repertoire (i.e., that the individual understands the goal-directed nature of gestural sequence). Hence, for the purposes of imitation, the mirror neurons appear to create simple input-output neuronal circuits that, at the level of the brain, appear to be reflexive in nature. The notion of imitation as fluent is of great importance to our perspective on stuttering. As we begin to explain the nature of choral speech and its derivatives, we will come to see that the choral speech phenomenon is really no more than a form of fluent imitation made possible by the presence of this simple input-output neural circuitry that are the mirror neurons.

Yet how did this this simple circuitry lead to the development of communication and language? Although the ability to imitate is at a relatively highly advanced cognitive level, it is not sufficient to explain our current linguistic abilities. In their account of how action recognition drove ability to communicate, Rizzolatti and Arbib's (1998) explanation fills in the blanks for us regarding this evolutionary progression. Although many forms of goal-directed actions might trigger mirror activity in an observer, we do not actively imitate every goal-directed action that we see, most likely due to some inhibition of the gestural representation at the level of the spinal cord (Baldissera, Cavallari, Craighero, & Fadiga, 2001). With the idea that mirror neuron circuitry can be activated via the observation and/or execution of specific actions, Rizzolatti and Arbib (1998) postulated that a "primitive dialogue" could be established when an individual recognizes a specific executed action via the mirror system (e.g., grasping) and the motor representation "leaks through" to elicit brief, condensed imitation of the same action. The original sender of the action recognizes the elicited condensed version of the action in the receiver and a simple connection is established between the two individuals, thus creating simple communication via a shared sensory and motor representation of a meaningful gesture.

Returning again to the evolutionary scheme, surely individuals who were able to connect with others had a clear advantage over those lacking this ability. Thus, Rizzolatti and Arbib (1998) postulated that this communicative advantage resulting from the presence of mirror neurons has been passed down from generation to generation and refined over millions of years to evolve into our current speech. For this to be possible, a number of factors must be considered. First, we must acknowledge the gestural nature of both the primitive communication described above and speech as it today according to motor theory. When a monkey reaches for an object in a grasping motion, it can be considered a goal-directed action. Similarly, when we change the configuration of our vocal tract to elicit a sequence of meaningful sounds, we are also producing a goal-directed gestural sequence. In other words, though evolution has shaped our primary mode of communication, elevating it from a gross brachio-manual (arm-hand) system to the intricate and precise speech mechanism we possess today (made it increasingly more efficient and effective along the way), it has essentially retained its gestural form. Over the years gestural communication has become increasingly more efficient and effective, with one gestural system gradually supplanting another.

Second, spurred by the mirror neuron advantage, the changes in gestural communication probably also coincided with anatomic, physiologic and cognitive changes resulting, in the evolutionary process (Lieberman, 1984; Lieberman, Crelin, & Klatt, 1972 ). The communication system of primates was thought to become more personalized as it moved to orofacial gestures. That is, gross brachio-manual gestures could be received by many, but movements of the mouth and face are more characteristic of one-to-one communication. Thus, gestures such as lip and tongue smacks, sucking, licking, and chewing sounds probably associated with feeding may have begun to take on communicative significance. In support of this, recent evidence exists of auditory-based mirror neuron activity for sounds associated with specific actions such as breaking a peanut and tearing paper (Fadiga & Craighero, 2003; Ferrari, Maiolini, Addessi, Fogassi, & Visalberghi, 2005; Kohler et al., 2002). In other words, the presence of mirror neurons responding to acoustic stimuli that represent a goal-directed action may have contributed to gestural communication progressing from brachio-manual to orofacial gestures. It is also speculated that to achieve a larger range of communicative function and meaning that could be achieved by each system in isolation, brachio-manual and orofacial gestures may have been combined in a complementary manner (Rizzolatti & Arbib, 1998). Thus, as manual gestures became paired with vocalized sounds, the door was opened for acoustic representations of the gestures themselves to take on greater meaning.

However, it was not until about 300,000 years ago that our species had undergone sufficient anatomic development to produce the repertoire of vocal gesture that we use today. At this point, the larynx had descended, creating a longer and more versatile vocal tract capable of producing a larger array of acoustically rich gestures in an almost infinite number of combinations. Individuals began to share the meanings associated with the different combinations of gestural forms, creating the highly efficient and effective form of gestural communication that we now possess. As well as being related to the refinement of the mirror system, the advancement in linguistic ability must also have been accompanied by increased cognitive abilities that necessitated the need for improved communication as well as fine-tuning of the language centers in the brain for both producing and processing rapidly changing sequences of gestures. Thus, it is not surprising that neuroimaging techniques have revealed more highly specialized patterns of activation in the auditory cortices for receiving speech as opposed to nonspeech sounds. The auditory centers of the brain have even been shown to be active in the processing of silently lipped speech (Calvert & Campbell, 2003), suggesting that these centers have become specialized for processing speech gestures, regardless of the modality of input.

If we return to motor theory we can see how the presence of mirror neurons accounts for the specialized dual nature of speech. During speech perception and production, we are simply sharing common gestures via a process that is innately human and has undergone specialization over millions of years of evolution to meet the increasingly demanding communicative needs of our species. With this view of the evolutionary course, we can also understand why it is very difficult to separate speech from language and, thus, why Liberman and Mattingly (1985) also expanded their notion of a "phonetic" module to that of "linguistic" module. Regardless of the name, the mirror neuron system seems to hold special importance in making this specialized modularity possible, making speech perception and production one and the same at the neural level.

Although speech continues to be the primary mode of human communication, the kinship to more primitive communication forms is readily evident and cannot be ignored. Humans convey volumes of information through body language, facial expressions, and hand gestures as well as in the prosodic aspects of speech that can serve to communicate emotion and grammatic function. The human communication mechanism undoubtedly extends beyond the sending and receiving of acoustic representations of vocal tract configurations. Current literature suggests hands and speech system are linked at a central level that is possibly mediated by Broca's area. For example, mirror neurons in Broca's area have been found to be stimulated during observations of hand actions in humans (Avikainen, Forss, & Hari, 2002; Hari et al., 1998; Rizzolatti, Fogassi, & Gallese, 2002). In a reciprocal manner, linguistic tasks (e.g., reading silently, reading aloud, and spontaneous speech) have been found to induce stimulation of motor neurons of the hand (Floel, Ellger, Breitenstein, & Knecht, 2003; Meister et al., 2003), and corticospinal tracts of the hand and arm (Tokimura, Tokimura, Oliveiro, Asakura, & Rothwell, 1996). Perhaps the evolutionary course has simply allowed one system to be overlaid on top of its predecessor as the primary modality for communication (Daniloff, Fritelli, Buckingham, Hoffman, & Daniloff, 1986). This neural tie between the hands and oral mechanism may also be important in understanding a possible purpose to the secondary stuttering behaviors involving manual movements, but more on that in the next chapters.

The advancement in human communication and the rich neural interconnections between manual and oral gestural systems seem to allow humans flexibility to use the hands as channels for communication, either independently or in concert with the speech system, as it may have occurred during the evolutionary process. When used in concert, the hands can provide a rich complement to speech information. When used independently from speech (e.g., in some hearing-impaired populations), the hands can be used as a primary modality for communicating a full range of linguistic information. When a particular modality is partially or completely closed, as in hearing-impaired populations, alternative communicative modalities may come to dominate. In manually signed languages such as ASL and British

Sign Language the dynamic spatial and temporal relationships among hand movements are highly structured linguistic systems, complete with phonologic, morphologic, and syntactic levels. They are highly encoded in the visual-spatial instead of acoustic-temporal changes found in spoken languages, such that foreign accents can even be detected among manual signers (Hickok, Kirk, & Bellugi, 1998). Furthermore, during early linguistic development, signed languages are even characterized by a babbling stage, analogous to that found in spoken languages (Larkin, 2000).

## Mirror Neurons and Language Development in Children

Infant development throughout the first few years of life is truly a wonder to behold. The rapid advancement in cognitive, linguistic, and motor skills that characterize these first years are a continual source of amazement for parents and scientists alike. Of most importance to us, is the proficiency with which communication develops. From birth, the immediate bond that parents form with their child may mesmerize parents. Even in the first few weeks of life infants can display the ability to track and imitate facial gestures such as tongue or lip movements (Meltzoff & Moore, 1977). In addition, infants as young as 18 weeks of age also have been shown to be able to match the prosodic patterns of their caregivers (Kuhl & Meltzoff, 1996). Again it should be noted that these imitated goal-directed gestural forms, early signs of a specialized communication system that is about to flourish, are produced fluently (Skoyles, 1998). Thus, fluent imitation is evident in what we have referred to as "prelinguistic" populations. It is innate, primitive, with a clearly communicative goal, and requires no training to elicit, suggesting that it truly is a precursor to what we have often considered truly linguistic (Bekkering, Wohlschlaeger, & Gattis, 2000).

Much like the early communicative bonds found in our ancestors, these reflexively imitated action sequences may be evolutionary adaptations that are paramount to the infant's early survival. They seem to be evidence of prelinguistic gestural bases for requesting food or nurturing, or even indicating the presence of danger (Rizzolatti & Arbib, 1998). During this initial period of communicative development, mirror neuronal-based communicative links seem to be strengthened via the continued observation-action pairing and the desired outcomes (e.g., receiving food or nurturing). Simply stated, the observation comes to elicit the initiation of the action (Rizzolatti & Arbib, 1998; Rizzolatti, Fadiga, Gallese, & Fogassi, 1996; Skoyles, 1998). This could explain why two- to three-month-old infants have been found to increase the amount of sucking on electronic pacifiers when they witnessed gestural syllabic productions (Karzon & Nicholas, 1989). This specialized behavior is a natural wonder of infancy and displays our natural predisposition to imitate oral gestures as a precursor to formal language (Rizzolatti & Arbib, 1998; Liberman & Whalen, 2000). However, as most parents have witnessed, as soon as "motorically possible," this newborn infant will not only suckle to the observation of gestural speech productions, but will attempt to imitate them (Kalinowski & Saltuklaroglu, 2003a). Mirror systems can endow children with gestural maps that will later emerge as recognizable speech, once the motor system develops sufficiently to be able to accurately produce these gestural representations. Thus, even early patterns of speech babbling are considered to be meaningful productions of representations found in a rapidly developing gestural repertoire (Kuhl, 1994, 2000). In support of this notion, Dehaene-Lambertz, Dehaene, & Hertz-Pannier (2002), using fMRI found evidence of activation patterns in three-month-old infants that resembled those of adults for processing both forward and acoustically reversed speech, suggesting that precursors for adult cortical language centers were active prior to development of meaningful speech production. That is, speech development does not seem to be hindered as much by the immaturity of gestural representations (i.e., perception) in an infant communicative repertoire, but more so by the development of the motor system for execution. An immature motor system cannot keep up with the rich realm of communicative intentions that infants begin to acquire from birth. Thus, as infants begin to gain higher levels of control of their oral motor mechanism, speech gestures have already been "primed" for production. They are already on the tips of infant tongues and waiting to be released into their parents' ears. As such, it is not uncommon for parents to observe a sudden "explosion" in their child's speech production, when their vocabulary seems to expand at an almost exponential rate for a period of time.

According to renowned developmental psychologist Jean Piaget (1963), cognitive development can be divided into a series of stages. The first stage is termed "sensorimotor" and is primarily characterized by being reflexive and imitative. We suggest adding that, in terms of communicative development, it is a period of fluency. We have yet to hear normally developing infants stuttering while babbling, imitating prosodic patterns, saying their first words, or reproducing other familiar gestural sequences. Perhaps this stage is simply dominated by mirror neuron engagement creating strong links between perception and action to allow numerous motor, cognitive, and linguistic skills to become adequately ingrained in the developing child. The strong presence of mirror neurons may ensure that the goal-directed gestural sequences, including speech, are both adequately recognized and faithfully replicated (Kalinowski & Saltuklaroglu, 2003a, 2003b). This period of fluent imitation occurs at the most basic level and, thus, does not appear to be dependent on higher cognitive functioning, again providing evidence that the mirror system is an innate mechanism for action recognition inherited from our predecessors. Thus, assuming that a gestural sequence in question is adequately represented within the child's gestural repertoire, it should be reproducible if the motor capacity is sufficient. For speech, this means that because infants and adults have human vocal tracts, if they are normally developing, they should be able to eventually reproduce all speech gestures common to the language they are learning. Such appears to be the power of these simple mirror neuronal input-output circuits. Thus, if gestures with the same meaning are produced in millions of different human vocal tracts, ranging in size from infant to adult and across genders, it is not surprising that they are produced differently and show different acoustic and kinematic features. As such, it is not surprising that motor theory claims that the only invariance in these gestures is at the neuronal levels of perception and production, creating the link between the two processes (Liberman, 1998; Liberman & Mattingly, 1985; Liberman & Whalen, 2000).

When gestures become symbolic (as in speech) and are exchanged between individuals we have language, often considered the defining characteristic of our species (Liberman, 1998; Liberman & Mattingly, 1985; Liberman & Whalen, 2000). Thus, the early engagement of mirror neurons appears to be instrumental to an infant's ability to imitate and acquire formal language, in a manner not unlike the one we described for the evolution of language, with a progression from simple manual and orofacial gestures to the efficiently produced symbolic speech gestures. In fact, Wohlschlager and Bekkering (2002) stated "imitation is probably the oldest and most important means to transmit memes between individuals and thus represents a fundamental aspect of cultural evolution," hinting toward the importance of mirror neurons in the evolution of different cultural rituals as well as language (Arbib, 2001). Thus, infants perform simple gestural encoding and decoding, leading to the reflexive and fluent imitation of speech gestures that continue to develop at an exponential rate into a complete system for gestural interchange, which is language. In summary, it may be that as we watch a child's linguistic skills mature over the course of a few short years, we may be seeing a reflection, albeit an accelerated one, of millions of years of linguistic evolution.

## Mirror Neurons and the Onset of Stuttering

Imitative forms that may be considered evidence of strong mirror neuron contributions mark the initial stage of language development. This stage of language development is also a period of fluency. It seems, therefore, that any predisposition for stuttering is unlikely to emerge until children begin to relinquish imitative linguistic forms and begin to independently assemble different representations from their gestural repertoire to produce more complex linguistic forms consistent with their cognitive development. In other words, in normally developing children, linguistic forms go beyond the level of imitation so that the child can develop other functions for communication. Along with an increase in vocabulary, new grammatic, syntactic and morphologic forms emerge so that during interactions, gestural information is not necessarily replicated, but exchanged for efficient and effective communication. Although mirror neurons have been implicated in normal speech production (Miall, 2003), as the process of imitation is relinquished during language development, it seems likely that their mediation over speech production diminishes. Therefore, any child with a predisposition to stutter may begin to exhibit symptoms after speech as expressive language begins to assume longer and more complex forms.

It may be fair to state that if language development in children never surpassed the imitative stage, stuttering might not emerge, due to the constant use of mirror systems for fluent imitation. Simply put, at the early stages of development, mirror systems seem to keep stuttering in check. If we compare when language development generally surpasses the imitative stage and when stuttering begins to surface in children, the similarity in time course is not easily ignored. Stuttering generally begins between the ages of 2 and 6 years, which loosely corresponds with the relinquishing of imitative forms in favor of more complex expressive language. In terms of Piaget's developmental stages, it may loosely correspond to the transition from the sensorimotor to the preoperational stage. Though it is difficult to ascertain this point empirically, and a great deal of further investigation is needed, we have spoken with many parents who have stated that stuttering began to manifest in their child at a time when their expressive language skills were beginning to thrive.

## Mirror Systems and Fluency Enhancement

As stuttering does not exist in early infancy due to the engagement of mirror neuronal systems meeting imitative linguistic needs, it is suggested that the re-engagement of these systems is the most efficient and effective way of bestowing fluent speech upon those who stutter. Primordial systems have power and precedence over later-developing systems. For example, since the dawn of time, our innate, primordial drive to feed and reproduce seems to overpower any cognitive, religious, spiritual, behavioral, psychoanalytic, or other psychologic needs that have been created. In the same vein, choral or imitated speech engages mirror neurons and invariably overrides the central involuntary stuttering block, as mirror systems were innately present prior to the onset of the pathologic condition. Simply put, gestural imitation has preceded the disorder of stuttering in children and supplants the disorder, at least to some significant degree. In the case of choral speech, engagement of mirror neuronal systems easily inhibits stuttering and establishes fluency. However, the inhibition lasts for the duration of the choral speech signal. Upon termination of the signal, stuttering relapses to its previous levels.

## Choral Speech and the Mirror System

If we look at what is happening during choral speech, we can see that it is really no more than a form of direct imitation. Two people are simply copying each other's gestural speech output. There are really no roles assigned as to who is leading and who is copying. Both speakers appear to be speaking at the same time and can be thought to be copying each other. However, the concept of choral speech is in fact misleading. True unison speech is very difficult to achieve, even by those who have received intensive training to do so, such as professional singers. In other words, when two people speak together their speech gestures are never quite matched up. But that is a good thing. It affords the system some "flexibility" for achieving fluency. Although the two speakers may never achieve true synchrony and may take turns slightly leading or lagging during an utterance, choral speech maintains its strong fluency-enhancing capabilities, which suggests that there is some temporal leeway in the system. We examine this temporal flexibility and the flexibility for accommodating different linguistic material in more detail in the next chapter as we look at "second speech signals."

We are the first to have claimed that the power of choral speech lies in the engagement of mirror neurons. Choral speech is no more than a form of direct gestural imitation. If we return to our pipeline analogy, having an externally presented (or exogenous) speech signal that is nearly perfectly matched to the intended utterance is the optimal condition for keeping the pipeline open and free-flowing. The flow of speech simply cannot be impeded when appropriate gestural stimuli are being introduced to the neural speech pipeline. In the presence of a choral speech signal, mirror neurons may once again become engaged to allow for fluent imitation of speech gestures (Kalinowski & Saltuklaroglu, 2003a; 2003b; Kalinowski et al., 2004; Saltuklaroglu et al., 2003).

Although mirror systems appear to play their largest role in language development during the initial critical period of acquisition, it appears that they may be recruited at almost any point in one's life to help learn new skills. Even at later stages of life people learn by imitating each other's actions (Arbib, 2001). This is evident in athletic, musical, and artistic endeavors, as well as learning foreign languages. We learn by watching others, imitating their motor sequences until we become proficient. Although second languages can be learned to some extent in classrooms or via books and tapes, most people acknowledge that they become most proficient when immersed in another culture. This is when second language gestural models are present and mirror neurons can be engaged to proficiently replicate them. Thus, for people who stutter, having a mirror system that can be exploited for fluent imitation of speech gestures allows them a means of accessing fluent speech by overriding the involuntary neural block. We have suggested that during choral speech conditions, a gestural mirror is provided. It inhibits or overrides the neural block, keeps the speech pipeline completely open, and functions via direct and immediate transposition of speech percept to speech product (i.e., motor theory).

Again in accordance with motor theory, stuttering inhibition under choral speech is "special." The mirror neuron system is primitive and reflexive, so it is not dependent on higher levels of cognition. Stuttering is inhibited "in parallel" with speech production. That is, the person talks while listening to the unison speaker and becomes fluent—all at the same time. In addition, no motor control is imposed upon the speech system. No one is asked to speak in a certain way or listen in a certain way. All that is required is a neural gestural pipeline that can engage the mirror systems for fluent goal-directed gestural imitation.

Stuttering inhibition via the re-engagement of mirror systems using choral seems logical. The mirror system appears to exist at a more primordial neural level than stuttering. It was seen in our early ancestors and is apparent in children from birth. In contrast, although the predisposition for stuttering may exist from birth, symptoms of the pathology do not manifest until later. Thus, it is not surprising that engaging mirror systems can supplant the involuntary neural block and overrride stuttering even in the most severe cases. Primordial systems seem to take precedence over later-developing systems in humans and animals. Logically this makes sense as these primordial systems are tied to basic survival skills. Likewise, when we hear someone saying the words we want to say it is natural and easy to simply join in and speak fluently. A common phenomenon is finishing a sentence for someone when they are experiencing a long speech block. Oftentimes, people who stutter do so on an important word in a sentence and the listener feels obligated to finish the sentence for them, even though they may have been told that it is not polite to do so. Even so, the simple urge to finish another's sentence when we know what the word is appears to be evidence of mirror neurons creating the communicative bond between sender and receiver and generating a prefix of a gestural action via perception.

It is not surprising that people who stutter feel invulnerable to stuttering under choral speech conditions. This hallmark is probably created by the presence of mirror neurons. Instead of having to step into the unknown during speech and risk perpetual breakdown, under choral conditions, those who stutter are provided a "gestural mirror" of their own speech that opens the channels for forward flowing and fluent speech production. All controls and covert behaviors can be released because the neural mechanism for fluency is engaged. For those who stutter this is an unbelievable sensation and one that needs to be continually recreated via therapeutic interventions in order for those who stutter to become indistinguishable from normally fluent speakers. Given the invulnerable nature of the derived fluency under choral speech conditions and our view that therapeutic interventions should strive to meet this benchmark, the next chapter delves into further understanding the power of choral speech, its relationship to other inhibitory conditions, and, thus, our goal of uncovering functional applications of choral speech.

# Additional Notes on Mirror Neurons

Having stumbled upon what we believe to be a common mechanism for explaining a wide array of gestural conditions that inhibit stuttering, we have followed with considerable interest numerous other areas in which mirror neuron systems have been implicated. First we became interested in how mirror neurons may be related to other communicative disorders. Autism spectrum disorders are characterized by language deficits, especially in areas related to social interaction. Much like stuttering, the etiology of autism has been subjected to much debate and is still essentially unknown. However, scientists are now implicating mirror neuronal deficiencies in autism (Williams, Massaro, Peel, Bosseler, & Suddendorf, 2004; Williams, Whiten, Suddendorf, & Perrett, 2001) and milder forms such as Asperger's syndrome (Avikainen, Wohlschlager, Liuhanen, Hanninen, & Hari, 2003). If mirror neurons help create a link between sender and receiver for gestural exchange, a deficit in this system may be expected to compromise this link and create social interaction difficulties. Recently, the role of mirror neurons in compensating for pantomime deficits in aphasia have also been examined (Saygin, Wilson, Dronkers, & Bates, 2004). The results suggested that areas of the brain that are important in expressive language can also be recruited for the purposes of comprehension. Our preliminary clinical investigations also suggest that taking advantage of the mirror system may provide therapeutic options for a number of communicative disorders. However, adopting a "mirror" perspective in the field of communication disorders is still in its infancy.

Most humans are able to understand the emotions of others. We can read facial expression, we can derive emotional content from the prosody of others' speech, we can even make sense of body language to some extent. According to the theory of mind (ToM), we can develop understanding of the emotions of others because we can experience this emotions ourselves (Gallese, Keysers, & Rizzolatti, 2004), again implying a perception-production relationship. It is suspected that mirror neurons allow us to make this empathetic connection with others. If we see somebody's eyes and they convey surprise, it is probably because if we were surprised, our eyes would emit the same message to others. Baron-Cohen et al., (1997) have shown that most adults are capable of assigning mental states to individuals simply by looking at the eyes. Not surprisingly, autistic children appear to perform more poorly on this task. The ability to understand the emotions of others seems to transcend direct interactions. If we see someone suffer an injury or even hear about an injury, we can feel the pain. For us, when we see a child stuttering, it evokes a great deal of emotion as we have been there before ourselves and know the pain they are experiencing. In addition, we enjoy watching movies and sporting events, as well as reading novels because we can get caught up in the emotional content. Some people cry in movies because they feel they are experiencing the sadness of the characters. We cheer on our favorite sporting team because we get caught up in experiencing the emotions of the players on the team. Thus, even in areas of human emotion, perception and production appear to be linked via mirror neurons, even to the point that a motor theory of empathy has been developed (Leslie, Johnson-Frey, & Grafton, 2004), suggesting that much like speech, empathy is a truly human characteristic that is "hardwired" into normally developing brains and possibly driven by mirror systems.

Mirror neuron systems are also beginning to have an impact on the field of robotics (Tani, Ito, & Sugita, 2004; Wermter & Elshaw, 2003). With rapid advances in technology, robots are being created to perform a variety of tasks. However, it makes sense that advances in artificial intelligence may be derived from a perception-production link. In other words, rather than just producing robots that can move in certain preordained manners, these mechanical beings may become more versatile if they can also "perceive" and make "on-line" adjustments to their motor functioning by the sensory input they are receiving. Though it is a little scary (and has been the subject of many science fiction books and movies) to imagine the possibilities of endowing robots with a mirror system that works as efficiently as the one we have, with a better understanding of our mirror system and continued technologic advancements, these possibilities may not be so far-fetched.

# References

Andrews, G., Howie, P. M., Dozsa, M., & Guitar, B. E. (1982). Stuttering: Speech pattern characteristics under fluency-inducing conditions. *Journal of Speech and Hearing Research, 25,* 208–216.

Arbib, M. A. (2000). Warren McCulloch's search for the logic of the nervous system. *Perspectives in Biology and Medicine, 43,* 193–216.

Arbib, M. A. (2001). Co-evolution of human consciousness and language. *Annals of New York Academy of Sciences, 929,* 195–220.

Avikainen, S., Forss, N., & Hari, R. (2002). Modulated activation of the human SI and SII cortices during observation of hand actions. *NeuroImage, 15,* 640–646.

Avikainen, S., Wohlschlager, A., Liuhanen, S., Hanninen, R., & Hari, R. (2003). Impaired mirror-image imitation in Asperger and high-functioning autistic subjects. *Current Biology, 13,* 339–341.

Baldissera, F., Cavallari, P., Craighero, L., & Fadiga, L. (2001). Modulation of spinal excitability during observation of hand actions in humans. *European Journal of Neuroscience, 13,* 190–194.

Baron-Cohen, S., Wheelwright, S., Jolliffe, T. (1997). Is there a "language of the eyes"? Evidence from normal adults, and adults with autism or Asperger syndrome. *Visual Cognition, 4,* 311–331.

Bekkering, H., Wohlschlaeger, A., & Gattis, M. (2000). Imitation of gestures in children is goal-directed. *Quarterly Journal of Experimental Psychology, 53,* 153–164.

Calvert, G. A., Brammer, M. J., & Iversen, S. D. (1998). Crossmodal identification. *Trends in Cognitive Sciences, 2,* 247–253.

Calvert, G. A., & Campbell, R. (2003). Reading speech from still and moving faces: The neural substrates of visible speech. *Journal of Cognitive Neuroscience, 15,* 57–70.

Campbell, R. (1998). Speechreading: Advances in understanding its cortical bases and implications for deafness and speech rehabilitation. *Scandinavian Audiology, 49*(Suppl.), 80–86.

Campbell, R., MacSweeney, M., Surguladze, S., Calvert, G., McGuire, P., Suckling, J., et al. (2001). Cortical substrates for the perception of face actions: An fMRI study of the specificity of activation for seen speech and for meaningless lower-face acts (gurning). *Cognitive Brain Research, 12,* 233–243.

Cherry, C., & Sayers, B. (1956). Experiments upon the total inhibition of stammering by external control and some clinical results. *Journal of Psychosomatic Research, 1,* 233–246.

Craig, A. R., & Hancock, K. (1995). Self-reported factors related to relapse following treatment for stuttering. *Australian Journal of Human Communication Disorders, 23,* 48–60.

Daniloff, J. K., Fritelli, G., Buckingham, H. W., Hoffman, P. R., & Daniloff, R. G. (1986). Amer-Ind versus ASL: Recognition and imitation in aphasic subjects. *Brain and Language, 28,* 95–113.

Dayalu, V. N., & Kalinowski, J. (2001). Re: Stuttering therapy results in pseudofluency. *International Journal of Language and Communication Disorders, 36,* 405–408.

Dayalu, V. N., & Kalinowski, J. (2002). Pseudofluency in adults who stutter: The illusory outcome of therapy. *Perceptual and Motor Skills, 94,* 87–96.

Decety, J., Chaminade, T., Grezes, J., & Meltzoff, A. N. (2002). A PET exploration of the neural mechanisms involved in reciprocal imitation. *Neuroimage, 15,* 265–272.

Dehaene-Lambertz, G., Dehaene, S., & Hertz-Pannier, L. (2002). Functional neuroimaging of speech perception in infants. *Science, 298,* 2013–2015.

Di Pellegrino, G., Fadiga, L., Fogassi, L., Gallese, V., & Rizzolatti, G. (1992). Understanding motor events: A neurophysiological study. *Experimental Brain Research, 91,* 176–180.

Eisenson, J., & Wells, C. (1942). A study of the influence of communicative responsibility in a choral speech situation for stutterers. *Journal of Speech Disorders, 7,* 259–262.

Emerick, L., & Haynes, W. (1986). *Diagnosis and evaluation in speech pathology.* Englewood Cliffs, NJ: Prentice-Hall.

Fadiga, L., & Craighero, L. (2003). New insights on sensorimotor integration: From hand action to speech perception. *Brain and Cognition, 53,* 514–524.

Fadiga, L., Craighero, L., Buccino, G., & Rizzolatti, G. (2002). Speech listening specifically modulates the excitability of tongue muscles: A TMS study. *European Journal of Neuroscience, 15,* 399–402.

Ferrari, P. F., Maiolini, C., Addessi, E., Fogassi, L., & Visalberghi, E. (2005). The observation and hearing of eating actions activates motor programs related to eating in macaque monkeys. *Behavioural Brain Research, 161,* 95–101.

Floel, A., Ellger, T., Breitenstein, C., & Knecht, S. (2003). Language perception activates the hand motor cortex: Implications for motor theories of speech perception. *European Journal of Neuroscience, 18,* 704–708.

Gallese, V., Fadiga, L., Fogassi, L., & Rizzolatti, G. (1996). Action recognition in the premotor cortex. *Brain, 119,* 593–609.

Gallese, V., Keysers, C., & Rizzolatti, G. (2004). A unifying view of the basis of social cognition. *Trends in Cognitive Science, 8,* 396–403.

Grezes, J., Armony, J. L., Rowe, J., & Passingham, R. E. (2003). Activations related to "mirror" and "canonical" neurones in the human brain: An fMRI study. *Neuroimage, 18,* 928–937.

Guntupalli, V. K., Kalinowski, J., Saltuklaroglu, T., & Nanjundeswaran, C. (2005). The effects of temporal modification of second speech signals on stuttering inhibition at two speech rates in adults. *Neuroscience Letters, 385,* 7–12.

Hari, R., Forss, N., Avikainen, S., Kirveskari, E., Salenius, S., & Rizzolatti, G. (1998). Activation of human primary motor cortex during action observation: A neuromagnetic study. *Proceedings of National Academy of Sciences USA, 95,* 15061–15065.

Heiser, M., Iacoboni, M., Maeda, F., Marcus, J., & Mazziotta, J. C. (2003). The essential role of Broca's area in imitation. *European Journal of Neuroscience, 17,* 1123–1128.

Heyes, C. (2001). Causes and consequences of imitation. *Trends in Cognitive Sciences, 5,* 253–261.

Hickok, G., Kirk, K., & Bellugi, U. (1998). Hemispheric organization of local- and global-level visuospatial processes in deaf signers and its relation to sign language aphasia. *Brain and Language, 65,* 276–286.

Iacoboni, M,, Koski, L. M., Brass, M., Bekkering, H., Woods, R. P., Dubeau, M. C., Mazziotta, J. C., & Rizzolatti, G. (2001). Reafferent copies of imitated actions in the right superior temporal cortex. *Proceedings of National Academy of Sciences USA, 98,* 13995–13999.

Johnson, W., & Rosen, L. (1937). Studies in psychology of stuttering: VII. Effect of certain changes in speech pattern upon frequency of stuttering. *Journal of Speech Disorders, 2,* 105–109.

Kalinowski, J., Armson, J., Roland-Mieszkowski, M., Stuart, A., & Gracco, V. L. (1993). Effects of alterations in auditory feedback and speech rate on stuttering frequency. *Language and Speech, 36,* 1–16.

Kalinowski, J., Armson, J., & Stuart, A. (1995). Effect of normal and fast articulatory rates on stuttering frequency. *Journal of Fluency Disorders, 20,* 293–302.

Kalinowski, J., & Dayalu, V. N. (2002). A common element in the immediate inducement of effortless, natural-sounding, fluent speech in people who stutter: "The second speech signal." *Medical Hypotheses, 58,* 61–66.

Kalinowski, J., Dayalu, V. N., Stuart, A., Rastatter, M. P., & Rami, M. K. (2000). Stutter-free and stutter-filled speech signals and their role in stuttering amelioration for English speaking adults. *Neuroscience Letters, 29,* 115–118.

Kalinowski, J., Noble, S., Armson, J., & Stuart, A. (1994). Naturalness ratings of the pretreatment and post-treatment speech of adults with mild and severe stuttering. *American Journal of Speech Language Pathology, 3,* 61–66.

Kalinowski, J., & Saltuklaroglu, T. (2003a). Speaking with a mirror: Engagement of mirror neurons via choral speech and its derivatives induces stuttering inhibition. *Medical Hypotheses, 60,* 538–543.

Kalinowski, J., & Saltuklaroglu, T. (2003b). Choral speech: The amelioration of stuttering via imitation and the mirror neuronal system. *Neuroscence and Biobehavioral Reviews, 27,* 339–347.

Kalinowski, J., Saltuklaroglu, T., Guntupalli, V., & Stuart, A. (2004). Gestural recovery and the role of forward and reversed syllabic repetitions as stuttering inhibitors in adults. *Neuroscence Letters, 363,* 144–149.

Kalinowski, J., Stuart, A., Rastatter, M. P., Snyder, G., & Dayalu, V. N. (2000). Inducement of fluent speech in persons who stutter via visual choral speech. *Neuroscience Letters, 281,* 198–200.

Kalinowski, J., Stuart, A., Sark, S., & Armson, J. (1996). Stuttering amelioration at various auditory feedback delays and speech rates. *European Journal of Disorders in Communication, 31,* 259–269.

Karzon, R. G., & Nicholas, J. G. (1989). Syllabic pitch perception in 2- to 3-month-old infants. *Perception and Psychophysics, 45,* 10–14.

Kohler, E., Keysers, C., Umilta, M.A., Fogassi, L., Gallese, V., & Rizzolatti, G. (2002). Hearing sounds, understanding actions: Action representation in mirror neurons. *Science, 297,* 846–848.

Kuhl, P. K. (1994). Learning and representation in speech and language. *Current Opinion in Neurobiology, 4,* 812–822.

Kuhl, P. K. (2000). A new view of language acquisition. *Proceedings of the National Academy of Sciences USA, 97,* 11850–11857.

Kuhl, P. K., & Meltzoff, A. N. (1996). Infant vocalizations in response to speech: Vowel imitation and developmental change. *Journal of the Acoustical Society of America, 100,* 2425–2439.

Larkin, M. (2000). Speech and sign language trigger similar brain activity. *The Lancet, 356,* 1989.

Leslie, K. R., Johnson-Frey, S. H., Grafton, S. T. (2004). Functional imaging of face and hand motion: Towards a motor theory of empathy. *Neuroimage, 21,* 601–607.

Liberman, A. M. (1993). Some assumptions about speech and how they changed. *Haskins Laboratories Status Report on Speech Research, 113,* 1–32.

Liberman, A. M. (1998). When theories of speech meet the real world. *Journal of Psycholinguistic Research, 27,* 111–122.

Liberman, A. M., Cooper, F. S., Shankweiler, D. P., & Studdert-Kennedy, M. (1967). Perception of the speech code. *Psychological Review, 74,* 431–461.

Liberman, A. M., & Mattingly, I. G. (1985). The motor theory of speech perception revised. *Cognition, 21,* 1–36.

Liberman, A. M., & Whalen, D. H. (2000). On the relation of speech to language. *Trends in Cognitive Science, 4,* 187–196.

Lieberman, P. (1984). *The biology and evolution of language,* Cambridge, MA: Harvard University Press.

Lieberman, P., Crelin, E. S., & Klatt, D. H. (1972) *American Anthropology, 74,* 287–307.

Mataric, M. J., & Pomplun, M. (1998). Fixation behavior in observation and imitation of human movement. *Brain Research Cognitive Brain Research, 7,* 191–202.

McGurk, H., & MacDonald, J. (1976). Hearing lips and seeing voices. *Nature, 264,* 746–748.

Meister, I. G., Boroojerdi, B., Foltys, H., Sparing, R., Huber, W., & Topper, R. (2003). Motor cortex hand area and speech: Implications for the development of language. *Neuropsychologia, 41,* 401–406.

Meltzoff, A. N., & Moore, M. K. (1977). Imitation of facial and manual gestures by human neonates. *Science, 198,* 74–78.

Miall, R. C. (2003). Connecting mirror neurons and forward models. *Neuroreport, 14,* 2135–2137.

Netsell, R. (1981). The acquisition of speech motor control: A perspective with directions for research. In R. Stark (Ed.), *Language behavior in infancy and early childhood* (pp. 127–153). Amsterdam: Elsevier-North Holland.

Nishimura, H., Hashikawa, K., Doi, K., Iwaki, T., & Watanabe, Y. (1999). Sign language "heard" in the auditory cortex. *Nature, 397,* 116.

Nishitani, N., & Hari, R. (2000). Temporal dynamics of cortical representation for action. *Proceedings of National Academy of Sciences USA, 97,* 913–918.

Nishitani, N., & Hari, R. (2002). Viewing lip forms: Cortical dynamics. *Neuron, 36,* 1211–1220.

Orr, B., Friedman, H. L., & Williams, J. C. (1965). Trainability of listening comprehension of speeded discourse. *Journal of Educational Psychology, 56,* 148–156.

Packman, A, & Onslow, M. (2002). Searching for the cause of stuttering. *Lancet, 360,* 655–656.

Piaget J. (1963). *The origins of intelligence in children.* New York: Basic Books.

Pickett, J. M. (1980). *The sounds of speech communication: A primer of acoustic phonetics and speech perception.* Baltimore: University Park Press.

Remez, R. E., Rubin, P. E., Pisoni, D. B., & Carrell, T. D. (1981). Speech perception without traditional speech cues. *Science, 212,* 947–949.

Rizzolatti, G., & Arbib, M. A. (1998). Language within our grasp. *Trends in Neuroscience, 21,* 188–194.

Rizzolatti, G., & Craighero, L. (2004). The mirror-neuron system. *Annual Reviews of Neuroscience, 27,* 169–192.

Rizzolatti, G., Fadiga, L., Gallese, V., & Fogassi, L. (1996). Premotor cortex and the recognition of motor actions. *Cognitive Brain Research*, *3*, 131–141.

Rizzolatti, G., Fogassi, L., & Gallese, V. (2001). Neurophysiological mechanisms underlying the understanding and imitation of action. *Nature Review Neuroscience*, *2*, 661–670.

Rizzolatti, G., Fogassi, L., & Gallese, V. (2002). Motor and cognitive functions of the ventral premotor cortex. *Current Opinion in Neurobiology*, *12*, 149–154.

Saltuklaroglu, T., Dayalu, V. N., & Kalinowski, J. (2002). Reduction of stuttering: The dual inhibition hypothesis. *Medical Hypotheses*, *58*, 67–71.

Saltuklaroglu, T., Dayalu, V. N., Kalinowski, J., Stuart, A., & Rastatter, M. P. (2004). Say it with me: Stuttering inhibited. *Journal of Clinical and Experimental Neuropsychology*, *26*, 161–168.

Saltuklaroglu, T., & Kalinowski, J. (2002). The end-product of behavioural stuttering therapy: Three decades of denaturing the disorder. *Disability and Rehabilitation*, *24*, 786–789.

Saltuklaroglu, T., Kalinowski, J., Dayalu, V. N., Guntupalli, V., Stuart, A., & Rastatter, M. P. (2003). A temporal window for the central inhibition of stuttering via exogenous speech signals in adults. *Neuroscience Letters*, *349*, 120–124.

Saltuklaroglu, T., Kalinowski, J., & Guntupalli, V (2004). Towards a common neural substrate in the immediate and effective inhibition of stuttering. *International Journal of Neuroscience*, *114*, 435–450.

Sams, M., Aulanko, R., Hamalainen, M., Hari, R., Lounasmaa, O.V., Lu, S.T., et al. (1991). Seeing speech: Visual information from lip movements modifies activity in the human auditory cortex. *Neuroscience Letters*, *127*, 141–145.

Sams, M., Mottonen, R., & Sihvonen, T. (2005). Seeing and hearing others and oneself talk. *Cognitive Brain Research*, *23*, 429–435.

Saygin, A. P., Wilson, S. M., Dronkers, N. F., & Bates, E. (2004). Action comprehension in aphasia: Linguistic and non-linguistic deficits and their lesion correlates. *Neuropsychologia*, *42*, 1788–1804.

Skoyles, J. R. (1998). Speech phones are a replication code. *Medical Hypotheses*, *50*, 167–173.

Spehar, B., Tye-Murray, N., & Sommers, M. (2004). Time-compressed visual speech and age: A first report. *Ear and Hearing*, *25*, 565–572.

Stuart, A., & Kalinowski, J. (2004). The perception of speech naturalness of post-therapeutic and altered auditory feedback speech of adults with mild and severe stuttering. *Folia Phoniatrica et Logopedia*, *56*, 347–357.

Tani, J., Ito, M., & Sugita, Y. (2004). Self-organization of distributedly represented multiple behavior schemata in a mirror system:

Reviews of robot experiments using RNNPB. *Neural Networks, 17,* 1273–1289.

Tokimura, H., Tokimura, Y., Oliviero, A., Asakura, T., & Rothwell, J. C. (1996). Speech-induced changes in corticospinal excitability. *Annals of Neurology, 40,* 628–634.

Tuomainen, J., Andersen, T. S., Tiippana, K., & Sams, M. (2005). Audio-visual speech perception is special. *Cognition, 96,* B13–B22.

Warren, R. M. (1976). Auditory perception and speech evolution. *Annals of New York Academy of Sciences, 280,* 708–717.

Warren, R. M., Obusek, C. J., Farmer, R. M., & Warren, R. P. (1969). Auditory sequence: Confusion of patterns other than speech or music. *Science, 164,* 586–587.

Wermter, S., & Elshaw, M. (2003). Learning robot actions based on self-organising language memory. *Neural Networks, 16,* 691–699.

Williams, J. H., Massaro, D. W., Peel, N. J., Bosseler, A., & Suddendorf, T. (2004). Visual-auditory integration during speech imitation in autism. *Research in Developmental Disabilities, 25,* 559–575.

Williams, J. H. G., Whiten, A., Suddendorf, T., & Perrett, D. I. (2001). Imitation, mirror neurons and autism. *Neuroscience and Biobehavioral Reviews, 25,* 287–295.

Wingate, M. E. (1976). *Stuttering theory and treatment.* New York: Irvington Publishers, Inc.

Wohlschlager, A., & Bekkering, H. (2002). Is human imitation based on a mirror-neurone system? Some behavioural evidence. *Experimental Brain Research, 143,* 335–341.

Yairi, E. & Ambrose, N. G. (1999). Early childhood stuttering I: Persistency and recovery rates. *Journal of Speech Language Hearing Research, 42,* 1097–1112.

# 6

# Second Speech Signals: Sources of Gestural Redundancy

> *"It is impossible to transcend the laws of nature. You can only determine that your understanding of nature has changed."*
>
> —*Nick Powers*

Choral speech or speaking in unison is the most powerful and immediate means of inhibiting the involuntary stuttering block and keeping the neural speech pipeline free from neural obstruction. We have suggested that this benchmark fluency enhancer, which usually induces 90 to 100% elimination of overt stuttering symptoms (Andrews, Howie, Dozsa, & Guitar, 1982; Cherry & Sayers, 1956), works by engaging the "monkey see, monkey do" mirror neuron system, predisposed for fluently imitating gestural sequences such as speech. Although the operation of this stuttering inhibitory mechanism is becoming increasingly clearer to us, and we are now attempting to pass this understanding on to our students, it took a great deal of time, experimentation, reading, and collaboration to arrive at this paradigmatic viewpoint. The author's (JK) own series of experiments began in the early 1990s, with investigations into the effects of altered auditory feedback (see below) on stuttering, at Dalhousie University in Halifax, Nova Scotia. This early line of investigation led to later work at East Carolina University, where he and Dr. Andy Stuart continued their previous work from Dalhousie looking at "second speech signals" to inhibit stuttering and produce natural-sounding speech. The initial notions were relatively simple: to examine the depth and breadth of the signal optimization for stuttering inhibition. But it soon turned to the question of identifying the mechanism responsible. The second author (TS) began his doctoral studies in the fall of 2000, when some of these notions were coming to fruition. The importance of gestures in the perception and production of speech was essential reading at Haskins Labs, home of the motor theory, where the author (JK) had worked as a research assistant during his doctoral studies.

While it seemed "second speech signals" or supplementary gestures were responsible for stuttering inhibition in choral speech, shadow speech, visual choral speech, delayed auditory feedback (DAF), and frequency altered feedback (FAF), questions remained as to what neural mechanism they might be engaging. Insights and answers came from the expected (scientific conferences and articles) and the unexpected (scientific reporters). Alison Motluk at *New Scientist* talked to us about the discovery of mirror neurons and how they might relate to our work, and then more than a year later at a conference on the evolution of language at Harvard it became clear to us that this might be the mechanism of engagement. Since then, we have been able to look at stuttering inhibition and recovery in children via our gestural/mirror neuronal perch, interpret all the data we have collected, and previous data pertaining to the inhibition of stuttering.

The problem is that, while the nature of choral speech and its power for nearly eliminating all overt stuttering symptoms is undisputed and sometimes gives the person who stutters a "sense of invulnerability" to stuttering rarely achieved via therapy (Kalinowski, Saltuklaroglu, Guntupalli, & Stuart, 2004), its functionality in its true "raw" form is fairly limited. Perhaps if clinicians had a means of harnessing its power and making it available for a wide variety of speaking situations, choral speech may have seen more clinical application over the years. However, enlisting the services of another person to continually speak in unison with a person who stutters would be highly impractical, dysfunctional, expensive, and would draw a great deal of unwanted attention— probably much more than stuttering itself. So, beyond demonstrating the ability of a person who stutters to speak fluently, choral speech has never received a great deal of airplay in clinical circles.

However, the answer was staring us in the face. The effects of choral speech can be functionally captured by using "second speech signals" which, like choral speech, provide strong sources of "gestural redundancy," which is the amount of salient gestural information that the speaker receives per unit time. It turned out that mirror neuronal systems have the power to make these effects possible because of their intricate ties with language, fluency, and immediate imitation. During choral speech, the two speakers are in unison or near unison. The speech gestures produced by one person are the same that the other produces. This imitative process seems to optimize mirror neuronal engagement. Because the speech being produced by the person who stutters is the same as that produced by the accompanist, the person who stutters receives the highest levels of "gestural redundancy." That is, all the gestures produced are readily available via perception, allowing them to be easily used as the incoming signal, and reproduced via imitation. This keeps the "neural pipeline open" and free from "neural blocks," thus immediately overriding any chance of stuttering. Mirror neurons bridge the gap between incoming speech gestures and the production of fluent speech, thus temporarily restoring the integrity of the neural pipeline that is compromised during central stuttering blocks (Kalinowski & Saltuklaroglu, 2003a, 2003b). The question now is how to recreate these effects in functional manners so we get a better understanding of the disorder, its inhibition, and, most importantly, provide feasible therapeutic options for those who stutter.

## Second Speech Signals

When receiving a choral speech signal, those who stutter are not asked to change their manner of speaking or assume any form of motor control over the speech output. As such, we attribute the powerful inhibition of stuttering to the sensory input, which in the case of true choral speech is a linguistic match to what the speaker is producing. However, we stated that choral speech is never completely synchronized. One speaker always seems to lead or lag the other, usually without any detrimental effect on stuttering inhibition. So, there seem to be some flexibility within this gestural input-output system. The question is whether "permutations" of choral speech exist that also produce powerful inhibitory effects. Or, how flexible is this system for inhibiting stuttering via gestural redundancy?

There are essentially three main parameters that can be examined with respect to the flexibility of this inhibitory mechanism. The first is the "temporal" parameter: how well do the two sets of speech gestures need to be synchronized in time to produce strong stuttering inhibition? Some flexibility may exist here considering the lack of perfect synchrony during choral speech. Another condition that demonstrates the temporal flexibility is shadowed speech. Whereas during choral speech two speakers speak in unison, shadowed speech is a direct imitation of another speaker. Thus, when shadowing, the second speech signal precedes the intended utterance. Shadowed speech is a close relative of choral speech, the only difference being the relatively consistent temporal lag between the two signals (i.e., the leader and the shadowed signal), making shadowing a slightly delayed imitative task. Not surprisingly, the levels of stuttering inhibition that shadowing induces are similar to those induced by true choral speech (Andrews et al., 1982; Cherry & Sayers, 1956; Healey & Howe, 1987; Johnson & Rosen, 1937; Kondas, 1967). The importance of the temporal flexibility in the choral effect surfaces again in both the other two forms of second speech signals, where we argue that the use of delayed auditory feedback (DAF) is simply "reversed shadowing," and the production of syllabic repetitions is simply endogenous or "self-shadowing" that seems to aid in rendering the approximately 80% recovery among incipient stutterers (Bloodstein, 1995; Kalinowski, Saltuklaroglu, Dayalu, & Guntupalli, 2005; Saltuklaroglu & Kalinowski, 2005; Yairi & Ambrose, 1999). In stuttering, the person with neural block creates a short syllabic nucleus with energy bursts that are repetitive in nature to alleviate the neural block; thus, we have endogenous shadowing (Kalinowski et al., 2004).

Linguistic content is the second parameter that can be examined for its flexibility with respect to stuttering inhibition. The question is whether the linguistic content of the incoming supplementary speech signal needs to match the one being produced to inhibit stuttering. Coarticulated speech gestures contain a wealth of gestural information, a great deal of which may be shared by other coarticulated gestures. In other words, two linguistically distinct utterances may share a great deal of gestural information. If this is the case, then, it may be possible for two speakers to be saying completely different things while stuttering is still being inhibited, due to the redundancy of gestural content across speech signals and the same shared functional goal (speaking) for engaging mirror neurons (Iacoboni et al., 2005). The important characteristic of the phonetic module, in this case, is its specialization for extracting the relevant gestural information that can be used to engage mirror systems and inhibit stuttering. Therefore, even if two different utterances are being produced, it may still be possible to extract the relevant gestural information from the sensory speech signal for the purposes of inhibiting stuttering. The third parameter is the modality of presentation. The "visual choral" study described below shows how speech does not need to travel through the ears for it to be useful for stuttering inhibition.

Prior to the Dalhousie studies, a great body of literature already existed examined the effects on stuttering frequency by such phenomena as altered auditory feedback and various sensory inputs. However, the Dalhousie studies presented serious challenges to the then current perspective on the effects of altered auditory feedback on stuttering and we came to realize that altering auditory feedback was but one way of creating a second speech signal for stuttering inhibition. In other words, it was just one permutation of choral speech, in which the temporal relationship between two sets of similar gestures was altered. Hence, understanding the gestural nature of human speech perception led to the behavioral research that has allowed us to better understand the parameters of choral speech involved in stuttering inhibition and how we can functionally manipulate them. We created a line of research investigating the effects of various second speech signals on the frequency of stuttering. Each of our group's experiments have provided additional insight into the flexibility within this inhibitory mechanism, and perhaps, most importantly, what this inhibitory mechanism tells us about the nature of stuttering.

By broad definition, a "second speech signal" exists when (1) a person perceives another speech signal in addition to his own speech (e.g., choral speech or unison speech, shadowed speech, etc.), (2) when one's own speech is electronically altered to create the illusion of another speech signal (e.g., delayed auditory feedback [DAF], frequency altered feedback [FAF], etc.), or (3) when a person's own speech is voluntarily or involuntarily modified to provide additional gestural information without changing linguistic content (e.g., overt stuttering behaviors, pseudostuttering, prolonged speech) (Guntupalli, Kalinowski, Saltuklaroglu, & Nanjundeswaran, 2005). In each of these cases, we are increasing the amount of "gestural redundancy" when producing speech, whether this is achieved via external (another speaker) or internal (one's own voice), or a combination of the two (e.g., altered feedback). This broad definition covers a range of conditions that have been empirically proven to inhibit stuttering. At first glance, these three types of second speech signals may seem to be reducing stuttering in different manners. However, the purpose of describing them all as second speech signals is that we believe they all can engage mirror systems for stuttering inhibition and, thus, in some manner they are all related. (It seems highly improbable that every condition that effectively reduces stuttering works differently.) We make the argument that although these powerful inhibitors of stuttering may seem to operate differently at the proximal or peripheral level (i.e., eyes, ears, and vocal tract), at the distal level of the brain, they all operate by engaging mirror systems (Saltuklaroglu, Kalinowski, & Guntupalli, 2004). The common element of all second speech signals is that they provide a source of gestural redundancy, which simply means that the phonetic module (according to motor theory) is being provided with supplementary gestural information to help in the transposition between perception and production (Guntupalli et al., 2005; Kalinowski, Dayalu, Stuart, Rastatter, & Rami, 2000; Kalinowski et al., 2004; Kalinowski & Saltuklaroglu, 2003a, 2003b; Saltuklaroglu, Kalinowski, Dayalu, Guntupalli, Stuart, & Rastatter, 2003).

The types of second speech signals described above are categorized according to the "source" of the second signal. Thus, according to how the second speech signal is created, we can also name three types of signals: exogenous, endogenous-exogenous, and endogenous, respectively.

## Exogenous Second Speech Signals

The term "exogenous" means outside the body. An exogenous second speech signal exists outside the body, or, in this case, the vocal tract, of the person who stutters. Simply put, it can exist independently of a person who stutters and is not affected by his or her speech output, regardless of whether it is fluent or stuttered. The best example of an exogenous speech signal is choral speech. During choral speech, the two speech signals are generated from two different sources. Even if one person stutters or falters in some way, the other speech signal can carry on unimpeded, as the two signals are not dependent on one another. Although the person who stutters may be reliant on the second signal to become more fluent, his or her speech can still exist without the presence of the second signal. This independent nature of the exogenous second speech signal has both practical advantages and disadvantages relative to the other types of signals, which are discussed in the next chapter.

Acoustically presented choral speech is the prototypical exogenous second speech signal, yet other exogenous speech signals are nearly as powerful and immediate with respect to their inhibitory powers over stuttering. What follows are some brief descriptions of several of our controlled experiments that have examined the robust effects of exogenous second speech for inhibiting stuttering relative to "control" conditions, during which no second speech signals were provided.

## Auditory Second Speech Signals

The first experiment in this paradigm consisted of playing different configurations of auditory speech gestures to people who stutter while they read passages (Kalinowski, Dayalu, et al., 2000). The speech signals selected for this first experiment comprised normal continuous speech, normal interrupted speech, stuttered continuous speech, and stuttered interrupted speech, a continuous vowel /a/, looping /a-i-u/ vowel trains, a continuous consonant /s/, and looping /s-f-sh/ consonant trains.

This extensive experiment provided some very valuable information. First, the overall high levels of stuttering inhibition obtained (61–78%) using most of the second speech signals in this experiment told us that as long as we are perceiving speech via audition, it does not need to be matched to the intended utterance for stuttering inhibition to occur. This finding demonstrated that the choral speech effect is linguistically flexible, probably due to the redundancy of shared speech information between the two speech signals. Second, introducing random intermittent short silences to the second speech signal did not affect its potency for stuttering inhibition, suggesting that the fluency induced via second speech signals may be amenable to some carryover effects following the removal of signal. We investigated this phenomenon further in a later experiment (Saltuklaroglu et al., 2003). Third, hearing the stutter-filled and stutter-free speech samples yielded the same high levels of stuttering inhibition, which told us that the fluency of the second signal does not factor into its potential as a stuttering inhibitor, as long as it does not interrupt the signal for too long, as may be the case if the stuttered speech consisted of long silent blocks. Fourth, and perhaps most importantly, the consonants and consonant trains did not yield significant levels of stuttering inhibition. These were the only second speech signals used in this study that did not contain voicing. If we interpret this finding from a gestural viewpoint, it becomes clear that the presence of voicing in a sensory signal is a powerful indicator of gestural information (Dayalu, Saltuklaroglu, Kalinowski, Stuart, & Rastatter, 2001). When voicing is present, there is little doubt that a signal is from a glottal source being filtered in a human vocal tract. In the absence of voicing and contextual information, voiceless fricatives may be perceived as originating from another source (i.e., outside the human vocal tract) or having "gestural ambiguity" (Kalinowski, Saltuklaroglu, et al., 2004). That is why a continuous /s/ may sound like it is being produced by a snake. Levels of gestural encoding in classes of sounds such as stops (closure, opening, release, and aspiration—movements), affricates (stops, plus fricatives—movements), approximants (movements), and vowels (voicing and formants) may be thought of as being higher than the levels of encoding found in voiceless fricatives, probably the least encoded of all speech sounds. We suggest that, because of this ambiguity, hearing these isolated continuous fricatives may fail in sufficiently activating the "phonetic module" for the presence of speech and, hence, decrease the potential for stuttering inhibition via mirror neuron engagement.

## Visual Choral Speech

During a clinical session, a patient with quite a severe stutter was having difficulty reciting "The Pledge of Allegiance" via the use of behavioral strategies (e.g., slowed speech, continuous phonation). The use of auditory choral speech was used to reduce stuttering, which, as expected, it did almost immediately. After a recitation or two, the clinician wanted to observe whether just the use of behavioral strategies would be sufficient for communication of the "Pledge" with the success of choral speech. However, the behavioral strategies were unsuccessful in this case and the patient reverted back to severe stuttering immediately. It was at this point that the author (JK) suggested that the patient watch his mouth gesture as he (JK) silently mouthed the words to "The Pledge of Allegiance." This was initially done in an attempt to wean the patient from auditory choral speech and allow the behavioral strategies to take over. Surprisingly, the patient immediately became fluent without auditory stimuli and a "visual choral speech" experiment was conceived (Kalinowski, Stuart, Rastatter, Snyder, & Dayalu, 2000). Instead of weaning the client off choral speech, that day we found a new modality for presenting the choral signal. Thus, we varied the modality of presentation of the choral signal. Instead of the stuttering participants receiving speech gestures through audition (i.e., hearing), the unison speaker silently mouthed the same text as the participants read. As described above, participants only watched movements of the experimenter's lips, silently. Remarkably, in the group of participants tested, this visual analog of choral speech brought about an 80% reduction in stuttering. Since then, these findings have been replicated both by us (Saltuklaroglu, Dayalu,

Kalinowski, Stuart, & Rastatter, 2004) and by others (Bothe, Taylor, Everett, 2003).

These findings were of utmost importance to our "gestural" perspective of speech and stuttering inhibition. To the best of our knowledge, this was the first time that a visual stimulus had resulted in such high levels of stuttering inhibition, presumably via the gestural nature of the sensory input. Prior to that, other visual stimuli (e.g., flashing lights) presented to stutterers had resulted in only marginal levels of stuttering inhibition (Kuniszyk-Jozkowiak, Smolka, & Adamczyk, 1996, 1997; Smolka & Adamczyk, 1992). This visual effect showed that an auditory second speech signal was not necessary for powerful stuttering inhibition, as long as the people who stuttered could visually perceive relevant gestural information.

In a follow-up to this experiment, we examined what would happen to the levels of stuttering inhibition when the second speaker silently mouthed different material from that being produced by the stuttering participants (Saltuklaroglu, Dayalu et al., 2004). For example, if the target utterance for the participant was "The radio was invented by . . . ," the experimenter may be simultaneously silently mouthing "At the beginning of human history . . . " At this point we had already conducted some experiments showing that linguistically different exogenously presented acoustic speech (e.g., continuous speech and steady-state vowels—see below) signals had the power to substantially inhibit stuttering, and we thought the same range of flexibility might be possible for visually presented second speech signals. However, it turned out that when the silently lipped material was different from the target utterance, stuttering was only reduced by 35%, substantially lower than the level achieved by other second speech signals. We concluded that although speech gestures can be transmitted by vision, audition is still the optimal modality. This is probably because audition provides a great deal more gestural information. Manner, place, voicing features, formant frequencies, and their transitions, are all encoded within the acoustic signal, representing configurations of the entire vocal tract within this sensory modality, whereas visual signals only contain gestural information produced at a surface level (i.e., the lips and front of the tongue). Thus, without substantial transitory or gestural information beyond that found at the very front of the oral cavity, it is much more difficult for the phonetic module to take visual gestural information and use it to inhibit stuttering, increasing the necessit of the linguistic match. The visual sensory modality simply does not contain the wealth or redundancy of information found in acoustic modality. The difficulty in acquiring ges-tural information from visual speech is also exemplified in lip reading, which has been found to be only about 30% accurate, even in accomplished lip readers (Spehar, Tye-Murray, & Sommers, 2004).

## A Temporal Window

In the experiment described above we noted that listening to a continuous vowel /a/ was sufficient to inhibit stuttering and also that a second speech signal need only be intermittently presented to be effective. However, it seemed intuitive that there were limits to the durations of silence that could be introduced into second speech signals before we would begin to observe degradation in their stuttering inhibition. Although the previous experiment inserted silences between 1 and 5 seconds in duration into the second speech signals, they were inserted randomly and it was impossible to tell the overall effect of any particular length of silence. Thus, we conducted another experiment on this "temporal window," as it was likely to provide valuable information regarding carryover inhibition via the mirror systems (Saltuklaroglu et al., 2003).

We created four different second speech signals: a continuous vowel /a/, a looping 1-second /a/ followed by a 1-second silence, a looping 1-second /a/ followed by a 3-second silence, and a looping 1-second /a/ followed by a 5-second silence. Thus, as longer silences were introduced following the 1-second /a/, the relative amount of speech in the signal was decreased and the "intermittency" of the signal was increased. We found that listening to the continuous /a/ and the looping 1-second /a/ with the 1-second silence both significantly reduced stuttering by about 65%. However, when the duration of silence was increased to 3 seconds and 5 seconds, the levels of stuttering inhibition dropped off to about 30%. From these data, we surmised that when using a 1-second /a/ as stimulus the "temporal window" for inhibition is somewhere between 1 and 3 seconds. In hindsight, we probably should have tested the effects of a 2-second silence to gain a more accurate picture. However, the fact that we had empirical evidence that the signal only needed to be present for 50% of the time (i.e., 1-second /a/ + 1-second silence) showed us that the inhibitory mechanism had some temporal flexibility in that the second speech signal does not need to be present all the time for it to be an effective stuttering inhibitor. We likened hearing the looped 1-second /a/ with 1-second silence to hearing syllabic repetitions, and hearing a continuous /a/ to hearing prolongations.

When endogenous second speech signals are produced (i.e., repetitions and prolongations), via overt stuttering behaviors they engage mirror systems and inhibit the central stuttering block allowing difficult sounds or words to pass through the neural pipeline unimpeded. Listening to a continuous and intermittent /a/ accomplishes the same thing without the production of disruptive stuttering behaviors. In other words, if people who stutter perceive a second speech signal, the act of communication remains relatively unimpeded as stuttering inhibition occurs "online." When people who stutter produce repetitions and prolongations to actively break through the neural block, they have to go "off- line" which presents an interruption to the communicative act (Saltuklaroglu et al., 2003). Although disruptive in nature, the power of repetitions and prolongations to eventually allow for forward-moving speech is indisputable and is the reason for simulated use in many therapeutic pro-tocols. Sheehan, Van Riper, Johnson and many others used the inhibitory power of repetitions in their programs. Johnson used bounce techniques, Van Riper embraced pseudostuttering and desensitization, and Sheehan incorporated voluntary stuttering, but they were simply using repetitions with different names. Prolongations have been integrated into every therapy since the beginning of time. Any time one tells a person who stutters to prolong a sound they are using a natural biological design to release a neural block and move forward. The more a person who stutters prolongs, or the more unnatural they sound, the more invulnerable they typically feel toward uncontrolled moments of stuttering.

## Reversing the Second Speech Signal

We conducted another experiment to test the boundaries of gesturally based stuttering inhibition (Kalinowski, Saltuklaroglu, et al., 2004). In this one, the second speech signal consisted of fluent speech and artificially stuttered speech characterized by evenly spaced syllabic repetitions on every word. However, we added another twist. As well as using fluent and stuttered speech as normal, forward-flowing second speech signal, we used some computer software to reverse the signals. This can also be done by playing a tape recorder in reverse.

Reversing an acoustic speech signal has very interesting consequences. First, as you listen to it, there is still no doubt that it is speech but its intelligibility is obviously compromised. The speech signal contains voicing and formant transitions, powerful cues of speech, but they are reversed. Our articulators are accustomed to moving in manners that are consistent with a normal, forward flow of speech. Therefore, much like energy or matter, speech has "entropy" for flowing in one direction—forward. This is in contrast to alphabets or ciphers that can be interpreted in either direction. We perceive coarticulatory relationships that are forward flowing, yet are not serial relationships, or beads on strings, that can travel forward or backward. Thus, when we hear a reversed acoustic speech signal, it may be representative of the vocal tract operating in reverse, achieving dynamic articulator configurations and acoustic signals that are quite abnormal as they represent violations to the normal manner in which speech is meant to be produced. Thus, we expected that reversing the second speech signals might not result in high levels of stuttering inhibition because some of the acoustic information might not be perceived as recognizable speech gesture due to the breakdown in natural coarticulatory gestural relationships.

Consistent with our previous results we found that both the fluent and stuttered forward-flowing second speech signals resulted in about 65% stuttering inhibition. We also managed to achieve a similar level from the reversed stuttered speech. The only second speech signal that resulted in a significantly lower level of inhibition was the reversed fluent speech. How is this possible? The advantage of stuttered speech, especially the type we used in this experiment which consisted of syllabic repetitions, is that it still contains higher levels of "gestural redundancy." Even when reversed, syllable repetitions were salient and obvious to the listener. Gestural information is repeated and becomes more symmetric and recognizable with the addition of this repetitive quality. In other words, overt stuttering creates "gestural redundancy," which for stuttering inhibition, means more of the second gesture available for stuttering inhibition. Thus, if we apply the speech perception-production link here, when people who stutter produce gestural repetitions or prolongations, they are simply creating their own gestural redundancy, or an endogenous second speech signal, which we will examine shortly.

## Compressing and Expanding the Second Speech Signal

The notion of "gestural redundancy" led us to manipulate the exogenous second speech signal in yet another way (Guntupalli et al., 2005). It is implied that for gestural redundancy to occur, more gestural speech information is being fed into the phonetic module per unit of time. Therefore, by temporally compressing or expanding speech via computer software, we manipulated the amount of gestural information delivered in second speech signals per unit of time.

The basic second speech signal used was a normally fluent speaker reading a series of passages. Different passages were compressed and expanded at rates of 20%, 40%, 60%, and 80%. When the second speech signals were expanded, they were still quite intelligible and sounded much like different rates of droned or prolonged speech. The compressed speech sounded as if it was "sped up." When it reached a level of 80% compression, its intelligibility was compromised. Two experiments were conducted under these premises. The main findings were as follows: the unaltered signals, all the expanded signals, and the 20% compressed signals all produced significantly high levels of stuttering inhibition relative to the control condition. However, compression rates of 40%, 60%, and 80% failed to yield significant levels of stuttering inhibition. It should be noted that two speech rates were tested (normal and fast), yet speech rate did not play a significant role in stuttering frequency.

This was the first time that second speech signals had *not* been found to be effective for inhibiting stuttering. It had been suggested that these findings might be attributed to the decrease in intelligibility with increased rates of compression, so we collected intelligibility data on the compressed stimuli. We found that the intelligibility of the spoken passages was not completely compromised until the signal was compressed by 80%. Thus, lower levels of compression were needed to degrade the inhibitory properties of the second speech signals than to degrade the intelligibility of the signal. In other words, the reduction in stuttering inhibition found at the higher levels of compression had to be attributed to something other than intelligibility and we returned to our gestural model of inhibition. We suggested that although we seem to have a phonetic module that is specialized for speech perception/production tasks, its processing capacities may have some limits. It may be that when speech is compressed at rates of 40% or higher, we begin to exceed the "temporal resolution" of the phonetic module for translating between perception and production for stuttering inhibition. In other words, the phonetic module is only able to process a certain amount of gestural information per unit of time. Once this capacity is exceeded, it appears that the relevant goal-directed gestural information is not able to be efficiently extracted from the incoming signal for the purposes of mirror neuron engagement and stuttering inhibition.

If speeding up the rate at which gestural information is introduced into the phonetic module tested its temporal resolving capacities resulting in decreased inhibition, then we may have expected the opposite effect when the speech gestures were expanded. However, this was not the case. Expanded and unexpanded second speech signals both induced approximately the same levels of stuttering inhibition (52–70%). Based on all our data, we believe that when second speech signals are used that are not linguistically matched to the intended utterance, the limits for stuttering inhibition may be around 70%. Even though this level is substantial and may have some functional use in a generic second speech signal, it appears that some sort of linguistic synchrony between the intended utterance and the second set of speech gestures is necessary for optimal level of inhibition (e.g., as in choral speech).

Thus, the relationship between the second speech signal and the intended speech is shown in the cogwheel analogy

Speech production          Incoming sensory signal

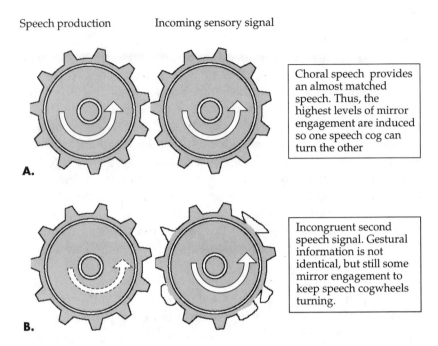

Choral speech provides an almost matched speech. Thus, the highest levels of mirror engagement are induced so one speech cog can turn the other

**A.**

Incongruent second speech signal. Gestural information is not identical, but still some mirror engagement to keep speech cogwheels turning.

**B.**

**Figure 6–1.** Second speech signals help propagate the intended utterance by providing gestural information to be "grabbed onto." The left cogwheel is the intended utterance and the right cogwheel is the second signal. **A.** When true choral signals are presented the gestural information is closely matched so the teeth (gestural information) on the two cogs are similarly configured. In this case, the second speech signal presents the best gestural match to help turn the intended utterance cogwheel, resulting in the highest levels of mirror neuron engagement and stuttering inhibition. **B.** The gestural information in the second speech signal is different from the intended utterance (linguistically asynchronous) so the gestures are configured differently, and the second speech signal may not continuously provide a gestural fit to help propagate the intended utterance. However, the redundancy of vocal tract information within gestures still allows for some mirror neuron engagement and turning of the intended utterance cog (i.e., stuttering inhibition). *(continues)*

(Figure 6–1) where the teeth on the cogs represent gestural information. Simply put, two speech signals presented simultaneously can help propagate each other by the redundancy of gestural information.

Speech production       Incoming sensory signal

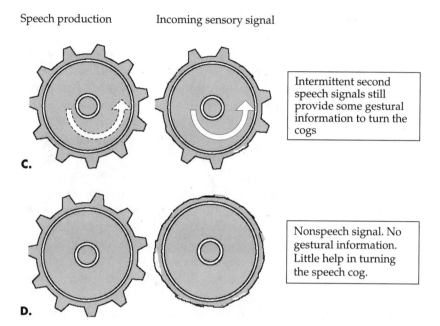

Intermittent second speech signals still provide some gestural information to turn the cogs

**C.**

Nonspeech signal. No gestural information. Little help in turning the speech cog.

**D.**

**Figure 6–1.** *(continued)* **C.** The gestures in the second speech signal are presented intermittently so fewer teeth are found on the second speech cogwheel. Although this second speech signal may not continuously provide gestural information, if the temporal window is not exceeded there may still be sufficient gestural information for stuttering inhibition. **D.** When a nonspeech signal is presented, there is no gestural information in the sensory signal and, therefore, it is not depicted as a cogwheel with teeth. It is not a second speech signal and does not engage mirror systems that help turn the cog of the intended utterance.

## Sine Wave Analogs of Second Speech Signals

In our discussion on speech perception in the previous chapter, we described how a few carefully synchronized sine waves could substitute for formants and produce acoustic sequences that could be perceived as speech. According to our second speech signal hypothesis, we thought it might also be possible for these sine wave analogs to serve as stuttering inhibitors if they were presented simultaneously with speech production. We suspected that if gestural speech information could be extracted from the sine wave speech, as with fluent speech, it might be degraded upon its reversal. Thus, the second speech signals in this experiment consisted of forward and reversed fluent speech, as well as forward and reversed renditions of the sine wave sentences available on the Haskins Web site (http://www.haskins .yale.edu/haskins/MISC/SWS/SWS.html).

We found that in addition to the expected stuttering inhibition derived from a normal forward-flowing, fluent second speech signal, sine wave analogs of forward-flowing speech could also significantly inhibit stuttering. In contrast, the reversed counterparts of both the speech and the sine wave analogs did not induce significant levels of stuttering inhibition. These data appear to support the original study by Remez, Rubin, Pisoni, and Carrell (1981) that suggested speech perception can exist in the absence of traditional cues. Our data suggest that, for the purposes of stuttering inhibition, gestural information can be extracted from forward-flowing sine wave analogs of speech. In addition, much like normal speech, reversing a sine wave analog of the speech signal appears to change any perceived gestural relationships, rendering the signal of little use for stuttering inhibition.

## Endogenous-Exogenous Second Speech Signals

Endogenous-exogenous second speech signals have two sources. Generally, one is the human vocal tract and the other is an external mechanism that alters the manner in which a person hears his or her own voice. The general idea is that by using some external device to alter the way one's own voice sounds, we can create the illusion of a second speaker producing unison speech and, hence, emulate the choral speech effect. This external device may be as simple as speaking in a church, hall, or stadium that echoes. Some people have told about speaking into a well. Even speaking into a hollow tube or "passive resonator" has empirical support for the inhibition of stuttering, approximately 30% (Stuart, Miller, Kalinowski, & Rastatter, 1997). However, much more sophisticated technology exists in the form of digital signal processors (DSPs) that can offer a wide range of altered auditory feedback (AAF) effects. They alter the temporal and spectral domains of a speech signal in innumerable ways, and in so doing, trick the brain into perceiving the presence of a second speaker. The two effects most commonly known to inhibit stuttering are delayed auditory feedback (DAF) and frequency altered feedback (FAF), which we now discuss in some detail.

## Delayed Auditory Feedback

Delayed auditory feedback (DAF) refers to a condition in which a person hears his own voice with slight temporal delay, similar to an echo. In the 1950s researchers began investigating the effects of DAF on speech of both people who stutter and normally fluent speakers. What is interesting about DAF is that it sometimes seemed to produce a disruptive effect on the speech of normal speakers and an ameliorative effect on the speech of those who stutter. Some have made the simple assumption that DAF was able to make stutterers out of nonstutterers and vice versa. This simplistic notion led to years of "wandering" and theories regarding an interplay between the auditory system and speech-producing mechanism and how unaltered auditory feedback from speech may be somehow compromised in those who stutter. Although we have witnessed hundreds of people who stutter achieving immediate and natural-sounding fluent speech under the effects of DAF, we seriously challenge the notion that DAF induces true stuttering behaviors in those who are normally fluent. We first address the role of DAF in stuttering amelioration.

Early researchers used what we now consider to be long auditory delays in the range of 200 to 600 ms. One-fifth of a second may not seem like a long time, but consider that speech is often produced at about four to six syllables per second, and one begins to realize the time scale we are working in with respect to our speech production-perception system. Delays of this magnitude create a significant phonemic lag in information from what is produced and what is perceived. As this happens, these long delays in auditory feedback are highly effective in reducing stuttering. The author (JK) fondly recalls his first experiences with

DAF when stuttering and receiving stuttering therapy at the University of Connecticut:

> For 3 hours a week. I was allowed to use this magical delayed auditory feedback (DAF) machine to slow down my speech. It was pure magic. I was fluent. My speech was slow and droning, yet fluent, when the machine was set to delays as long as 225 ms. However, I was fluent at short delays of 25 ms and 50 ms too without slowing down my speech rate! Using this device, not thinking about the "correct" form of speech production was required. It simply allowed me to produce unbridled and unadulterated fluent speech, in much the same way it is produced by those who do not stutter. For me, this was simply unbelievable—a source of renewed hope. However, strangely enough, when I spoke at a normal speech rate under these short delays my speech therapist always told me to slow down, even though I was still fluent, for they wanted me to speak slowly and fluently, rather than just fluently. The "experts" had led the therapists to believe that the two were interdependent, and therefore did not believe that I should be able to speak quickly and fluently under DAF (Kalinowski, 2003, p. 108).

However, these long delays also brought with them an unforeseen consequence. People who stutter and normal speakers naturally slow down their speech as a result of the feedback of speaking under auditory feedback with long temporal delays. Simply put, speech rate and delay in feedback covary. As the delay is increased, speech rate drops. It has been hypothesized that people who stutter want to "slow down" their rate of speech so that the auditory feedback can "catch up" to the words being produced. Furthermore, instruction to reduce one's speech to match the cadence of the DAF was reported to virtually eliminate stuttering (Andrews et al., 1982). Others discounted the feedback notions of DAF and suggested it was the reduced rate or the imposed byproduct of using DAF that was the "Holy Grail" of stuttering inhibition (Costello-Ingham, 1993; Goldiamond, 1965). No experimenter tried to differentiate rate from DAF at that time. That is, nobody tried to have a speaker read at fast and normal rates under DAF in 1965 and solve the mystery of its effects once and for all. Goldiamond (1965) implemented therapy that used DAF within a rigid behavioral protocol. The role of DAF was simply to induce prolonged speech. Once fluency was established using the bulky analog double-head tape-looped DAF machine, it was time to transition to the outside world. At this stage the use of DAF ceased for two reasons: the machines were big and bulky, and speech therapists believed that only the prolonged speech was necessary to maintain fluency. However, the transition was not generally as smooth as the therapists expected, resulting in tenuous and unstable speech patterns that we normally associate with traditional behavioral therapies.

Regardless, the behavioral school of thought was beginning to dominate and therapists decided that as the goal of therapy was to instate rate control, it was probably best to start with that goal initially, rather than trying to wean from the DAF. Why not simply "teach" people who stutter how to use prolonged speech and let them experience fluent speech without the use of an external "crutch." The view of independence from external mediating influences (e.g., medications or devices) permeates many therapeutic processes (e.g., depression, attention deficit disorder, alcoholism, dyslexia) but sometimes may be misplaced, especially when the etiology of the disorder is unknown and its management is often inefficient and filled with pain. As therapists, we should recognize that we are not here to build character, but to alleviate suffering and make life for those with the pathology more like that of those without. This is not a Puritan battle of will and character (i.e., Psychiatrist Peter Kramer's argument in *Listening to Prozac*) but simply a battle against a neural.

Furthermore, arguments were being posited to discount the role of DAF in stuttering. Borden (1979) proposed an open-loop model of speech production that suggested little or no role for auditory feedback as it was too "too slow" for on-line corrections of speech production. Simply put, by the time you perceived, processed, analyzed, and corrected for any short event, a speaker would be producing gestures further down the speech stream. It was proposed that hearing and auditory feedback was essential for speech and language acquisition skills but auditory feedback was less essential than internal models. Or, it seemed, ears were nothing more than something to hang your glasses on regarding stuttering inhibition. Later, Costello-Ingham (1993) clearly stated

" . . . the functional variable in regard to the reduction of stuttering is not DAF, but prolonged speech, and the latter can be produced without reliance on a DAF machine" (p. 30). If she and others (e.g., Perkins, 1979; Wingate, 1970, 1976) had been correct about the limited role of DAF, this reasoning would have been logical. It made sense to eliminate the use of DAF if possible, especially because at this time devices that induced DAF were very large, bulky, required the use of large headphones, and drew a great deal of unwanted attention to themselves (Stuart, Xia, Jiang, Jiang, Kalinowski, & Rastatter, 2003; Kalinowski et al., 2004). We now affectionately refer to them as "goober devices," not because of the effects they provided, but because of the stigma they were bound to induce if anyone ever attempted to use them outside the clinical milieu, which was the intended setting of use. Considering that people who stutter try to look and sound the same as everyone else, the outside use of such conspicuous devices would truly have been counterproductive to this goal.

Needless to say, the use of DAF was essentially abandoned in favor of behavioral therapeutic protocols that taught what were considered to be fluent speech patterns based on the use of prolonged speech. We now realize the flaw in this line of thinking. But to make this realization took a great deal more investigation into the effects of DAF and the confirmation of an anomaly that could not be accounted for by those who solely espoused prolonged speech protocols over the use of DAF in conjunction with such protocols. In 1993, Kalinowski, Stuart, and colleagues began to cast doubt onto the preconceived notions of DAF's role in stuttering inhibition. They created a series of experiments examining the role of endogenous-exogenous second speech signals fast and normal speech rates. The group posed a simple query. If rate reduction is necessary for DAF to be effective in reducing stuttering, then surely asking people who stutter to speak at a fast rate while under DAF should have no ameliorative effect. Surprisingly, it was found that while under the effects of DAF, people who stutter were nearly fluent while speaking both at normal and fast rates of speech. Furthermore, stuttering could be reduced with much shorter delays in auditory feedback. Delays of 50 to 75 ms were found to best inhibit stuttering (approximately 80%) during a reading task, but even extremely short delays of 25 ms were found to have an inhibitory effect (see Figure 6–2 below).

These findings are far reaching and have sown the seeds for our current view of stuttering and the most effective and efficient means of inhibiting it. The data clearly suggest that DAF need not induce changes in speech rates and that even the smallest changes in auditory feedback may have an inhibitory effect on stuttering. It has become evident that the inhibition of stuttering is not reliant upon motoric changes in speech production, such as the use of prolonged speech. As discussed in chapter 3, years were spent looking for invariant motor changes as results of therapy, but to no avail. Armson and Kalinowski and colleagues (1994) showed that comparisons of perceptually fluent pre- and post-therapeutic speech were confounded and like comparing apples to oranges. It is not surprising that after

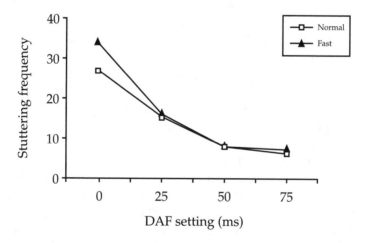

**Figure 1:** Mean stuttering frequencies as a function of auditory and speech rate.

**Figure 6–2.** The effects of various auditory delays on stuttering frequency at two speech rates. (Reprinted from Kalinowsk, J., Stuart, A., Sark, S., & Armson, J., [1996]. Stuttering amelioration at various auditory feedback delays and speech rates. *European Journal of Disorders in Communication, 31,* 259–269, with permission from Taylor and Francis [http://www.tandf.co.uk]).

3 weeks of therapy post-therapeutic speech showed a difference in displacement amplitude, peak velocity, voice onset tine, and vowel durations relative to its pretherapeutic counterpart (Mallard & Kelley, 1982; Mallard & Westbrook, 1985; Metz, Onufrak, & Ogburn, 1979; Metz, Samar, & Sacco, 1983; Onufrak, 1980; Ramig, 1984; Robb, Lybolt, & Price, 1985; Samar, Metz, & Sacco, 1986; Shenker & Finn, 1985; Story, 1990). These findings were simply artifacts of the motor techniques being used. Perceptually fluent pretherapeutic speech may be more natural sounding (Franken, Boves, Peters, & Webster, 1992; Kalinowski, Noble, Armson, & Stuart, 1994) even though it may also contain subperceptual stuttering. Post-therapeutic speech is perceptually, acoustically, and kinematically different from the fluent speech of nonstutterers. Regardless, we are comparing apples to oranges as they are different speech entities and, therefore, we can never identify a motor strategy responsible for stuttering inhibition. In contrast, if stuttering can be inhibited via an auditory speech signal at a relatively increased speech rate, it seems likely that prolongation is *not* necessary for stuttering inhibition. Simply put, at least one truly inhibitory agent must be the auditory second speech signal itself.

More recent research has also suggested that there are direct neural connections between phonation and audition that allow our auditory systems to "kick in" much faster when we begin to speak, so that sound does not have to travel from our vocal tract to our ears for us to feel its presence in the auditory cortex. It has been speculated that this direct phonation-audition connection may help the brain know what gestural information is forthcoming. This priming or the ability of the brain to predict the future has been called an "efferent copy" (Hari, Levanen, & Raij, 2000), and a compromise in this mechanism has even been associated with the central stuttering block (Curio, Neuloh, Numminen, Jousmaki, & Hari, 2000). If this is the case, then the use of DAF or other second speech signals appears to recruit mirror neurons to help restore the brain's ability to prime the neural pipeline for the production of fluent speech, which is the inhibition of stuttering. It is this process that probably explains why most stuttering occurs on the initial syllables, before speech is self-primed and the mirror neurons can become engaged. That is why we attempt to inhibit stuttering as quickly as possible and maintain the source of inhibition. If we can start speech fluently, we may be able to continue fluently. If we begin to stutter, we may need to produce more stuttering. The adage that fluency begets fluency and stuttering begets stuttering seems true. Thus, in our attempt to make increasingly more potent sources of inhibition, we have implemented second speech signals designed to inhibit stuttering prior to speech initiation. The exogenous and endogenous forms of these signals are discussed in the next section.

With regard to the induction of stuttering in normal speakers using DAF, Stuart, Kalinowski, Rastatter and Lynch (2002) found that normal speech patterns were only very mildly disrupted at both normal and fast rates until delays reached 200 ms. It was only at this longer delay that speech disruptions were more pronounced. This was attributed to the fact that recognition of running speech seems to be possible only following at least 200 ms after production (Marsen-Wilson & Tyler, 1981, 1983) so that peripheral feedback mechanisms could impact central speech production. Furthermore, distinct differences exist between the speech disruptions of nonstutterers and stutterers. Whereas stuttered speech disruptions are characterized by part-word repetitions, prolongations, and postural fixations, speech disruptions of normally fluent speakers under DAF seem to be characterized by misarticulations, hesitations, and slurred syllables. These findings seem to suggest that the disfluencies produced by normal speakers under DAF are poor analogs of stuttering (Stuart et al., 2002). They may be slightly disfluent, but normally fluent people under DAF do not suffer from multiple repetitions, long prolongations, silent blocking for extended periods, head jerks, fist pounding, fear of sounds or words, struggle, avoidance, or expectancy characteristics of those who truly stutter. In other words, people who do not stutter cannot be made to stutter by altering auditory feedback. As Wendell Johnson also discovered, aside from neurogenic (caused by trauma to the brain) and a few psychogenic (generally spontaneously occurring following an emotional trauma) cases of stuttering, we cannot create this pathology in those who are not so predisposed simply by exposing them to auditory stimuli.

## Frequency Altered Feedback

While under DAF, a person's voice is perceived with a slight delay. FAF on the other hand, creates a perceived change in the pitch of one's own voice (Howell, El-Yaniv, & Powell, 1987; Kalinowski et al., 1993). The pitch change can be either up or down relative to one's own speaking voice. From our clinical trials and teaching classes of student clinicians about the effects of DAF and FAF on stuttering, we have observed that the first time anyone experiences FAF they are often amused or bewildered when they hear their frequency-shifted voice. When the frequency shift is in the negative direction and people hear their voice with a lower pitch, they often say that they sound like "Darth Vader" of *Star Wars* fame. Conversely, when the frequency is shifted upward, in a positive direction and people hear their own voice with a higher pitch, it has been described as sounding like Mickey Mouse or a chipmunk. However, more importantly, when people who stutter speak under FAF, they have described it as sounding as if someone was speaking in unison along with them, begging the comparison to choral speech. (Hargrave, Kalinowski, Stuart, Armson, & Jones, 1994).

Unlike DAF that previously could be created via the delayed playback of magnetic analog recordings, FAF was not technologically available until sounds could be recorded digitally and then changed via digital signal processing. For this reason, investigation into the effects of FAF on stuttering did not begin until 1987 when Howell, El Yaniv, and Powell (1987) reported a series of experiments that investigated the effects of FAF relative to DAF and masking (high intensity white noise—to be discussed) on stuttering frequency. They found all three conditions to be inhibitory to stuttering, but found FAF to be the most powerful stuttering inhibitor of the three, followed by DAF, and then masking. Howell and colleagues tended to view FAF as simply another feedback condition to be used for achieving attendant motor consequences (e.g., prolonged speech) thought necessary to reduce stuttering under the reigning behavioral paradigm (Howell, 1990). In contrast, Kalinowski et al. (1993) also found all three altered feedback conditions to be inhibitory to stuttering but found DAF and FAF to be especially powerful. No statistical difference in stuttering inhibition was found between the DAF and FAF conditions, suggesting that FAF and DAF may be almost equally potent stuttering inhibitors (72–87%). These investigators also found FAF to be effective at fast rates of speech. Furthermore, Hargrave et al. (1994) found that the direction or magnitude of the frequency shift does not have a significant bearing on the levels of derived stuttering inhibition (i.e., all shifts induced approximately 80% stuttering inhibition). That is, frequencies could be shifted either up or down, either half an octave or a full octave, and the degree of stuttering inhibition was stable (Hargrave et al., 1994; Stuart et al., 1996) (see Figure 6–3).

Based on our current research, and clinical observations using FAF, we now believe that FAF would remain a powerful fluency enhancer even if the limits of intelligibility of the frequency-shifted voice are pushed to the edge. FAF has been found to be

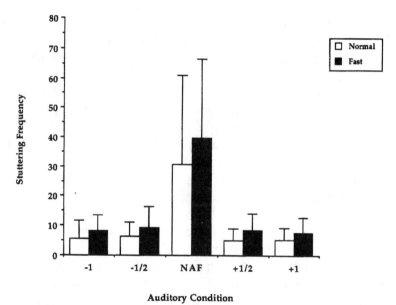

FIGURE 1. Mean stuttering frequencies as a function of auditory and speech rate conditions (*n* = 14). Error bars represent plus one standard deviation.

**Figure 6–3.** Mean stuttering frequency as a function of auditory and speech rate conditions. Error bars represent plus one standard deviation. (From Hargrave, S., Kalinowski, J., Stuart, A., Armson, J., & Jones, K. [1994]. Stuttering reduction under frequency-altered feedback at two speech rates. *Journal of Speech and Hearing Research, 37,* 1313–1320. Reprinted by permission from the American Speech and Hearing Association.)

an effective stuttering inhibitor (e.g., 70–90%) in situations that are generally the most difficult for most people who stutter, such as speaking in front of audiences of 2, 4, and 15 people (Armson, Foote, Witt, Kalinowski, & Stuart, 1997) or when making 200-syllable scripted telephone calls to businesses (Zimmerman, Kalinowski, Stuart, & Rastatter, 1997), suggesting to us, that it is truly a powerful emulator of choral speech.

## DAF and FAF Combinations

DAF and FAF act on different parameters of speech. DAF alters the perception of one's own voice in the temporal domain, while FAF makes changes in pitch perception. With digital signal processing, these changes can be made independently or in combination. Logically it makes sense that in combination, these effects of DAF and FAF on stuttering frequency would be more powerful than if either effect were independently presented, as it may be argued that they create a more powerful illusion of the second speaker. However, to the best of our knowledge, only two studies exist that examine the additive effects of DAF/FAF combination on stuttering frequency. Surprisingly, Macleod, Kalinowski, Stuart, and Armson (1995) found that while both DAF and FAF significantly inhibited stuttering, the combination of the two did not provide any significant further reduction. However, this may be attributed to a "floor effect," meaning there was little room for improvement relative to using either feedback condition independently. To tease out the additive effects, they suggested using more severe stutterers who would not demonstrate optimal fluency enhancement using each feedback condition independently. In addition, the measures of stuttering were taken from reading tasks, which for many people who stutter are not as challenging as spontaneous conversation tasks, speaking on the telephone, or to an audience. Therefore, we would also suggest changing the task to create higher baseline levels of stuttering and more room for improvement. By doing this we may be able to observe an increased effect of combining the two forms of altered auditory feedback. A combination of effects reportedly is usually what most people prefer to help them through silent blocks when using these portable devices.

Based on all the data supporting the use of altered auditory feedback to inhibit stuttering, many of our group's early publications included statements regarding the necessity of "all-in-the-ear" inconspicuous altered auditory feedback devices for functional, everyday stuttering inhibition. Upon arriving at East Carolina University, the author (JK), in collaboration with Andrew Stuart, searched the country, contacting hearing aid companies and engineering departments in major universities for someone to produce such a device. For about six years their requests were unanswered. Then, in February 2001, Dr. Stuart made a trip to Chengdu, China on a teaching endeavor. There, one of his Chinese colleagues at Micro-DSP knew of our work and suggested that his company's innovative and creative engineers might be able develop our patented design of an "all-in-the-ear" device. One month later the first prototype was shipped to the United States. What followed has dramatically altered the view of stuttering treatment across the country and more than likely will have a similar effect across the globe.

The advent of the SpeechEasy™ device in July 2001 opened a new, viable, and exciting therapeutic avenue for people who stutter. In this therapeutic modality the primary goal was to ensure that the second speech signal was presented in a relatively inconspicuous device that could allow the person who stutters to minimize the notice brought to the disorder or any supportive device. The SpeechEasy™ device is currently available in three models: behind-the-ear (BTE), in-the-canal (ITC), and completely-in-the-canal (CIC). Figure 6–4 shows these three devices.

Interestingly, the behind-the-ear (BTE) device is not usually a good seller as per our limited knowledge of early sales, because of its conspicuous nature. The same type of sales patterns is true in the hearing aid industry with the high-end in-the-canal (ITC), and completely-in-the-canal (CIC) aids comprising the vast majority of sales. The current version of the SpeechEasy™ is capable of producing frequency shifts (FAF) up to 2000 Hz, both up or down, in increments of 500 Hz and is capable of producing temporal delays (DAF) of up to 220 ms. These DAF and FAF shifts can be applied individually

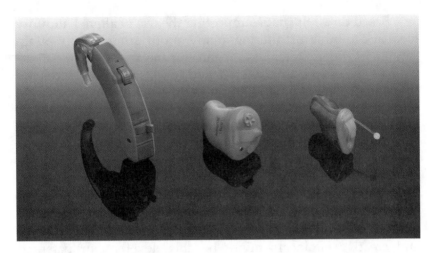

**Figure 6–4.** Three SpeechEasy™ models. From left to right: behind-the-ear (BTE), in-the-canal (ITC), and completely-in-the-canal (CIC).

or simultaneously to provide a wide range of combinations of effects. For a full description of this device see Stuart et al. (2003). Most users of the SpeechEasy™ report the most significant benefits when using combinations of DAF and FAF, especially during silent blocks. Stuart, Kalinowski, Rastatter, Saltuklaroglu, and Dayalu (2004) reported a recent efficacy study that followed eight SpeechEasy™ users over 4 months. Initial findings showed that by using both DAF and FAF, participants showed approximately 85% stuttering reduction in reading and 80% reduction of stuttering in conversation, while following a simple protocol constructed by the authors. The protocol advised some users to intermittently prolong vowels, a time-tested technique of behaviorists, to help engage mirror neurons to ensure that the signal would engage via silent periods and create sufficient inhibition. Follow-up data were collected on these clients after 4 months (Stuart et al., 2004) and after one year (Stuart et al., in press). At both extended testing intervals, the clients continued to speak with similar high levels of fluency as in the initial fitting when they wore the device. When the device was not worn, their levels of stuttering regressed, suggesting that this treatment method is not curative in nature and, aside from anecdotal reports of carryover fluency, stuttering returns when the device is removed.

Long-term use of altered feedback and techniques examining the plasticity of the brain need to be studied, especially in the youngest of those who stutter. Also of considerable importance in these efficacy studies were the levels of naturalness attained. Naïve listeners rated the speech of the users to be significantly more natural sounding when stuttering was inhibited using the SpeechEasy™ than when speaking without it. This is in contrast to ratings achieved by Kalinowski et al. (1994) that post-therapeutic speech after traditional therapies, although relatively free from overt stuttering, is considerably less natural sounding than its pretherapeutic counterparts. Perhaps of most importance were ratings on the Perceptions of Stuttering Inventory (PSI). After 1 year of continued SpeechEasy™ use, participants in the efficacy study reported significantly lower levels of struggle, avoidance, and expectancy associated with stuttering. These data suggest that using the SpeechEasy™ device helped reduce covert stuttering behaviors as well as the overt behaviors and is truly having a positive impact on people's lives. To further these notions, a "self-report" efficacy study was conducted (Kalinowski, Guntupalli, Stuart, & Saltuklaroglu, 2004), in which 105 participants who had been using the SpeechEasy™ device for at least 6 months reported improvements on the following speech related parameters: overall stuttering frequency, use of avoidances, speech naturalness, stuttering on the telephone, frequency of telephone use, and stuttering in conversation (see Figure 6–5).

They also reported an overall high satisfaction level with the SpeechEasy™ device. It should be noted that the device is no cureall still has limitations (discussed in the next chapter with ideas on how to compensate for these limitations). However, for those that it helps, the effects are dramatic and powerful. This tells us much about the nature and amelioration of the disorder of stuttering. The SpeechEasy™ device is worn monaurally (in one ear) so as not to interfere with everyday listening tasks. Before recommendations for a monaural device were made, testing was conducted to see whether the effects of altered auditory feedback were diminished if the effects were presented either

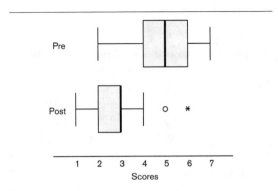

Box plots showing the pre and post ratings of overall stuttering
frequency on a seven-point rating scale.

**A.**

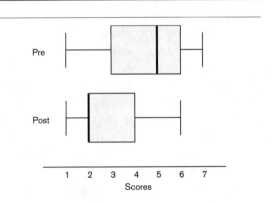

Box plots showing the pre and post ratings of overall use of avoidances
on a seven-point rating scale.

**B.**

**Figure 6–5.** Box plots showing reported improvements on a 7-point
scale (lower numbers indicate a more positive response) across 5 speaking parameters by 105 SpeechEasy™ users after at least 6 months of
use. (Reprinted from Kalinowski, J., Guntupalli, V., Stuart, A., & Saltuklaroglu, T., Self-reported efficacy of an ear-level prosthetic device that
delivers altered auditory feedback for the management of stuttering.
*International Journal of Rehabilitation Research, 27*, 167–170. with permission from Lippincott Williams & Wilkins [2004].) *(continues)*

monaurally or binaurally (in both ears). Although the monaural
presentation was not quite as powerful as the binaural presentation for stuttering inhibition, it still produced robust reductions
in stuttering frequency (Stuart, Kalinowski, & Rastatter, 1997).

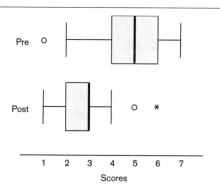

Box plots showing the pre and post ratings of speech naturalness on a seven-point rating scale.

**C.**

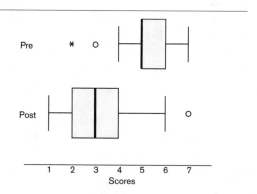

Box plots showing the pre and post ratings of frequency of stuttering over the telephone on a seven-point rating scale.

**D.**

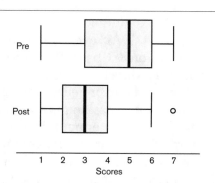

Box plots showing the pre and post ratings of frequency of telephone usage on a seven-point rating scale.

**E.**

## Figure 6–5. *(continued)*

## Masked Auditory Feedback

We cannot leave the topic of altered auditory feedback without discussing the use of masking noise to inhibit stuttering. Masking noise is "hissing" or "white" noise similar to that produced when your radio or television is not tuned properly. It is a crude, nongestural form of altered auditory feedback that needs to be presented at high intensities (e.g., 90 dB) to "drown out" or ablate the normal airborne feedback produced from one's own speech. Masking noise has been used to inhibit stuttering for several decades (Cherry & Sayers, 1956; Maraist & Hutton, 1957; Shane, 1955; Van Riper, 1965), and has repeatedly proven to reduce stuttering frequency though to a lesser extent than DAF and FAF in experimental conditions. Before portable versions of DAF and FAF were available, the Edinburgh masker became a fairly popular means of providing altered auditory feedback for everyday use. To the best of our knowledge, only one documented study exists regarding the long-term effects of AAF in the amelioration of stuttering, that conducted using the Edinburgh Masker. Dewar, Dewar, Austin, & Brash (1979) found that 82% of long-term users reported continued "considerable" or "great" benefit from the masker, despite its suboptimal fluency enhancing capacities, its bulky conspicuous nature, and the discomfort provided by high-intensity masking noise required to "drown out" one's own speech.

Although masking has proven to inhibit stuttering (Cherry & Sayers, 1956; Maraist & Hutton, 1957; Murray, 1969; Shane, 1955; VanRiper, 1965; Yairi, 1976), even when presented intermittently (Murray, 1969; Sutton & Chase, 1961; Webster & Dorman, 1970) its effects cannot be directly attributed to the inducement of gestural redundancy and mirror neuron engagement. Relative to the use of gestural stimuli, masking is a less efficient and less effective means of reducing stuttering. It is less efficient as high intensities are required thus making it almost impossible to hear one's own speech while listening to the masking, and making it almost impossible to hear any other external sounds. The portable masker needed to be turned on and off to allow the speaker to hear the other person speaking. That is why portable masking devices have never caught on, as they depend on this manual restart of the masking signal throughout conversations. It is less effective as it generally does not inhibit stuttering to the same extent as gestural stimuli. No one is quite sure how masking operates to inhibit stuttering. Bloodstein (1995, p. 347) claims that it is a distracter, along with anything else that reduces stuttering. We are of the impression that by taking a "shotgun" approach to the entire auditory/neural system, the neural stuttering block can be circumvented. However, using masking, this type of neural reorganization is accomplished in a highly inefficient and ineffective manner. Such inhibition can be accomplished just as easily with a 50 ms temporal delay. It also may be possible that when people are unable to hear their own speech because of the intensity of masking, they may make some motoric compensations that may possibly derive a Lombard effect or other kinesthetic or proprioceptive feedback that slightly alters the manner of speaking and endogenously contributes to the enhanced levels of fluency.

## Endogenous Second Speech Signals: The Importance of Vowels

Our third type of second speech signal for stuttering inhibition is endogenous, or one that is self-generated by the person who stutters. At first, this may sound somewhat like a misnomer. How can the person who stutters create his own second speech signal to help him overcome the central stuttering block? The object of a second speech signal is to create gestural redundancy so as to allow the mirror system to engage stuttering inhibition (Kalinowski, Saltuklaroglu, et al., 2004; Saltuklaroglu et al., 2003; Saltuklaroglu, Kalinowski, & Guntupalli, 2004). In the absence of an exogenous second speech signal, people who stutter must resort to using their own speech system to derive gestural redundancy. The importance of vocalic gestural information for stuttering inhibition was revealed to us in our exogenous second speech signal studies, whereby vocalic second (e.g., continuous /a/, vowel trains) speech signals had almost twice the inhibitory power of nonvocalic signals (e.g., continuous /s/, voiceless fricative trains) (Kalinowski, Dayalu, et al., 2000). The same concept applies to endogenous second speech signals, except in this case, the person who stutters generates a higher level of vocalic gestural information in speech relative to what would normally be generated. What seems imperative is keeping the neural pipeline from closing for long periods of time, and to do this endogenously, we must use vowels as endogenous sources of gestural energy for mirror neuron engagement. Van Riper saw the sanctity of the vowel when he suggested (1971) that "stutterers are likely to be conspicuously free of their disorder when doing nothing more than phonating (p. 291). Thus, the importance of vowels in stuttering inhibition is probably also related to the finding that voiceless consonants (especially fricatives) are stuttered more often than voiced sounds (Jayaram, 1983), as the production of voiced sounds is intrinsic to the inhibition of the pathology. In this section, we focus on how self-generated vocalic gestural redundancy can be achieved both voluntarily via therapy techniques and other motoric speech manipula-tions, and involuntarily via the production of overt stuttering behaviors. As you read this section, you will notice how closely some forms of pseudostuttering can resemble incipient invol-untary syllabic repetitions and how therapeutically induced prolongations can resemble involuntary advanced stuttering behaviors. The structures of all the motoric manipulations appear to be simply tied to their inhibitory characteristics and the relative amount of derived inhibition seems to be tied to the added vocalic content in the resultant speech output.

Endogenous second speech signals can be extremely powerful for stuttering inhibition. Not only can they induce the near-perfect levels of stuttering inhibition derived via choral speech and the attendant invulnerability to stuttering (e.g., via droning or singing), but they also allow the inhibition to carry-over beyond the time frame in which the gestural redundancy is generated. For example, in therapy, if someone uses vowel prolongations for a short period of time as a source of inhibition, they often stop using the prolongation and speak fluently and naturally for some time afterward. This carryover inhibition is of considerable importance for two reasons. First, it provides clues to the plasticity of the system, which is an essential part of future research, especially when trying to uncover the neurophysiology of recovery from stuttering. Second, endogenous second speech signals cannot be created without deviations from normal speech. In fact, the greater the deviation (i.e., increase in vocalic content), the greater the amount of inhibition that is derived and the more unnatural the speech sound (Saltuklaroglu, Kalinowski, & Guntupalli, 2004). Therefore, being able to access an endogenous mechanism that carries over and keeps the mirror system engaged for a period of time after its use is relinquished can help impart an added degree of naturalness in the resulting speech.

These therapeutic implications are discussed further in the next chapter with ideas on how to combine various second speech signals for optimal fluency and naturalness in the resultant speech. We are not the first to suggest this type of integration. However, we are probably the first to suggest that combining second speech signals merely taps into synergistic resources for creating gestural redundancy, mirror neuronal engagement, and stuttering inhibition.

## Incipient Syllabic Repetitions

Typically, the first signs of stuttering in children are the involuntary productions of tension-free, evenly spaced syllable repetitions, each of which contains a salient vocalic nucleus (Yairi & Ambrose, 1999; Zebrowski, 1995) of the initial syllable of words (e.g., "buh-buh-buh-balloon"). Although these disruptive speech behaviors present a source of concern to parents and speech pathologists, we believe that they are simply nature's first-generation second speech signal and an attempt to compensate for the neural block, remove the blockage from the speech pipeline, and put children's speech back on a fluent course. What is the evidence for this? Of primary importance are the natural recovery rates. With an 80% success rate irrespective of therapeutic intervention, Mother Nature offers a powerful healing balm to children who stutter. The repeating syllable nuclei can be inherently powerful in overcoming overt stuttering behaviors and promoting recovery, which appears to be why nature selected syllable repetitions as the incipient form of self-shadowed endogenous second speech signal. The vowel nuclei have the ability to convey gestural information making syllables the fundamental acoustic units of speech (Studdert-Kennedy, 2000). In other words, although at the neural level, the individual units of speech are gestures, aside from the production of voiceless fricatives (the least encoded of all speech sounds); most gestures cannot exist acoustically in units smaller than syllables. Therefore, these basic units may be the simplest forms of complete gestures that can be most easily processed by the phonetic module and fluently shadowed, making their structure "Mother Nature's" logical choice. Simply put, syllabic repetitions are the shortest speech forms that can be self-shadowed and seem to allow the quickest release from the involuntary neural block.

Unlike the other second speech signals that we have discussed so far, the production of syllabic repetitions typically occurs prior to the intended utterance. Incipient stutterers often produce syllabic repetitions on the initial syllable and then go on to speak the rest of the utterance fluently. Again, it is not surprising that we see most stuttering on the initial syllable (Brown, 1945), as subsequent blocks may be inhibited after producing syllabic repetitions. In contrast, the exogenous and endogenous-exogenous second speech signals operate "on-line," in conjunction with speech production. Thus, we observe the carryover stuttering inhibition from the initial syllable forward. We have conducted three studies investigating the inhibitory power of similar endogenous and exogenous second speech signals prior to speaking, each of which increased our understanding of endogenous inhibitory mechanisms.

## Producing and Perceiving the Vowel /a/ Prior to Speaking

First we investigated the effects on stuttering inhibition of both producing and perceiving a continuous vowel /a/ prior to speaking (Dayalu et al., 2001). Four experimental conditions were created in which participants either listened to or produced a four-second /a/, either immediately prior to or four seconds prior to speaking. Relative to a control condition of reading text normally, the only condition that showed any significant inhibitory effect was producing the four-second /a/ immediately prior to speaking, which produced about 30% inhibition. This was not as strong as those previously found when using exogenous or endogenous-exogenous second speech signals, which typically ranged from 60 to 80% inhibition. However, it was achieved prior to speaking and this relatively low yet significant level of stuttering inhibition provided initial clues as to how endogenous mechanisms could be used to maintain speech flow through the neural pipeline and how other vowel concentrated techniques such as gentle onsets, continuous phonation, and light articulatory contacts could allow the neural pipeline to stay open. This experiment also showed that endogenous second speech signals are characterized by temporal and linguistic flexibility. However, it also taught us some limitations. The inhibition derived via producing an /a/ prior to speaking was less than typical. In addition, it did not carry over more than 4 seconds and the vowel /a/ was not effective in its passive perceived form prior to speaking. Considering that syllabic repetitions are produced prior to an intended utterance and are so powerful in remitting the pathology in children, we suspected that we could create endogenous second speech signals that better emulated this powerful self-shadowing effect.

## Pseudostuttering

The next form of endogenous second speech signal that we examined was pseudo- or artificial stuttering. Pseudostuttering is wonderful to study because of its history of useful application in the protocols of pioneers (e.g., Johnson, Van Riper, & Sheehan). Its ameliorative effects were usually attributed to reducing the covert fear associated with stuttering or in desensitizing people to their stuttering. However, this "fear reduction" hypothesis was not tested rigorously even though early studies (e.g., Fishman, 1937; Meissner, 1946) had shown that pseudostuttering (using syllabic repetitions) could produce dramatic reductions in stuttering. Automatically it was assumed that fear could be a causal agent for stuttering events, or at least a source of exacerbation, which formed the basis of Johnson's (bouncing) and Van Riper's (desensitization) pseudostuttering therapeutic regimes. Nobody thought to test the power of pseudostuttering for reducing true stuttering when fear levels were thought to be reduced or elevated. Even so, the available physiological data do not seem to support a direct link between a reduction in fear and increased fluency levels. Autonomic responses that are often associated with fear (e.g., skin conductance, heart rate and pulse) have not been known to increase in people who stutter under normal speaking conditions (Janssen & Kraaimaat, 1980; Peters & Hulstijn, 1984), nor decrease under conditions that are associated with stuttering inhibition (Adams & Moore, 1972; Gray & Brutten, 1965; Reed & Lingwall, 1976,1980; Ritterman & Reidenbach, 1975). Furthermore, significant differences have not been found in self-reported levels of anxiety between stuttering and nonstuttering groups (Blood, Blood, Bennett, Simpson, & Susman, 1994; Kraamaat, Janssen, & van Dam-Baggen, 1991). Although methodologies for collecting physiological data are imperfect, we suspected that pseudostuttering's powerful ameliorative effects could not be accounted for only by fear reduction, but were probably also due to the creation of gestural redundancy.

These notions about pseudostuttering coupled with our already established notions of a gestural perception-production link and an observation made by the second author (TS) led to another series of experiments. In the fall of 2000, the SpeechEasy™ had not yet come to fruition and the first author (JK) was stuttering quite severely at times. The second author noticed that in their discussions, he seemed to become much more fluent when listening to these gestural conflagrations. This experiential stuttering inhibition is difficult to explain but happens all the time to those of us who stutter. It is a pronounced shift in stuttering levels. This shift occurred by simply listening to the severe stuttering produced by the first author. Thus, the second author demonstrated a shift in levels in stuttering levels that was "passively" induced (i.e., via perception). When he reported to the first author, the first author confirmed that he had also experienced a similar shift when speaking with those stuttering more severely than himself. That experience and confirmation tells us something about the experiential nature of stuttering and the strong perception and production link. It was as if simply seeing and hearing strong overt repetitions and prolongations being produced by the first author inhibited stuttering in the second author and allowed him to speak more fluently. If overt stuttering was the peripheral solution or release mechanism for the central stuttering block, then it may be possible that the perception-production link may to some extent allow one person to stutter so another person does not have to. Thus, we created an experiment with four conditions in which participants actively produced (via shadowing) or passively watched and listened to either pseudostuttered (using syllable repetitions) or fluent speech prior to producing target utterances (Saltuklaroglu, Kalinowski, Dayalu, Stuart, & Rastatter, 2004). We found that both the active production tasks prior to speaking resulted in approximately 40% stuttering inhibition, which was not surprising as the neural speech pipeline in the target utterances probably remained somewhat open, as with stuttering inhibition carrying over from the fluent shadowing of the stimuli. The interesting finding, however, was that simply listening to pseudostuttered speech prior to speaking also resulted in the same significant degree of inhibition. This seemed to be evidence of overt stuttering behaviors in one person producing gestural redundancy for the other person. In other words, the speech perception-production link seemed to again be employed to inhibit stuttering via mirror neuronal engagement. Not surprisingly, listening to fluent speech before speaking did not have a significant inhibitory effect, as without the pseudostuttered syllabic repetitions it did not contain the high levels of gestural redundancy necessary to inhibit stuttering prior to speaking.

These two experiments that yielded approximately 30% and 40% levels of stuttering inhibition provided valuable information, yet they did not reach the same levels of inhibition reported in the two early studies. We suspected that the possible difference might be in the nature of the stimuli used. In our experiments we had used continuous vowels and connected pseudostuttered speech as our primary stimuli. If syllable repetitions were Mother Nature's answer then we thought it would be appropriate to conduct another experiment that examined the inhibitory powers of elementary syllables, again both in passive perception and active production tasks (Saltuklaroglu, Kalinowski, Dayalu, et al., 2004). This time we constructed syllabic stimuli that were either matched or unmatched to the intended utterance. Rather than shadowing connected speech, participants were required only to shadow elementary syllables consisting of a vocalic nucleus, with the repeating vocalic nuclei providing high levels of endogenous stuttering inhibition. The levels of inhibition derived were substantially powerful when any configuration of syllabic repetitions was produced prior to speaking. Even when simply perceived prior to speaking, syllables matched to the intended utterance could produce high levels of inhibition. The observed endogenous flexibility for accommodating different gestural configurations (as long as the vowel nucleus was present) may provide clues to how the pathology can progress to other forms as the system attempts to provide more powerful inhibitory sources when syllabic repetitions fail to remit.

## Involuntary Prolongations

If the involuntary production of syllabic repetitions can be a source of release from a neural stuttering block, then it also follows that the involuntary production of gestural prolongations, which are also core stuttering behaviors, can also act as endogenous sources of block release. Prolongations may be even more powerful sources of release than syllabic repetitions. Syllable repetitions have transitory vocalic energy bursts and are produced before an utterance, whereas prolongations are extended vocalic gestures with high levels of continuous acoustic vowel energy that are present during speech production. Therefore, the higher levels of acoustic energy combined with the better temporal synchronization of the release mechanism to the block makes for a more potent stuttering inhibitor. This is probably why most contemporary behavioral therapy procedures are controlled emulations of involuntary prolongations, (e.g., Van Riper, Sheehan, rate control) rather than repetitions (e.g., Johnsonian bounce). It should be noted, however, that as prolongations become more potent sources of release, with increasing duration and intensity, they also become more conspicuous in nature.

If we examine the production of gestural prolongations with reference to the progression of stuttering, we can begin to see how the need for more potent endogenous inhibitory sources arises. Syllabic repetitions do not appear to be powerful enough to completely remit stuttering in about 20% of incipient stutterers. In this unremitted population, syllabic repetitions may continue to provide some temporary sources of release, yet the natural tendency of the system seems to make it want to seek out other more potent endogenous forms of inhibition. Hence, involuntary gestural prolongations start to emerge that contain more acoustic energy and gestural redundancy in portions of the intended utterance. Though perceived to be more severe forms of the disorder. They may provide increasingly powerful means of releasing neural blocks to keep the neural speech pipeline open.

## Prolongation and Other Behavioral Techniques

Prolongation, gentle onsets, continuous phonation, airflow techniques, and anything else we can do to manipulate the gestural output via changes in vowel energy create an endogenous second speech signal. Every "motoric" technique produces deviation (i.e., vocalic distortion) in the way one perceives the gestural output. It is the relative amount of distortion that creates the endogenous second speech signal. In other words, the saliency of the second speech signal is found in its increase in vocalic energy and the relative lack of speech naturalness. For example, if someone is using prolongation at a rate of a syllable per second, the endogenous second speech signal is found in the droned nature of the speech. This is simply the voluntary and controlled counterpart to a long involuntary struggle-filled prolongation. However, from a functional systemic viewpoint, the goal of achieving gestural redundancy is the same.

As discussed in chapter 3, motoric techniques do not compensate for some flaw in the speech motor periphery. Instead they seem to be just another means of engaging mirror systems and inhibiting stuttering. This seems logical, as the use of any technique is really an imitative process, continually striving to replicate acoustic and kinesthetic sensations associated with a speech "target." In this case, the imitative behavior seems to initiate the mirror neuron engagement, which is then probably maintained via priming of the auditory cortices (i.e., efferent copies). One technique that may be especially effective for this purpose is the use of "gentle onsets," which are small amplitude envelopes that grow in size, providing vocalic gestures as the most appropriate corkscrew to keep the neural pipeline open. This method of speech initiation provides an immediate and powerful source of stuttering inhibition that often has the potential to carry over into the remainder of the utterance, especially if the motor machinations are greatly exaggerated. Thus, vowel prolongation via starched speech, gentle onsets, light articulatory contacts, and continuous phonation all help maintain mirror neuron engagement and keep the speech pipeline open. Yet, any time an endogenous method is used, speech naturalness seems to be compromised. It is most likely because of this that stuttering begins to return when trying to make therapeutic speech sound more natural. Simply put, when we make speech sound more natural, we are removing a portion of the endogenous second speech signal.

The creation of endogenous second speech signals via the use of therapy techniques has proven to be a powerful method of inhibiting stuttering. Much like using choral speech, when speech is droned at prolongation rates of one syllable per second or slower, it is almost impossible to stutter. At these slow rates, the sense of invulnerability to stuttering can be almost as powerful as the one derived from choral speech. This may be expected as the same mirror neuron mechanism appears to be engaged to keep the speech pipeline open, and probably to similar extents. Yet the use of endogenous methods is fundamentally constrained by the extended effort and compromises to speech naturalness that are required to use them. When a person who stutters is required to generate his or her own second speech signal, the very goal of creating the illusion of a second speaker forces the resultant speech product to be conspicuous and unnatural.

Besides being high in vocalic content, another reason that endogenous prolongations are powerful is because, similar to choral speech, they inhibit stuttering while the intended target speech utterances are being produced. This differs from the production of syllabic repetitions and the endogenous second speech signals described in the experiments above, whereby the stuttering inhibition is generally derived prior to producing the speech targets, and it had to carry over into the target utterances. Therefore, if the inhibition is derived during speech production, it can be more closely synchronized to when neural blocks occur, making it a more powerful source of stuttering inhibition, especially for more severe cases. Thus, the temporal relationship between the source of inhibition and the possible occurrence of the involuntary block also may help explain how stuttering begins to progress in children who are not spontaneously remitted by the early production of syllabic repetitions. As the pathology becomes stronger, they may need more powerful sources of inhibition that are more temporally aligned to the occurrences of stuttering blocks.

Most people who stutter have little difficulty singing fluently (Andrews, Craig, Feyer, Hoddinott, & Nelson, 1983; Bloodstein, 1950; Johnson & Rosen, 1937; Reid, 1946). Perhaps the most famous case is country music crooner Mel Tillis, who was known to be quite a severe stutterer, but never had any difficulty singing to audiences of millions on television. Over the years numerous explanations have been offered for this powerful effect. Wingate (1969) suggested that it may be due to altered vocalization, a notion that has also been supported by Colcord and Adams (1979), who found increased durations of voiced segments while singing. Others (e.g., Starkweather, 1982) have suggested that it may be due to the imposed rhythm that singing naturally induces. Healey, Mallard, & Adams (1976) attributed the effects of singing to a combination of altered vocalization and familiarity with the lyrics. Similarly, Andrews, Craig, Feyer, Hoddinott, and Nelson (1983) suggested that the effects of singing may be caused by the reduced linguistic demands, which they also used to explain the effects of choral and shadowed speech.

To further investigate the effects of singing on stuttering frequency, Glover, Kalinowski, Rastatter, and Stuart (1996) asked stuttering participants to sing passages at both normal and fast rates of speech. No imposed melody was provided and the participants were unfamiliar with the passages. Compared to control conditions, in which the participants read the passages normally at slow and fast rates, stuttering was reduced by about 75% in both singing conditions. These results showed that for singing to effectively reduce stuttering, it was not necessary for participants to know the lyrics, nor was it necessary for them to use a preimposed melody or use a specific rate so as to volitionally extend voiced segments. All that was necessary was the instruction to sing. The authors suggested that singing may "involve alternate neural pathways or activate interactions among neuromechanisms that govern fluency" (p. 520). According to our current understanding, this may be the mirror neuron system. The simple act of being asked to sing creates a significant deviation from normal speech, as the speech produced is easily identified as singing rather than speaking. Therefore, a self-imposed melody is sufficient for mirror neuronal engagement and stuttering inhibition. Singing makes use of continuous phonation (i.e., high vocalic gestural content) that is systematically manipulated to achieve the desired melody. This seems imperative in preventing the neural pipleline from closing for long periods of time.

## Whispering and Foreign Accents

Whispering and the purposeful use of foreign accents are the last two types of endogenous second speech signals that we discuss. Both of these motoric manipulations have been reported to reduce the frequency of stuttering (Bloodstein, 1950). In the case of whispering, documented empirical support also exists for its powerful inhibitory effects (Perkins, Rudas, Johnson, & Bell, 1976). These authors interpreted their findings as evidence that stuttering was related to breakdown in the coordination between phonation, articulation, and respiration. They saw whispering, which eliminated the phonatory task, as a means of facilitating the coordination between the speech subsystems and, hence, reducing stuttering. Findings such as these also contributed to the notion that the source of stuttering was in the larynx (see chapter 3). As a final word on this matter, if stuttering truly originated in the larynx, then there should be no stuttering in anyone who has undergone a laryngectomy. Even though these cases are rare and can be difficult to identify, there has been evidence to support occurrences of stuttering in laryngectomy patients (e.g., Bachman, 1980). From Thomas Kuhn's (1962) paradigmatic standpoint, these findings are overwhelming anomalies that cannot be explained by those who have viewed stuttering as a laryngeal disorder, and call for a re-examination of the evidence.

Many people who stutter (including the author [TS]) have reportedly implemented foreign accents to hide or reduce their stuttering. We have even heard about cases of people who stutter adopting entirely new personas to accommodate different accents in an effort to reduce stuttering. Obviously, this can be exhausting, but in some ways it is no more exhausting than whispering all the time or maintaining the use of therapy techniques. The common element is that all these alternative speech forms require motoric deviations from normal speech. They allow the person who stutters to perceive his or her own speech differently, and, hence, create an endogenous second speech signal for gestural redundancy and stuttering inhibition.

## Nonspeech Signals and the Distraction Hypothesis

Bloodstein (1950) compiled a fairly extensive list of conditions that seem to reduce stuttering frequency to some extent, including speaking while dancing, speaking when in pain, and speaking when intoxicated. His textbook (Bloodstein, 1995), lists 192 studies that all seem to show some capacity for reducing stuttering. Thus, in an effort to make sense of the almost infinite number of conditions that reduce stuttering to some extent, Bloodstein created his "distraction hypothesis" (Bloodstein, 1995; 1999) which simply states that any condition that reduces stuttering, is simply a distracter. However, there are a number of problems with this theory. First, it is unscientific, calling for "post hoc" or "after the fact" analyses. That is, if a person stutters, it is assumed that they were not sufficiently distracted. If they do not stutter, they must have been distracted. from their stuttering. Is this not the same type of logic that Johnson used to explain his diagnosogenic theory?

In addition to the post hoc analysis, Bloodstein's distraction theory does a poor job in explaining the different levels of stuttering inhibition that can be achieved. This is where our gestural interpretation of stuttering inhibition has considerably stronger explanatory power. When we examine the range of sensory and motoric conditions that can inhibit stuttering while speaking, we note that, with the exception of masking noise which requires a person's own speech to be "drowned out," and highly compressed second signals that seem to exceed the phonetic module's limits for temporal resolution, conditions that have high gestural content are the ones that show the highest levels of stuttering inhibition. Presenting flashing lights or listening to pure tones while speaking are sensory inputs which by any standard can be considered "distracting." However, the levels of stuttering inhibition achieved are substantially lower, generally not exceeding

40 to 50%. It does not make sense to us that choral speech which induces 90 to 100% inhibition can be more distracting than listening to pure tones, which is how the distraction theory would explain differences in stuttering inhibition between these conditions.

However, even within our gestural frameworks, hierarchies of inhibition exist. When we use exogenous second speech signals, as a general rule, the more closely aligned the two speakers are with respect to time, linguistic content, and availability of gestural information, the more likely it is that gestures in a second speech signal can be recovered, culminating in the gold standard set by choral speech. When we use altered feedback, although all FAF signals appear about equal, optimal levels of DAF (50–75 ms), consistently produced about 70 to 85% inhibition.

When using endogenous second speech signals such as those created by prolongation, singing, and whispering the level of stuttering inhibition achieved seems to be proportional to the deviation from natural-sounding speech. Thus, of considerable importance in our studies are the differential effects that we have obtained. In every one of our experiments, the differential effects can be explained in terms of the availability of relevant and redundant speech gestures for extraction in the phonetic module and stuttering inhibition via mirror neuron engagement. Thus, we see this interpretation as being among the most parsimonious for explaining the bulk of data related to decreases in stuttering frequency.

## Synopsis

When stuttering is inhibited, the neural speech pipeline is kept open as mirror systems relay speech gestures back and forth between perception and production. Second speech signals can be used to meet this demand with their effectiveness increasing as they begin to most closely emulate a true auditory choral signal (see Table 6–1). The auditory modality is the most powerful for receiving gestural information and in all our auditory second speech signals, we observe a common thread in effective stuttering inhibition: the highlighting of vocalic gestures for mirror neuronal engagement.

**Table 6-1.** Summary second speech signal experiments conducted by the author (JK) and colleagues

| Second Speech Signal | Type | Levels of Stuttering Inhibition | Interpretation | Reference |
|---|---|---|---|---|
| Matched visual choral speech | Exogenous | ~80% | Stuttering inhibition is gestural in nature. | Kalinowski, Stuart, Rastatter, Snyder, & Dayalu, 2000 |
| Stutter-free, stutter-filled, continuous, and intermittent speech, continuous vowels, vowel trains, continuous consonants, consonant trains | Exogenous | 61–78% from voiced signals, ~30–50% from voiceless signals. | • Linguistic match is not necessary.<br>• Choral speech phenomenon is temporally and linguistically flexible.<br>• Complete gestures (source and filter information) are most powerful for stuttering inhibition. | Kalinowski, Stuart, Rastatter, Snyder, & Dayalu, 2000 |
| Matched and non-matched visual choral speech | Exogenous | 35–70% | • Linguistic match needed for visual signal<br>• Audition is probably a better gestural conduit for stuttering inhibition | Saltuklaroglu, Dayalu, Kalinowski, Stuart, & Rastatter, 2004 |
| Continuous and intermittent /a/ | Exogenous | 30–60%, decreasing with intermittency of the signal | Temporal window for inhibition via vowels is between 1 and 3 seconds. | Saltuklaroglu, Kalinowski, Dayalu, Guntupalli, Stuart, & Rastatter, 2003 |

*(continues)*

**Table 6–1.** (continued)

| Second Speech Signal | Type | Levels of Stuttering Inhibition | Interpretation | Reference |
|---|---|---|---|---|
| Forward and backward stutter-free and stutter-filled speech | Exogenous | ~65% via fluent forward, stuttered forward, stuttered backward | Speech has forward entropy, but gestural redundancy can be found in reversed stuttered forms. | Saltuklaroglu, Kalinowski, Dayalu, Stuart, & Rastatter, 2004 |
| Temporally compressed and expanded speech | Exogenous | ~60% using expanded signals and compression rates up to 20% | Compression rates of 40% and beyond exceed temporal resolution of phonetic module—before intelligibility is affected. | Guntupalli, Kalinowski, Saltuklaroglu, & Nanjundeswaran, 2005 |
| Singing | Endogenous | 75% when asked to sing, at both normal and fast rates | Singing is a powerful fluency-enhancing strategy that functions without reliance on any motoric strategy or altered auditory feedback. | Glover, Kalinowski, Rastatter, & Stuart, 1996 |
| Producing vowel /a/ prior to speaking | Endogenous | 30% when 4 sec. vowel immediately precedes speech, no significant inhibition when 4 sec. of silence separates vowel from speech | Stuttering inhibition via self-generated vowel production prior to speech is significant, but short-lived. | Dayalu, Saltuklaroglu, Kalinowski, Stuart, & Rastatter, 2001 |

| Second Speech Signal | Type | Levels of Stuttering Inhibition | Interpretation | Reference |
|---|---|---|---|---|
| Pseudostuttered and fluent speech, produced prior to speaking target utterance | Endogenous | 40% for both fluent speech and speech that was pseudostuttered | Seeing and hearing other people pseudostutter can have an inhibitory effect over true stuttering. | Satluklaroglu, Kalinowski, Dayalu, Stuart, & Rastatter, 2004 |
| | Exogenous | 40% for passive audiovisual presentation of pseuostuttered speech | | |
| DAF | Exogenous-endogenous | Increase in disfluencies for normally fluent speakers speaking under DAF at 200 ms only | DAF induces disfluencies that are poor analogs of stuttering. | Stuart, Kalinowski, Rastatter, & Lynch, 2002 |
| FAF alone, and DAF alone | Exogenous-endogenous | 72% for DAF and 87% for FAF, no significant effect of speaking rate<br><br>Both DAF and FAF were more powerful than masking | Rate of speech is not a factor in stuttering inhibition under altered feedback. | Kalinowski, Armson, Roland-Mieszkowski, Stuart, & Gracco, 1993 |
| FAF alone, and DAF alone | Exogenous-endogenous | 60% monoaural<br>75% binaural | Bilateral input is optimal, but monoaural input is also highly effective for stuttering inhibition. | Stuart, Kalinowski, & Rastatter, 1997 |

(continues)

**Table 6–1.** *(continued)*

| Second Speech Signal | Type | Levels of Stuttering Inhibition | Interpretation | Reference |
|---|---|---|---|---|
| FAF alone, and DAF alone | Exogenous-endogenous | Normal and fast rates with various delay: decrease in stuttering at both rates at all DAF settings. ~40–50% for 25 ms delay ~70% for 50 ms and 75 ms | 50–75 ms appears to be optimal delay for stuttering inhibition. Even delays as low as 25 ms are effective. | Kalinowski, Stuart, Sark, & Armson, 1996 |
| FAF alone, and DAF alone | Exogenous-endogenous | 80% with FAF conditions: + or – ¼, ½, or 1 octave | Direction of frequency shift does not matter. FAF is a permutation of choral speech. | Hargrave, Kalinowski, Stuart, Armson, & Jones, 1994 Stuart, Kalinowski, Armson, Stenstrom, & Jones, 1996 |
| FAF | Exogenous-endogenous | 74% | Like choral speech, FAF is effective in front of audiences of various sizes. | Armson, Foote, & Witt, Kalinowski, & Stuart, 1997 |
| FAF alone, and DAF alone | Exogenous-endogenous | 55% and 60% for the FAF and DAF | Altered feedback is effective on the telephone. | Zimmerman, Kalinowski, Stuart, & Rastatter, 1997 |

| Second Speech Signal | Type | Levels of Stuttering Inhibition | Interpretation | Reference |
|---|---|---|---|---|
| FAF | Exogenous-endogenous | 85% across monitoring conditions while experiencing FAF | Knowledge of monitoring did not impede effects of FAF. | Kalinowski, Stuart, Wamsley, & Rastatter, 1999 |
| Combination FAF and DAF | Exogenous-endogenous | ~80% for all three conditions: DAF alone, FAF alone, and combination DAF/FAF | Combining effects of DAF and FAF did not provide additional inhibition in reading task. | Macleod, Kalinowski, Stuart, & Armson, 1995 |
| In-the-ear device providing FAF and DAF (60 ms delay, +500 Hz) | Exogenous-endogenous | ~90% during reading ~67% during monologue<br><br>Speech is judged to be natural-sounding | SpeechEasy™ protocol is effective after four months of continued use. | Stuart, Kalinowski, Rastatter, Saltuklaroglu, & Dayalu, 2004 |
| In-the-ear device providing FAF and DAF (60 ms delay, +500 Hz) | Exogenous-endogenous | ~85% during reading ~75% during monologue<br><br>Speech is judged to be natural-sounding | SpeechEasy™ protocol is effective after one year of continued use. | Stuart, Kalinowski, Saltuklaroglu & Guntupalli, in press |
| Passive resonator | Exogenous-endogenous | 30% | Even talking into a simple hollow tube can create a second speech signal. | Stuart, Miller, Kalinowski, & Rastatter, 1997 |

273

In the next chapter, we begin to explore how best to combine and manipulate the various signals so that this vocalic highlighting can assume a form that is stutter-free and as natural sounding as possible.

# References

Adams, M. R., & Moore, W. H., Jr. (1972). The effects of auditory masking on the anxiety level, frequency of dysfluency, and selected vocal characteristics of stutterers. *Journal of Speech and Hearing Research, 15,* 572–578.

Andrews, G., Craig, A., Feyer, A., Hoddinott, P., & Nelson, M. (1983). Stuttering: A review of research findings and theories circa 1982. *Journal of Speech and Hearing Disorders, 45,* 287–307.

Andrews, G., Howie, P. M., Dozsa, M., & Guitar, B. E. (1982). Stuttering: Speech pattern characteristics under fluency-inducing conditions. *Journal of Speech and Hearing Research, 25,* 208–216.

Armson, J., Foote, S., Witt, C., Kalinowski, J., & Stuart, A. (1997). Effect of frequency altered feedback and audience size on stuttering. *European Journal of Disorders of Communication, 32,* 359–366.

Bachman, G. G. (1980). An investigation into the prevalence of stuttering among the laryngectomized. *Journal of Speech and Hearing Disorders, 45,* 564.

Blood, G. W., Blood, I. M., Bennett, S., Simpson, K. C., & Susman, E. J. (1994). Subjective anxiety measurements and cortisol responses in adults who stutter. *Journal of Speech and Hearing Research, 37,* 760–768.

Bloodstein, O. (1950). A rating scale study of conditions under which stuttering is reduced or absent. *Journal of Speech and Hearing Disorders, 15,* 29–36.

Bloodstein, O. (1995). *A handbook on stuttering* (5th ed.). San Diego, CA: Singular Publishing Group, Inc.

Bloodstein, O. (1999). Altered auditory feedback and stuttering: A postscript to Armson and Stuart. *Journal of Speech and Hearing Research, 42,* 910–914.

Borden, G. J. (1979). An interpretation of research on feedback interruption in speech. *Brain and Language, 7,* 307–319.

Bothe, A. K., Taylor, H. R., & Everett, J. (2003). Effects of visual choral speech on stuttering frequency. *Asha Leader, 8,* 150.

Brown, S. F. (1945). The loci of stutterings in the speech sequence. *Journal of Speech Disorders, 10,* 181–192.

Cherry, C., & Sayers, B. (1956). Experiments upon the total inhibition of stammering by external control and some clinical results. *Journal of Psychosomatic Research, 1*, 233–246.

Colcord, R. D., & Adams, M. R. (1979). Voicing duration and vocal SPL changes associated with stuttering reduction during singing. *Journal of Speech and Hearing Research, 22*, 468–479.

Costello-Ingham, J.C. (1993). Current status of stuttering and behavior modification—I: Recent trends in the application of behavior modification in children and adults. *Journal of Fluency Disorders, 18*, 27–55.

Curio, G., Neuloh, G., Numminen, J., Jousmaki, V., & Hari, R. (2000). Speaking modifies voice-evoked activity in the human auditory cortex. *Human Brain Mapping, 9*, 183–191.

Dayalu, V. N., Saltuklaroglu, T., Kalinowski, J., Stuart, A., & Rastatter, M. P. (2001). Producing the vowel /a/ prior to speaking inhibits stuttering in adults in the English language. *Neuroscience Letters, 22*, 111–115.

Dewar, A., Dewar, A. D., Austin, W. T. S., & Brash, H. M. (1979). The long-term use of an automatically triggered auditory feedback masking device in the treatment of stammering. *British Journal of Disorders of Communication, 14*, 219–229.

Fishman, H. C. (1937). A study of the efficacy of negative practice as a corrective for stammering. *Journal of Speech Disorders, 2*, 67–72.

Franken, M. C., Boves, L., Peters, H. F. M., & Webster, R. (1992). Perceptual evaluation of the speech before and after fluency shaping therapy. *Journal of Fluency Disorders, 17*, 223–242.

Glover, H., Kalinowski, J., Rastatter, M., & Stuart, A. (1996). Effect of instruction to sing on stuttering frequency at normal and fast rates. *Perceptual Motor Skills, 83*, 511–522.

Goldiamond, I. (1965). Stuttering and fluency as manipulatable operant response classes. In L. Krasner., & P. L. Ullmann (Eds.), *Research in behavior modification*. New York: Holt, Rinehart & Winston.

Gray, B. B., & Brutten, E. J. (1965). The relationship between anxiety, fatigue, and spontaneous recovery in stuttering. *Behavior Research and Therapy, 2*, 251–259.

Guntupalli, V. K., Kalinowski, J., Saltuklaroglu, T., & Nanjundeswaran, C. (2005). The effects of temporal modification of second speech signals on stuttering inhibition at two speech rates in adults. *Neuroscience Letters, 385*, 7–12.

Hargrave, S., Kalinowski, J., Stuart, A., Armson, J., & Jones, K. (1994). Stuttering reduction under frequency-altered feedback at two speech rates. *Journal of Speech and Hearing Research, 37*, 1313–1320.

Hari, R., Levanen, S., Raij, T. (2000). Timing of human cortical functions during cognition: Role of MEG. *Trends in Cognitive Sciences, 1*, 455–462.

Healey, E. C., & Howe, S. W. (1987). Speech shadowing characteristics of stutterers under diotic and dichotic conditions. *Journal of Communication Disorders, 20,* 493–506.

Healey, E. C., Mallard, A. R., & Adams, M. R. (1976). Factors contributing to the reduction of stuttering during singing. *Journal of Speech and Hearing Research, 19,* 475–480.

Howell, P. (1990). Changes in voice level caused by several forms of altered feedback in fluent speakers and stutterers. *Language and Speech, 33,* 325–338.

Howell, P., El-Yaniv, N., & Powell, D. J. (1987). Factors affecting fluency in stutterers. In H. F. M. Peters & W. Hulstijin (Eds.), *Speech motor dynamics in stuttering* (pp. 361–369). New York: Springer-Verlag.

Iacoboni, M, Molnar-Szakacs, I, Gallese, V., Buccino, G., Mazziotta, J. C., & Rizzolatti, G. (2005). Grasping the intentions of others with one's own mirror neuron system. *Public Library of Science (PLoS) Biology, 17,* 273–281.

Janssen, P., & Kraaimaat, F. (1980). Disfluency and anxiety in stuttering and non-stuttering adolescents. *Behavioral Analysis and Modification, 4,* 116–126.

Jayaram, M. (1983). Phonetic influences on stuttering in monolingual and bilingual stutterers. *Journal of Communication Disorders, 16,* 287–297.

Johnson, W., & Rosen, L. (1937). Studies in the psychology of stuttering: VII. Effect of certain changes in speech patterns upon the frequency of stuttering. *Journal of Speech Disorders, 2,* 105–109.

Kalinowski, J. (2003). Self-reported efficacy of an all-in-the-ear-canal prosthetic device to inhibit stuttering during one hundred hours of university teaching: A case study. *Disability and Rehabilitation, 25,* 107–111.

Kalinowski, J., Armson, J., Roland-Mieszkowski, M., Stuart, A., & Gracco, V. L. (1993). Effects of alterations in auditory feedback and speech rate on stuttering frequency. *Language and Speech, 36,* 1–16.

Kalinowski, J., Armson, J., & Stuart, A. (1995). Effect of normal and fast articulatory rates on stuttering frequency. *Journal of Fluency Disorders, 20,* 293–302.

Kalinowski, J., & Dayalu, V. N. (2002). A common element in the immediate inducement of effortless, natural-sounding, fluent speech in people who stutter: "The second speech signal." *Medical Hypotheses, 58,* 61–66.

Kalinowski, J., Dayalu, V. N., Stuart, A., Rastatter, M. P., & Rami, M. K. (2000). Stutter-free and stutter-filled speech signals and their role in stuttering amelioration for English speaking adults. *Neuroscience Letters, 293,* 115–118.

Kalinowski, J., Guntupalli, V., Stuart, A., & Saltuklaroglu, T. (2004). Self-reported efficacy of an ear-level prosthetic device that delivers altered auditory feedback for the management of stuttering. *International Journal of Rehabilitation Research, 27*, 167–170.

Kalinowski, J., Noble, S., Armson, J., & Stuart, A. (1994). Naturalness ratings of the pretreatment and post-treatment speech of adults with mild and severe stuttering. *American Journal of Speech Language Pathology, 3*, 61–66.

Kalinowski, J., & Saltuklaroglu, T. (2003a). Speaking with a mirror: Engagement of mirror neurons via choral speech and its derivatives induces stuttering inhibition. *Medical Hypotheses, 60*, 538–543.

Kalinowski, J., & Saltuklaroglu, T. (2003b). Choral speech: The amelioration of stuttering via imitation and the mirror neuronal system. *Neuroscience and Biobehavioral Reviews, 27*, 339–347.

Kalinowski, J., & Saltuklaroglu, T. (2004). The road to efficient and effective stuttering management: Information for physicians. *Current Medical Research and Opinion, 20*, 509–515.

Kalinowski, J., Saltuklaroglu, T., Dayalu, V., & Guntupalli, V. (2005). Is it possible for speech therapy to improve upon natural recovery rates in children who stutter. *International Journal of Language and Communication Disorders, 40*, 349–358.

Kalinowski, J., Saltuklaroglu, T., Guntupalli, V., & Stuart, A. (2004). Gestural recovery and the role of forward and reversed syllabic repetitions as stuttering inhibitors in adults. *Neuroscience Letters, 363*, 144–149.

Kalinowski, J., Stuart, A., Rastatter, M. P., Snyder, G., & Dayalu V. (2000). Inducement of fluent speech in persons who stutter via visual choral speech. *Neuroscience Letters, 281*, 198–200.

Kalinowski, J., Stuart, A., Sark, S., & Armson, J. (1996). Stuttering amelioration at various auditory feedback delays and speech rates. *European Journal of Disorders in Communication, 31*, 259–269.

Kalinowski, J., Stuart, A., Wamsley, L., & Rastatter, M.P. (1999). Effect of monitoring condition and altered auditory feedback on stuttering frequency. *Journal of Speech Language and Hearing Research, 42*, 1347–1354.

Kondas, O. (1967). The treatment of stammering in children by the shadow method. *Behavioral Research and Therapy, 5*, 325–329.

Kraamaat, F.L., Janssen, P., & van Dam-Boggen, R. (1991). Social anxiety and stuttering. *Perceptual Motor Skills, 72*, 766.

Kuhn, T. (1962). *The structure of scientific revolutions* (1st ed.). Chicago: University of Chicago Press.

Kuniszyk-Jozkowiak, W., Smolka, E., & Adamczyk, B. (1996). Effect of acoustical, visual, and tactile reverberation on speech fluency of stutterers. *Folia Phoniatrica et Logopedica, 48*, 193–200.

Kuniszyk-Jozkowiak, W., Smolka, E. & Adamczyk, B. (1997). Effect of acoustical, visual, and tactile echo on speech fluency of stutterers. *Folia Phoniatrica et Logopedica, 49,* 26–34.

MacLeod, J., Kalinowski, J., Stuart, A., & Armson, J. (1995). Effect of single and combined altered auditory feedback on stuttering frequency at two speech rates. *Journal of Communication Disorders, 28,* 217–228.

Mallard, A. R., & Kelly, J. S. (1982). The precision fluency shaping program: Replication and evaluation. *Journal of Fluency Disorders, 7,* 287–294.

Mallard, R. R., & Westbrook, J. B. (1985). Vowel duration in stutterers participating in precision fluency shaping. *Journal of Fluency Disorders, 10,* 221–228.

Maraist, J. A., & Hutton, C. (1957). Effects of auditory masking upon the speech of stutterers. *Journal of Speech and Hearing Disorders, 22,* 385–389.

Marslen-Wilson, W. D., & Tyler, L. K. (1981). Central process in speech understanding. *Philosophical Transactions of the Royal Society Ser. B, 259,* 297–313.

Marslen-Wilson, W. D., & Tyler, L. K. (1983). Reply to Cowart. *Cognition, 15,* 227–235.

Meissner, J. H. (1946). The relationship between voluntary non-fluency and stuttering. *Journal of Speech Disorders, 11,* 13–23.

Metz, D. E., Onufrak, J. A., & Ogburn, R. S. (1979). An acoustic analysis of stutterers' fluent speech prior to and at the termination of speech therapy. *Journal of Fluency Disorders, 4,* 249–254.

Metz, D. E., Samar, V. J., & Sacco, P. R. (1983). Acoustic analysis of stutterers' fluent speech before and after therapy. *Journal of Speech and Hearing Research, 26,* 531–536.

Murray, F. P. (1969). An investigation of variably induced white noise upon moments of stuttering. *Journal of Communication Disorders, 2,* 109–114.

Onufrak, J. A. (1980, November). *A follow-up analysis of stutterers' speech after successful speech therapy.* Paper presented at the annual convention of the American Speech-Language-Hearing Association, Detroit, MI.

Perkins, W. H. (1979). From psychoanalysis to discoordination. In H. H. Gregory (Ed.), *Controversies about stuttering therapy* (pp. 97-127). Baltimore: University of Park Press.

Perkins, W. H., Rudas, J., Johnson, L., & Bell, J. (1976). Stuttering: Discoordination of phonation with articulation and respiration. *Journal of Speech and Hearing Research, 19,* 509–522.

Peters, H. F. M., & Hulstijn, W. (1984). Stuttering and anxiety: The difference between stutterers and nonstutterers in verbal apprehension and physiologic arousal during the anticipation of speech and non-speech tasks. *Journal of Fluency Disorders, 9,* 67–84.

Ramig, P. R. (1984). Rate changes in the speech of stutterers after therapy. *Journal of Fluency Disorders, 9*, 285–294.

Reed, C. G., & Lingwall, J. B. (1976). Some relationships between punishment, stuttering, and galvanic skin responses. *Journal of Speech and Hearing Research, 19*, 197–205.

Reed, C. G., & Lingwall, J. B. (1980). Conditioned stimulus effects on stuttering and GSRs. *Journal of Speech and Hearing Research, 23*, 336–343.

Reid, L. D. (1946). Some facts about stuttering. *Journal of Speech Disorders, 11*, 3–12.

Remez, R. E., Rubin, P. E., Pisoni, D. B., & Carrell, T. D. (1981). Speech perception without traditional speech cues. *Science, 22*, 947–949.

Ritterman, S. I. & Reidenbach, J. W., Jr. (1975). Inter-digital variability in the palmer sweat indices of adult stutterers. *Journal of Fluency Disorders, 1*, 33–46.

Robb, M. P., Lybolt, J. T., & Price, H. A. (1985). Acoustic measures of stutterers speech following an intensive therapy program. *Journal of Fluency Disorders, 10*, 269–279.

Saltuklaroglu, T. (2004). *The role of gestural imitation in the inhibition of stuttering.* Unpublished doctoral dissertation, East Carolina University, Greenville.

Saltuklaroglu, T., Dayalu, V. N., Kalinowski, J., Stuart, A., & Rastatter, M. P. (2004). Say it with me: Stuttering inhibited. *Journal of Clinical and Experimental Neuropsychology, 26*, 161–168.

Saltuklaroglu, T., & Kalinowski, J. (2005). How effective is therapy for childhood stuttering? Dissecting and reinterpreting the evidence in the light of spontaneous recovery rates. *International Journal of Language and Communication Disorders, 40*, 359–374.

Saltuklaroglu, T., Kalinowski, J., Dayalu, V. N., Guntupalli, V., Stuart, A., & Rastatter, M. P. (2003). A temporal window for the central inhibition of stuttering via exogenous speech signals in adults. *Neuroscience Letters, 349*, 120–124.

Saltuklaroglu, T., Kalinowski, J., Dayalu, V. N., Stuart, A. & Rastatter, M. P. (2004). Voluntary stuttering suppresses true stuttering: A window on the speech perception-production link. *Perception and Psychophysics, 66*, 249–254.

Saltuklaroglu, T., Kalinowski, J., & Guntupalli, V. (2004). Towards a common neural substrate in the immediate and effective inhibition of stuttering. *International Journal of Neuroscience, 114*, 435–450.

Samar, V. J., Metz, D. E., & Sacco, P. R. (1986). Changes in aerodynamic characteristics associated with therapy. *Journal of Speech and Hearing Research, 29*, 106–113.

Shane, M. L. S. (1955). Effect on stuttering of alteration in auditory feedback. In W. Johnson (Ed.). *Stuttering in children and adults.* Minneapolis: University of Minnesota Press.

Shenker, R. C., & Finn, P. (1985). An evaluation of effects of supplemental "fluency" training during maintenance. *Journal of Fluency Disorders, 10,* 257–267.

Smolka, E., & Adamczyk, B. (1992). Influence of visual echo and visual reverberation on speech fluency of stutterers. *International Journal of Rehabilitation Research, 15,* 134–139.

Spehar, B, Tye-Murray, N, Sommers, B. (2004). Time-compressed visual speech and age: A first report. *Ear and Hearing, 25,* 565–572.

Starkweather, C.W. (1982). *Stuttering and laryngeal behavior: A review.* (ASHA Monographs 21) Rockville, MD: American Speech-Language-Hearing Association.

Story, R. S. (1990). *A pre- and post-therapy comparison of articulatory, laryngeal, and respiratory kinematics of stutterers' fluent speech.* Unpublished doctoral dissertation, University of Connecticut, Storrs.

Stuart, A., Kalinowski, J., Armson, J., Stenstrom, R., & Jones, K. (1996). Fluency effect of frequency alterations of plus/minus one-half and one-quarter octave shifts in auditory feedback of people who stutter. *Journal of Speech and Hearing Research, 39,* 396–401.

Stuart, A., Kalinowski, J., & Rastatter, M. P. (1997). Effects of monaural and binaural altered auditory feedback on stuttering frequency. *Journal of the Acoustical Society of America, 101,* 3806–3809.

Stuart, A., Kalinowski, J., Rastatter, M. P., & Lynch, K. (2002). Effects of delayed auditory feedback on normal speakers at normal and fast speech rates. *Journal of the Acoustical Society of America, 111,* 2237–2241.

Stuart, A., Kalinowski, J., Rastatter, M., Saltuklaroglu, T., & Dayalu, V. (2004). Investigations of the impact of altered auditory feedback in-the-ear devices on the speech of people who stutter: Initial fitting and 4-month follow-up. *International Journal of Language and Communication Disorders, 39,* 93–113.

Stuart, A., Kalinowski, J. Saltuklaroglu, T., & Guntupalli, V. K., (in press). Investigations of the impact of altered auditory feedback in-the-ear devices on the speech of people who stutter: One-year follow-up. *Disability and Rehabilitation.*

Stuart, A., Miller, R.K., Kalinowski, J., & Rastatter, M. P. (1997). The effect of speaking into a passive resonator on stuttering frequency. *Perceptual and Motor Skills, 84,* 1343–1346.

Stuart, A., Xia, S., Jiang, Y., Jiang, T., Kalinowski, J., Rastatter, M. P. (2003). Self-contained in-the-ear device to deliver altered auditory feedback: Applications for stuttering. *Annals of Biomedical Engineering, 31,* 233–237.

Studdert-Kennedy, M. (2000). Imitation and the emergence of segments. *Phonetica, 57,* 275–283.

Sutton, S., & Chase, R. A. (1961). White noise and stuttering. *Journal of Speech and Hearing Research, 4,* 72.

Van Riper, C. (1965). Clinical use of intermittent masking noise in stuttering therapy. *Asha, 7,* 381.

Van Riper, C. (1971). *Speech correction: Principles and methods* (5th ed.). Englewood Cliffs, NJ: Prentice-Hall.

Webster, R. L., & Dorman, M. F. (1970). Decrease in stuttering frequency as a function of continuous and contingent forms of auditory masking. *Journal of Speech and Hearing Research, 13,* 82–86.

Wingate, M. E. (1969). Sound and pattern in "artificial" fluency. *Journal of Speech and Hearing Research, 12,* 677–686.

Wingate, M. E. (1970). Effect on stuttering of changes in audition. *Journal of Speech and Hearing Research, 13,* 861–873.

Wingate, M. E. (1976). *Stuttering theory and treatment.* New York: Irvington Publishers, Inc.

Yairi, E. (1976). Effects of binaural and monaural noise on stuttering. *Journal of Auditory Research, 16,* 114–119.

Yairi, E., & Ambrose, N. G. (1999). Early childhood stuttering I.: Persistency and recovery rates. *Journal of Speech, Language and Hearing Research, 42,* 1097–1112.

Zebrowski, P. M. (1995).The topography of beginning stuttering. *Journal of Communication Disorders, 28*(2), 75–91.

Zimmerman, S., Kalinowski, J., Stuart, A., & Rastatter, M. (1997). Effect of altered auditory feedback on people who stutter during scripted telephone conversations. *Journal of Speech Language and Hearing Research, 40,* 1130–1134.

# 7

# Therapy

We have presented our views on stuttering inhibition, gestural redundancy, and mirror neurons in a theoretical framework supported by a great deal of behavioral evidence. Some may argue against our perspective, but we suspect that with continued research, especially in the area of brain imaging, our ideas may prevail. We are blessed to live in an era of accelerated scientific advancement that offers newfound hope for several medical ailments. It is likely that we are on the cusp of a number of scientific breakthroughs, in which stem cells, DNA, proteomics, genetic engineering, and the pharmaceutical industry will change lives in unforeseen ways. These advancements may make the changes from the 17th to the 20th century seem relatively pale in comparison. Scientists are now able to map the human genome, and identify functional correlates in brain physiology to the overt manifestations of stuttering, schizophrenic behaviors, depression, and a number of other experiential pathologies. In the very near future we may be able to fight off the ravages of diabetes, cancer, Parkinsonism, and other debilitating neurologic pathologies.

However, stuttering is a unique pathology in that Mother Nature still offers a most potent solution to its involuntary manifestations. Even though no cure is in immediate sight, children, adolescents, and adults who stutter can still have access to different renditions of this biological ameliorative mechanism that works its magic on the neural pathway and keep it clear for speech flow. That is, unlike schizophrenia and depression and most other chronic neurologic pathologies, stuttering needs only the simple presentations of second speech signals to induce dramatic decreases in its pathologic manifestations (Kalinowski & Dayalu, 2002; Kalinowski & Saltuklaroglu, 2003a, 2003b; Saltuklaroglu, Dayalu, & Kalinowski, 2002; Saltuklaroglu, Kalinowski, & Guntupalli, 2004). The therapy espoused in this book attempts to put nature's biological inhibitory mechanism to best use. With this orientation in mind, metaphorically speaking, speech-language pathologists may be able to treat stuttering "going with the flow of the river" and "paddling against it." Plainly speaking, Johnson and Van Riper gave us techniques, such as bouncing and pullouts, that are simply controlled variations of the initial mechanism of producing syllabic repetitions in order to self-shadow.

Until this point, we have attacked previous therapy orientations and attempted to supplant the ideas behind them with our own. We have been explaining "why" we choose this particular orientation. Now we must reveal "how" to use this orientation to yield efficient and effective therapy for people who stutter. Without learning how to clinically apply the arguments previously presented, this textbook is of little use to those who stutter besides reinforcing the point that they truly cannot be blamed when this involuntary pathologic condition continues to manifest beyond the realm of voluntary control. By the same token, if readers have skipped over the previous chapters to this one with hopes of obtaining our "recipe" for stuttering treatment in this final chapter, they may be disappointed, as we are not prescribing recipes, but rather guidelines based on the theoretical perspective presented in the previous chapters.

## Nobody Can Be Blamed

The theoretical framework that we have pieced together allows us to focus on inhibitory goals via biological imitation mechanisms that seem predisposed to effectively and efficiently ameliorate stuttering (Kalinowski & Saltuklaroglu, 2003a; Saltuklaroglu, Kalinowski, & Guntupalli, 2004; ). It is based on scientific evidence and the notion that as therapists, we are there to alleviate the suffering of those who stutter and facilitate the communication process. Therefore, before proceeding further, we need to clearly separate our orientation from most others on the bases of culpability, shame, and guilt. Over the years, we have had the opportunity to see hundreds of patients from all over the world successfully treated using methods or combinations of the methods outlined below and we generally expect positive results. However, if those we treat are unable to achieve the results they desire in terms of producing fluent, natural-sounding, and effortless speech, they simply cannot be blamed or made to feel any shame about their stuttering. Regardless of the eventuality of speech outcomes, ours is a therapy approach whereby people who stutter are not castigated or made to feel responsible for failures to control stuttering.

No matter how our approach turns out from the standpoint of those who "count" overt behaviors, we will not allow our patients to be "shamed" into feeling a sense of failure. We cannot allow people who stutter to believe that if they overtly stutter it is because they are not using techniques properly, as some therapies may have them believe. This notion seems quite false, as stuttering and the use of behavioral techniques are not mutually exclusive. There is no empirical evidence to indicate that behavioral techniques always produce forward-flowing speech. That idea was simply "made up" to support the use of the techniques. The person who stutters (especially adolescents and adults) bring enough shame into their therapeutic process and there is no need to add to the self-hating and shame by creating a sense of failure. Therapy in the past has often had a surreal-like quality whereby the patient became immediately responsible for controlling the involuntary disorder once he or she was taught the magical techniques. That is, before the behavioral techniques were imparted, stuttering was accepted as being involuntary, yet after learning behavioral techniques, stuttering somehow became an event that could be controlled. Patients were only given the "grace period" to stutter before they learned the specific technique meant to induce "correct" speech. After that, stuttering was not accepted and the patients were told to go and practice the technique repeatedly until they could execute it properly without stuttering.

Amazingly, droned-speech is called "fluent" and applauded as such, when evidence has shown that it is perceived as being more unnatural than stuttered pretherapeutic speech (Dayalu & Kalinowski, 2002; Kalinowski, Noble, Armson, & Stuart, 1994; Stuart & Kalinowski, 2004). We cannot maintain this ruse and keep putting people who stutter in the "Catch-22" position of weighing the consequences of droned speech versus stuttering. Society punishes the person who stutters enough and the therapeutic arena must promise a comfort zone where the patient can be honest and open about what helps and what does not without being made to feel guilty or shameful. These ideas go back to the commercial schools of the 19th century that guaranteed cures. We must shed these ideas and change this surreal quality to one of reality in which we accept the shortcomings of techniques and the nature of the disorder while attempting to instill relatively fluent speech.

At all times during the course of therapy, we feel that it is imperative to remember the involuntary nature of this pathology. For behaviorally oriented clinicians who tend to be nonstutterers, this is not always easy to remember. While we strive to make advances in reaching an often elusive goal, we must acknowledge that there will be setbacks, occasionally big ones, that cannot be helped and are just part of the stuttering syndrome. There should be no blame cast by the clinician and no shame felt by the patient when this happens. It is simply part of the complex nature of this deep-rooted pathology. No matter how well a particular method works with one person who stutters, it may fail to produce effective stuttering inhibition in others for any number of reasons. The neural blocks we deal with are involuntary (Fox et al., 1996; Saltuklaroglu, Kalinowski, & Guntupalli, 2004) and sometimes highly unpredictable and powerful. Sometimes, anything short of true auditory choral speech cannot sufficiently engage the mirror systems to free the neural pipeline for continued flow. Simply put, the involuntary block occasionally wins over the inhibitory mechanism. This should not be surprising considering the history of relapse we have observed in the past and how deeply cemented this disorder can become ingrained in a person's psyche (Craig & Hancock, 1995).

When the desired speech outcomes are not achieved using a particular method or combination of second speech signals, it may simply be an indicator that for the intensity and pattern of neural block manifestations in question, the second speech signal combination being used is not optimal and different signal permutations should be tested. Unlike other therapies that hold the patient responsible for failing to implement techniques that are thought to be tried and true, our approach seeks to remove this responsibility from the patient, along with the attendant shame and guilt that comes from the failure. Similarly, the clinician cannot be blamed. If clinicians make use of a full repertoire of functional second speech signal combinations and are still unable to achieve the desired speech product over the long term, then we must again acknowledge the power and complexity of this pathology. There is no magic pill and sometimes the tools we have at our disposal for functionally achieving fluent speech are just not powerful enough. Nobody benefits when blame is cast for the failure of a particular method. The negativity experienced by the patient may make it more difficult to seek help elsewhere, possibly creating a sense of "learned helplessness." Similarly, the negativity experienced by clinicians may deter them from working with people who stutter in the future. In fact, many school-based speech-language pathologists with whom we have spoken have claimed an aversion for treating people who stutter based on the very limited successes they have experienced. Therefore, our therapy will not blame patient, parents, or speech pathologists and there will be no curative statements, even if natural recovery occurs, as it may in some children. In that case, we will be pleased, but cannot take credit due to the difficulty teasing out any therapeutic effects from natural biological developments.

## The Big Picture

We focus on the use of second speech signals helping people who stutter produce speech that is as fluent, natural-sounding, and effortless as the speech of those who are normally fluent (Kalinowski & Saltuklaroglu, 2004; Saltuklaroglu, Kalinowski, &

Guntupalli, 2004). In other words, the goal is to inhibit stuttering and keep the speech pipeline open to the greatest extent possible, while making as few deviations as possible from normal speech production. If we can achieve this type of potent inhibition of the central stuttering block, then we will be able to suppress most overt and covert stuttering behaviors. Having said that, we must acknowledge that overt stuttering behaviors are often more easily suppressed than the covert behaviors. Anyone who stutters beyond childhood will probably always have some remnants of covert stuttering behaviors, no matter how successful any intervention is for removing the overt behaviors. When it comes to treating the stuttering syndrome, we must apply the adage, "Rome wasn't built in a day" and accept the fact that simply providing those who stutter with more fluent speech forms does not immediately remove the scarring from a lifetime of stuttering that many patients have already endured. It may take a great deal of time and continued success, even after providing means of potent stuttering inhibition, for people who stutter to overcome their covert fears and begin to shed at least a layer or two of the psychologic scar tissue.

At the same time, the main impetus for our inhibitory orientation and this textbook was that previous therapy for those who stutter has essentially been relatively ineffective and inefficient. As a patient, the author (JK) can remember quite vividly trying to please all of his 11 graduate student clinicians at the University of Connecticut, one for every semester of his bachelor's degree. Inside his head was the notion that fluency was the goal and it could be achieved via droning during reading tasks and the use of covert strategies of substitution, circumlocution, and avoidance to hide what stuttering could not be inhibited. He could be relatively fluent for five minutes of monologue and conversation while attempting to "please the clinician at all costs," but now realizes that this approach is conducive to the use of covert avoidance strategies, simply to maintain the façade of fluency. The author called this stage of therapy the "perfume" stage, during which he went to therapy because it was the first time an attractive woman listened to him with an empathetic attitude about his stuttering. Attempting to please the clinician and feelings of transference are not uncommon in any clinical relationship and the author (JK) experienced this first-hand during his therapies. We now caution others not to mistake feelings of transference for speech improvements. Nonetheless, the therapy helped. Though his fluency levels continued to fluctuate, the author learned that he was able to inhibit stuttering behaviors to some extent by the use of some droning techniques. Seeing this new forward-flowing speech, he never wanted to return to previous levels of continued severe stuttering he endured prior to beginning his university studies.

From this experience, the author (JK) learned that gaining fluency is possible, but needs to be worth the price experientially. This is another difference that sets our approach apart from others. We are not a "fluency at all cost" approach. Accepting the idea that stuttering is an involuntary pathology means that we do not favor the use of inordinate means to suppress the expression of its symptoms via covert measures that simply improve the observer ratings yet can leave the person who stutters in a state of mental exhaustion. This is not a recovery program for addiction. We favor abandonment of the Puritan recovery program style of therapy, in favor of one that is more amenable to functionally suppress the symptoms of this chronic pathology using a variety of treatment modalities borne from experience and our understanding of neurologic underpinnings of the pathology. With this in mind, an examination of the experiential aspects of the disorder for those able to articulate those aspects of the disorder via self-report is essential.

Although long-term covert healing may take a substantial amount of time, it cannot happen without a catalytic spark for immediately providing substantial stuttering inhibition. When a person who stutters experiences a strong positive effect from a therapeutic method, he or she gains an immediate sense that something is different, that speech is easier to produce. This may approach the sense of invulnerability achieved via choral speech (Kalinowski & Saltuklaroglu, 2003a, 2003b; Kalinowski, Saltuklaroglu, Guntupalli, & Stuart, 2004). In our clinic, we have called this the experiential "click" of the brain activity switching from a stuttering to a fluent mode. With the right combination of second speech signals, the "click" can be achieved relatively quickly as the mirror system engages and stuttering is inhibited. It is similar to being "in the groove" when playing sports, but even better. People who stutter simply know when their speech cannot fail.

Successful therapy seems to reverse the course of the pathology to some extent, or move back the stuttering "set point."

In chapter 3 we provided our model of stuttering, showing how the possibility of central involuntary blocks can create the cascade of stuttering events, progressing from covert defenses to subperceptual stuttering, and to finally overt stuttering behaviors. The relatively small overt portion of the pathology is the part that simply "boils over" when covert strategies such as avoidances and substitutions fail, and the neural block erupts into observable repetitions and prolongations. Therefore, in order to reverse the course of the pathology, we start by attacking the observable overt symptoms. By continuing to inhibit the stuttering block, as evident by the observed fluent speech patterns, we can begin to chip away at the covert defense mechanisms, and in time remove some of their impact. However, if we keep in mind the 80:20 ratio that Sheehan suggested for covert to overt stuttering symptoms, we can begin to see that reverseal of the covert symtomatology can often be an uphill battle. The relationship between the pathologic manifestations and the therapeutic course can be observed in Figure 7–1.

Thus, when we see what we as clinicians are sometimes up against, we advocate against spending years using the same "recipe book" motoric techniques, in which improvements are incremental and relapse is anticipated for most (Bloodstein, 1995, p. 445–447; Craig & Calver, 1991; Craig & Hancock, 1995). Therapy should at least provide some relief as well as strategies that afford patients the luxury of never falling back to pretreatment levels. However, some interventions do not always meet this standard. Part of the problem is that though traditional therapy techniques make use of second speech signals, their potential for success is limited because they typically only employ the endogenous type and exclude potential synergistic sources of inhibition. As they try to make speech sound more natural, they attempt to wean people who stutter off the endogenous signal, which is often droned. Droning, not the "correction of the speech mechanism" can make almost anyone fluent via its strong vocalic energy the neural system seems to crave. When the droned quality is removed, patients are forced to rely on the carryover inhibition. Eventually, the carryover inhibition wears off and stuttering often returns, creating the therapy paradox that we previously discussed. In contrast, we advocate combining second speech signals to provide higher levels of stuttering

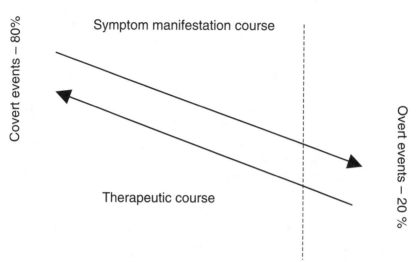

**Figure 7–1.** Graphic representation of the relationship between symptom manifestation and therapeutic course.

inhibition that can be supported while producing relatively natural-sounding speech. To do this, we have to acknowledge that everyone stutters differently, although certain general patterns exist. We attempt to provide some general guidelines on how some of the various stuttering patterns may best be treated using combinations of available second speech signals. However, before doing this, we discuss the functional advantages and disadvantages of the three second speech signals we have examined.

## Exogenous Signals

### Advantages

Second speech signals such as choral speech, continuously presented vowels, vowel loops, fluent speech, and stuttered speech exist independently from the speech of the person who stutters as they emanate from an outside source. This means that even if the person who stutters experiences an involuntary neural stuttering block that impedes the flow of speech, the second speech signal is always maintained, and the person who stutters can easily pick it up again. Thus, exogenous second speech signals are constant and unwavering, providing a continual source of gestural redundancy for the person who stutters to "grab onto" via the engagement of their mirror system (Kalinowski & Saltuklaroglu, 2003a, 2003b; Kalinowski, Saltuklaroglu, Guntupalli, & Stuart, 2004; Saltuklaroglu, Kalinowski, Dayalu, Guntupalli, Stuart, & Rastatter, 2003; Saltuklaroglu, Kalinowski, Dayalu, Stuart, & Rastatter, 2004).

In addition, when the source of gestural redundancy is external, there is often little need to make adjustments in speech production to achieve optimal levels of stuttering inhibition, with auditory choral speech being the prime example. The redundancy of gestural information in exogenous second speech signals allow for high levels of stuttering inhibition without the need to make endogenous changes. Therefore, relative to the other second speech signals in isolation, naturalness will probably be least compromised when using exogenous second speech signals.

## Disadvantages

Using an independent source to generate gestural redundancy can be both a blessing and a curse. The difficulty is finding a functional means continuously introducing an exogenous second speech signal that is portable, inconspicuous, and only engages when necessary, if it is to be worn in the "real world." If not, the problem then entails home practice with a conspicuous device to ensure carryover inhibition for "real-world" use. It is almost impossible to speak in unison with someone else constantly, even if we are not seeking to achieve linguistic synchrony between the two speakers. In addition, recreating the experimental effects of exogenous second speech signals in a functional manner may also be difficult. Devices that inconspicuously present vowels, vowel loops, or other speech forms as functional exogenous second speech signals have, to the best of our knowledge, not yet been developed, though they may be forthcoming.

# Endogenous-Exogenous Signals

## Advantages

Both delayed auditory feedback (DAF) and frequency altered feedback (FAF) have proven to be highly effective for inhibiting stuttering. Their primary advantage is that they allow the power of choral speech to be recreated without requiring an exclusively exogenous source. By perceiving one's own gestural output in a slightly delayed or spectrally shifted manner using digital signal processing, the brain seems to perceive the presence of an additional speaker. In most cases, users of DAF/FAF need only begin speaking in a normal and natural manner for this illusion to be created for immediate, on-line, and powerful stuttering inhibition. Although the potency of these effects has been known for some time, functional everyday use was previously limited by the bulky and conspicuous nature of older devices, as well as by those who believed that the effects were simply due to decreases in speech rate that sometimes coincide with longer delays (see chapter 6). With our new understanding of the effects of altered feedback (i.e., as permutations of choral speech) and the availability of inconspicuous, in-the-ear devices, we believe that AAF can be incorporated more readily into therapeutic protocols to provide a powerful source of ongoing gestural redundancy and stuttering inhibition. In addition, when someone can maintain an endogenous-exogenous second speech signal using his or her own speech, relatively few motoric manipulations generally are required. Hence, unlike behavioral therapies that call for gross deviations from normal speech production, stutter-free speech produced under altered feedback, is relatively natural-sounding (Stuart & Kalinowski, 2004; Stuart, Kalinowski, Rastatter, Saltuklaroglu, & Dayalu, 2004).

Another big advantage of altered feedback is that it is easily accessible and amenability to the effects can often be quickly tested. Besides the SpeechEasy™ device (www.speecheasy.com), a number of other altered feedback options exist. Casa Futura™ (www.casafuturatech.com) manufactures desktop and portable DAF/FAF devices that speech therapists can use in their practices (Figure 7–2).

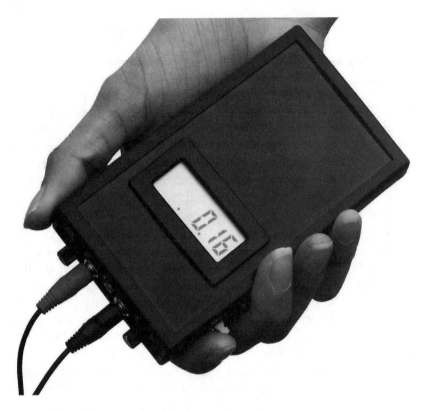

**Figure 7-2.** Casa Futura™ portable altered feedback device.

Companies such as Artefact LLC (www.artefactsoft.com) have created Windows™ based DAF/FAF software that can be downloaded onto personal computers and used by plugging in a headphone set and a microphone. They offer a free trial-period and a relatively inexpensive purchase price for the software. Other devices that may be used include the Facilitator by Kay Elemetrics (DAF), the Fluency Enhancer (DAF) by the National Stuttering Center, and the Digital Speech Aid (DAF and FAF) by Digital Recordings. Speech-language pathologists in possession of altered feedback devices or software can screen potential users quickly. Pre- and post-testing with and without altered feedback in reading, conversation, and natural settings can be done over a two- to three-hour period, taking inventory of overt stuttering decreases and the sense of improvement gained by the patient. Everyone who stutters knows when they feel that "click," often brought about by powerful emulations of choral speech. It should be noted, that initial screenings such as these do not always predict long-term success with altered feedback, but it can be an initial prognosticator. That is, a quick screen can help to quickly decide if AAF is a therapeutic option worth exploring in more depth. More details on thorough testing with altered feedback are provided later in this chapter.

Finally, altered feedback need not be used as a primary inhibitory modality. We generally find that altered feedback is best used constantly and in conjunction with other techniques; others suggest altered feedback be applied slightly differently. For example, the distributors of the Casa Futura™ suggest that the use of their larger devices can help with the transfer of endogenous fluency skills from the clinic to natural environments. In addition, Van Borsel, Reunes, and Van den Bergh (2003) conducted a study in which participants used the CasaFutura™ DAF models for an average of 260 minutes per week, over 3 months. At the completion of the study, participants' fluency levels without the use of DAF had improved by 50% in the five speaking conditions tested (automatic speech, conversation, picture description, reading aloud, and repeating). These authors also collected subjective experiential data regarding the participant's self-perceived fluency levels and overall emotional state. The data suggest that most participants felt both their fluency and emotional state improved as they participated in the experiment.

This synergistic and temporally flexible mechanism achieved via second speech signals is really the essence of ideas in this text. How we combine signals and to what extent they are used depends on each individual's needs, which are usually determined by type and severity of stuttering patterns, along with their propensity to inhibit stuttering in a manner that carries forward into ensuing utterances. The use of altered feedback is flexible in that it can be effectively used independently by some, combined continuously with motoric methods by others, and used only occasionally by those who prefer to use it for carryover inhibition and/or to support the continuous use of motor strategies.

## Disadvantages

Although many have found the power of DAF and FAF to be robust, there are some who stutter who receive less benefit from using such devices. If we examine the way in which endogenous-exogenous signals work, we can see why. Unlike exogenous second speech signals where gestural information is always present for stuttering inhibition, endogenous-exogenous signals require self-generation and cannot exist without the speech of the person trying to create them. That is, a person's own speech is necessary to create the altered feedback and drive the second speech signal (Guntupalli, Kalinowski, Saltuklaroglu, & Nanjundeswaran, 2005; Kalinowski, Saltuklaroglu, Guntupalli, & Stuart, 2004). Without the ability to initiate speech, no second speech signal is created. Therefore, for a person who has difficulty initiating speech or experiences long silent blocks during speech production, the use of altered feedback may not be immediately effective and may require the addition of endogenous techniques to generate a strong endogenous-exogenous signal. We have found that those who are highly amenable to the effects of altered feedback seem to almost anticipate the forthcoming inhibitory signal and have the ability to initiate speech relatively easily compared to others who constantly struggle to produce the first vowel.

We have discussed the power of the vowels in the inhibition of stuttering. This holds true for the use of DAF and FAF. Vocalic continuant sounds produced in our vocal tracts are the ones that create the salient gestural framework in endogenous-exogenous second speech signals via digital signal processing. Much like the use of exogenous speech signals, voiceless fricative provides little help (Kalinowski, Dayalu, Stuart, Rastatter, & Rami, 2000). In their continuous forms, they can sound more like a noisy hiss when perceived normally or through altered feedback. Therefore, those whose stuttering patterns include long prolongations of voiceless fricatives may have trouble initiating speech or maintaining a strong second speech signal under the effects of altered feedback. Though these types of overt stuttering behaviors may reduce the immediate effectiveness of altered feedback, we have been able to overcome these obstacles by using strategically placed endogenous vocalic supplementation (e.g., gentle onsets, vocalic gestural prolongations) to help compensate for the lack of vocalic feedback, as explained in more detail later.

Another complaint that we hear about the use of altered feedback devices does not pertain directly to their inhibitory effects. When worn outside the clinical environment, devices that produce altered feedback may also pick up background environmental noise. Therefore, in some noisy environments, it may be difficult to hear the endogenous-exogenous second speech signal coming through the device because of the background noise being picked up. For most users, this has been a relatively minor issue and the benefits of using altered feedback seem to far outweigh this noise issue. Measures are being taken to decrease the amount of background noise. Noise reduction algorithms in the software are continuing to improve and we anticipate that future generations of these devices will do more to combat this issue. However, considering the spectral overlap between speech and various sources of noise, we suspect that background noise may continue to be an irritation for some users, especially those who work in noise-filled environments.

## Endogenous Signals

### Advantages

Therapy techniques such as prolongation, gentle onsets, light articulatory contacts, continuous phonation, pseudostuttering, and so forth can all be powerful inhibitors of stuttering. They require no person speaking in unison or electronic device to alter perception. Under the right circumstances they can be implemented by anyone anywhere. In this way, they can be the most accessible forms of stuttering inhibitors. Table 7–1 provides information about a number of centers that train endogenous techniques.

Endogenous techniques can often be sufficiently powerful to not only release a neural block, but to inhibit or prevent the occurrence of subsequent blocks within a certain temporal window that varies with the severity of the block and the frequency, duration, and type of endogenous behaviors used.

**Table 7-1.** Table showing traditional therapy centers and the types of services offered

| Name of Therapeutic Protocol | Description of Intensive Program | Place and Person Who Offers It |
| --- | --- | --- |
| The Hollins Fluency System | An intensive 12-day therapy that emphasizes motor skill training and balanced attention to the cognitive and emotional aspects of stuttering. This program is substantially different from so-called "fluency-shaping" treatments. | Ronald Webster, Ph.D. Hollins Communications Research Institute 7851 Enon Dr. Roanoke, VA 24019 (540) 265-5650 admin@stuttering.org www.stuttering.org |
| Precision Fluency-Shaping Program | In this therapy program, the physical mechanisms used in the productions of speech are precisely and systematically retrained. It involves approximately 100–110 hours of therapy. | Ross Barrett, M.A., CCC-SLP Eastern VA Medical School 855 W. Brambleton Ave. Norfolk, VA 23510 (757) 446-5938 (757) 446-5911 PSFP@aol.com |
| Successful Stuttering Management Program | It is designed to assist the stutterer in learning to successfully manage and control the stuttering using "modification of stuttering symptoms approach." | Kim Krieger, M.S., CCC-SLP Workshop Director Eastern Washington University Dept. of Communication Disorders Cheney, WA 99004 (509) 359-2302 (509) 624-3271 kk505@aol.com www.ssmpmanual.com |
| Power Stuttering Center | SpeechEasy™ stuttering device and one-week intensive program with delayed auditory feedback (DAF) and rate control. | Mark Power, M.A., CCC-SLP 4010 Barranca Parkway, Suite 220 Irvine, CA 92604 (949) 552-5523 mpower@powerstuttering. com www.powerstuttering.com |

| Name of Therapeutic Protocol | Description of Intensive Program | Place and Person Who Offers It |
|---|---|---|
| The American Institute for Stuttering | This intensive treatment program is 100+ hours over a three- or four-week period which emphasizes teaching people how normal speech is produced by breaking it into parts and then practicing to rebuild the system into the coordinated movements that produce naturally fluent speech. | Catherine Otto Montgomery, M.S., CCC-SLP Executive Director 27 West 20th St, Ste 1203 New York, NY 10011 (877) 378-8883 toll-free ais@stutteringtreatment.org www.stutteringtreatment.org |
| The New England Fluency Program | The program integrates both stuttering modification and fluency-shaping strategies | Adriana Digrande, M.A., CCC-SLP Boston University Dept. of Communication Disorders 635 Commonwealth Avenue Boston, MA 02115 (781) 665-6623 digrande@bu.edu www.stutteringtherapy.org |
| Speech Foundation of Ontario Stuttering Centre | This program is based on the model of Precision Fluency Shaping and operates on the premise that stuttering is a speech motor behavior, which may be modified by learning a series of fluency facilitating techniques. The physical behaviors of speech, such as rate, respiration, articulation, and voicing are reconstructed through a systematic series of exercises | Robert Kroll 1210 Sheppard Ave. E, Suite 208 Toronto, Ontario M2K 1E5 (416) 323-3335 (416) 323-0516 (Fax) bob.kroll@utoronto.ca www.speechfoundation .org/SC.htm |

*(continues)*

**Table 7-1.** *(continued)*

| Name of Therapeutic Protocol | Description of Intensive Program | Place and Person Who Offers It |
| --- | --- | --- |
| Institute for Stuttering Treatment and Research (ISTAR) | Speech is modified through fluency skills relating to breathing, voice initiation, articulation, and speech rate. | Deborah Kully, M.S., CCC-SLP<br>3rd Floor, Aberhart Centre Two<br>8220-114 St.<br>Edmonton, Alberta T6G 2J3<br>(780) 492-2619<br>(780) 492-8457 (Fax)<br>www.istar.ualberta.ca |
| The Lidcombe Program (Australia) | It is a behavioral treatment program for young children who stutter. Parent (or caregiver) in the child's everyday environment administers the treatment program. It involves the parent commenting directly about the child's speech. | Mark Onslow<br>Australian Stuttering Research Centre<br>The University of Sydney<br>PO Box 1825<br>Lidcombe NSW 2141 Australia<br>61-2-9351-9061<br>www3.fhs.usyd.edu.au/ asrcwww/treatment/ lidcombe.htm |
| The Camperdown Program (Australia) | It is a treatment for stuttering in teenagers and adults. Prolonged speech to control stuttering is the basis of treatment. Camperdown program is a new way of teaching prolonged speech. The procedure does not involve pro-grammed instruction and is less time-consuming. | Australian Stuttering Research Centre<br>PO Box 170<br>Lidcombe NSW 1825, Australia<br>02 9351 9061<br>www3.fhs.usyd.edu.au/ asrcwww/treatment/ camperdown.htm |

These behaviors are not used to retrain the speech mechanism, but to engage the inhibiting mechanism of the neural system. To put this in perspective, the more vowel enhancing techniques such as prolongation or continuous phonation are used, the more flexible and wider the inhibitory window becomes afterward, even when the use of techniques is removed. That is, following intensive behavioral therapies, we have observed some inhibition lasting up to a month beyond the abandonment of techniques. The neural system seems to have assumed a state of extended inhibition. Many a client has gone home with this inhibitory fluency, giddy and free. It is as if making a substantial inhibitory "deposit" can pay remarkable dividends until it is time to deposit again. This acquired fluency is not from learning to speak again because the patient was most likely the most fluent on the first day when speaking at two seconds per syllable. It is from the extended period of droning, during which the central nervous system becomes almost impermeable to stuttering.

## Disadvantages

The price of using these techniques in isolation has been highlighted throughout this text. However, behavioral techniques, even with the problems highlighted, have been the "bread and butter" of stuttering therapy and for years were the only viable option available to those who stutter. Behavioral therapies have come with the promise of fluency via endogenous techniques, the Holy Grail of stuttering therapy. Most therapies even have a few videotapes of their most successful patients, espousing the virtues of therapy while in a state of fluent "Nirvana." Unfortunately, the odds seem to be against most people who stutter ever achieving such levels of fluency on a long-term basis. Thus, behavioral therapies used in isolation are probably not the answer for most people. If efficient and effective stuttering inhibition could be functionally accomplished over the long term by simple endogenous motoric changes, the stuttering problem would have been solved already.

## The Therapeutic Process

Although long-term decreases in severity may take time, the main initial focus is for all speech forms to become relatively fluent, natural-sounding, and effortless in all environments, as quickly as possible (Kalinowski & Dayalu, 2002). We believe that this is achieved via synergistic second signals and we cannot overstate this point. By using inhibitory methods, we try to continually lower the stuttering set point in all people who stutter, perhaps accelerating the recovery process in children who are so prone, and helping to alleviate the symptoms in everyone who stutters. Therapy from this orientation consists of speaking in multiple environments, increasing the complexity of the speech productions, and reducing the degree of clinical assistance. These are common therapeutic courses, but what makes our approach different is that we suggest using more than one set of tools to inhibit the stuttering. Rather than focusing on fluency, we focus on inhibition. Thus, we target the neural mechanism rather than the speech periphery. With effective inhibition of stuttering, the speech periphery takes care of itself. The general progression through stages of each parameter can be described as follows:

## Speaking Environment

We have made various references to the problems of assessing speech in the clinical environment and how measures of fluency, naturalness, and effort mean little in these environments. The goal should be to progress to more natural environments as quickly as possible. If we are using an altered feedback device, this includes a "road test" of the methods in use within the first clinical session. Unlike behavioral therapies that spend countless hours in the antiseptic therapeutic environment, where rapport is established, transference occurs, and "skills" are easy to use, we advocate the move to natural environments as quickly as possible. This helps to test the true efficacy of devices, allows people who stutter to gain the experiential sense of freedom in the outside world, and begins to immediately facilitate the transfer/maintenance phases of therapy.

Between doing basic exercises with the clinician and using the therapeutic methods in completely natural settings, the transfer of environments may include bringing friends or family into the clinical room for conversations as well as walking around the clinic, engaging in conversation with the clinician and others who may be present. The initial "road test" may include going to a shopping center and asking questions, talking to strangers, using the telephone, or ordering food in a restaurant. However, we do caution that during the initial road test, patients not be pushed into speaking situations in which they are not yet comfortable. Though many will be experiencing a true sense of freedom and be ready to "take on the world," others, especially the very severe cases, may require more time to adjust and may not feel as comfortable walking into situations they have consistently avoided for years. For these patients, we advocate that the road trip only entail speaking tasks that are within their comfort level, yet still allow the particular clinical method to be adequately experienced.

We also suggest that after the initial road test, once the method of treatment is established, patients continue to challenge themselves, seeking opportunities to test their speech in more difficult environments. Conquering fears of people, places, and situations will help to instill confidence and overcome the covert aspects of stuttering. Though it may take some time for patients to feel comfortable speaking to audiences, talking to people in authority, or calling strangers on the telephone, continued success in these types of situations can help long-term recovery. It is for this reason that we suggest extended trial periods when using altered feedback. Though patients may gain a sense of immediate improvement on the initial road test, they should be allowed to test the newfound fluency extensively on their own time, in situations that they perceive as being most representative of their speaking challenges. This will help determine how their speech will fare over the long term. Most patients we have seen have been provided with this opportunity and have been satisfied with the effects of the altered feedback for improving their speech (Kalinowski, Guntupalli, Stuart, & Saltuklaroglu, 2004).

## Complexity of Speech Productions

Many therapies begin by establishing skills at a syllable or word level. In the use of altered feedback, we use this initial level only to establish comfort with the particular method. We may ask a person to count, say the days of the week, or months of the year while listening to altered feedback. Except for very severe cases, most people are relatively comfortable in these sequential, automatic speaking tasks and this type of activity simply allows for some acclimatization to an altered auditory signal.

We try to move relatively quickly to sentence or paragraph reading tasks, which are the next level for two reasons. First, patients are not required to verbalize their own thoughts, a task that adds another level of complexity not needed during the initial therapeutic phase. Second, reading does not allow for substitution, avoidance, or circumlocution. Therefore, we can gain immediate knowledge of the impact of our methods, with reference to pretherapy measures during reading. In addition, we can begin to see the prevalent patterns of stuttering and gather ideas on how to incorporate various endogenous techniques to help supplement the altered feedback (to be discussed shortly). We use reading passages until we combine altered feedback with endogenous techniques so as to induce the levels of fluency, naturalness, effort, and comfort that the patient is seeking. Usually this will be an observable 70 to 80% reduction in overt stuttering, combined with the patient's account of the experiential sensation of ease of speech and naturalness. In addition, parents, family members, and friends who may be present may provide valid insights regarding the quality of the "new" speech during reading tasks before it is tested in more spontaneous monologue and conversational settings. Reading material can be used from various sources. We typically use junior-high level passages. Now random sentences can be generated using Web-based applications, which may also be useful. We suggest that clinicians have at their disposal a large amount of reading material and avoid repeated reading of the same material to prevent any potential adaptation effect.

Many AAF devices may yield positive results in your patients. The SpeechEasy™ DAF setting may be varied considerably depending on the needs of the client. Clinicians should experiment with a number of DAF settings, in about 30 ms increments (Kalinowski, Stuart, Saltuklaroglu, & Dayalu, 2003; Stuart, Kalinowski, Saltuklaroglu, & Dayalu, 2003). The Casa Futura™ device and Artefact software are also capable of producing these effects for this type of protocol. We have typically found that many patients perform well at the previously found "optimal" delays of 50 to 75 ms (Kalinowski & Stuart, 1996). However, some patients, especially those in the milder range, have reported not needing any significant delay, in which case the delay can be reduced. Conversely, some of the more severe cases, especially those with longer silent blocks, may benefit from longer delays to bridge the silences. These types of clients typically also benefit from the use of endogenous techniques, especially intermittent prolongations, which work well in combination with longer delay settings.

Following the basic sequence of the old GILCU program (Ryan & Van Kirk, 1974), monologue within the clinic generally precedes conversation. We ask the patients to maintain focus upon the altered speech signal while incorporating any endogenous techniques (i.e., vocalic highlighting) that may have proven useful. We ask patients to tell a story, usually recount a recent movie they have seen or book they have read. Providing patients with a series of monologue topics (e.g., jobs, education, family) can also be useful. We specifically ask patients to refrain from using covert strategies to avoid stuttering, as many patients are conditioned to avoid, substitute, and circumlocute, even when seeking help. Monologue allows patients the luxury of maintaining their own train of thought and producing continuous speech sequences. After monologues are successfully completed, we then progress to conversational tasks, which are the most natural in nature. They require the most stopping and starting of speech, which puts combinations of altered feedback devices and endogenous techniques to the best tests. Considering the difficulty with speech initiation that stutterers often encounter and the need to incorporate an endogenous technique such as a gentle onset, prolongation, or vocalic starter (e.g., "um," "ah," etc.), conversational speech often presents the most difficult task due to the constant turn-taking that requires much speech initiation by the person who stutters. If patients can adequately begin speech and initiate the altered feedback, they seem likely to succeed. If speech initiation continues to present difficulty, we suggest reverting back to reading tasks, using only sentences with adequate pause time in-between utterances. This allows patients an opportunity to practice initiating speech with strong vocalic gestures during the simpler task before once again resuming the more difficult conversational task.

## Level of Clinical Assistance

The final goal for patients is to be able to produce the speech they desire independently, without the help of cues from the clinician by using synergistic methods of inhibition. To best understand the role of the clinician in our therapy, we return to what our therapeutic intervention is trying to achieve. In all our patients, we are trying to replicate the effects of choral speech and engage the mirror system to the greatest level possible. Therefore, for any patient who has difficulty initiating or maintaining a second speech signal we can use true choral speech as our highest level of clinical assistance. Rather than using choral speech as a "parlor game," as other therapies did, we use it to show what the effects of altered feedback are trying to replicate. If patients realize that they can become fluent under true choral conditions, it can be easier to progress to the use of altered feedback, and then begin to add endogenous methods as necessary.

As we add endogenous techniques, the role of the clinician at first is to model appropriate use of the techniques and identify portions of utterances where the techniques can be most appropriately used. When the patient begins to incorporate the use of these techniques, the clinician may use a manual gesture to signal where an endogenous technique should be used. However, even this type of cueing is not generally used for long periods of time. Most patients begin to feel the synergistic effects of altered feedback with the endogenous techniques and begin to recognize how they can make use of the occasional vocalic prolongation, gentle onset, or syllabic repetition to enhance the effects of the altered feedback. At this point, the patient becomes his or her own second speech signal "manager" and the clinician's role is simply reduced to that of a passive monitor. This is also usually the point where the task is switched from reading to monologue and conversation as the patient becomes ready to take on more natural and challenging speaking situations.

## Combinations of Second Speech Signals

Providing those who stutter with combinations of second speech signals often provides the most potent inhibition of the central involuntary stuttering block. In the future, we expect to see therapeutic interventions that make use of all three forms of second speech signals discussed herein. However, currently the use of exogenous second signals for functional stuttering inhibition is limited. We hope to see this rectified in the future as the independence of exogenous second signals provides an immediate advantage as a framework for supporting fluent speech and may be of significant benefit to those who have difficulty initiating speech. The presence of an exogenous signal prior to speech may decrease the degree of endogenous motor adjustment currently necessary to begin speaking when stuttering is present.

Our most successful second speech signal combinations have been altered feedback with some motoric techniques for optimal mirror neuron engagement and stuttering inhibition. Our general approach to is let the altered feedback do as much of the work as possible (due to its effectiveness and efficiency) and add the motoric techniques as necessary to supplement its effects. For example, when someone who stutters adds some degree of prolongation to a vowel while under the effects of altered feedback, the inhibitory effects can be cumulative. The person is producing an endogenous inhibitor, receiving altered feedback, and receiving the endogenous inhibitor which is high in vocalic content through altered feedback, providing an extremely potent source of stuttering inhibition. Another advantage of such inter-mittent prolongations under altered feedback, is that they draw a person's attention to the auditory signal, allowing him to focus on what is making him fluent. This can be especially useful in children who sometimes need training to focus on the auditory signal. We recognize that stuttering is a chronic and involuntary pathology and often recommend the continued use of altered feedback as a source of inhibition rather than a crutch that one is "weaned off." However, as previously stated, others have used altered feedback only to train motoric techniques or as a means of "practicing" speech or generating some levels in inhi-bition that can carryover into real speaking events (Van Borsel et al., 2003).

Throughout this text we have stressed efficiency and effec-tiveness of therapy and this is where we put it to practice. We are trying to provide therapy that results in the best changes in the shortest amount of time. In many cases, the simple use of altered feedback provides users with at least an 80% decrease in overt stuttering, relatively effortless and natural-sounding speech, and an experiential sense of invulnerability to the disorder (Kalinow-ski & Saltuklaroglu, 2003a, 2003b). For everyone involved, this is usually considered highly efficient and effective management.

These types of patients are often happy with this level of fluency and require few motoric adjustments to their speech. We are not going to tell them they need to reach 99.9% fluency or the therapy has failed. An 80% reduction of an involuntary pathology with little time and effort expended is a marked improvement for many. However, these patients do need to be informed that if they choose to continue to work on their speech and seek higher levels of inhibition that it can be done and the price is relatively small. By intermittently making a few motoric changes, they are likely to be able to reach the highest levels of fluency that they desire. What these patients need to weigh in their own minds (not what we as therapists should decide for them), is whether the additional incremental gains are worth the added effort and the changes in production that may add traces of a therapeutic signature to their speech patterns. Our responsibility is not in forcing patients into making additional motoric changes, but rather to show them how to make them and what the results will be. As patients become more accustomed to using the altered feedback and their resulting speech patterns, they often learn to "play with the effects" and decide for themselves when to insert endogenous markers to supplement the effects. It may be that most of the time a person feels comfortable with an 80% improvement, and only requires the additional levels of inhibition at certain times. We are not the ones to judge. Everyone has his or her own speaking needs and we are simply there to provide the tools to achieve the desired results as quickly and effortlessly as possible.

Patients who immediately show an 80% or better improvement in both reading and conversational tasks under altered feedback can make our job relatively easy. However, a large group of patients also exist that do not obtain such pronounced immediate benefits from altered feedback. Typically, in our clinic, these patients have been adolescents or adults who are moderate to severe in severity and their stuttering is characterized by silent blocks, difficulty initiating, and prolongations of voiceless fricatives. These patients typically show about a 40% to 80% immediate decrease in observable stuttering behaviors using altered feedback. They typically report the experiential sense of feeling the added degree of fluency, sensing that speech is less of a struggle and their stuttering less severe. However, unlike those for whom the immediate benefit is more obvious, these patients are still looking for further improvements. It is this group with whom clinicians can usually provide the most assistance, examining their stuttering patterns for the most appropriate loci for inserting endogenous techniques to supplement the altered feedback. Clinical sessions with the patient focus upon weighing signal optimization using the combinations of second speech signals with the resultant speech naturalness (as reported by the patient, family, and friends) and ease of use.

We have also observed a handful of patients for whom the use of AAF is simply not an option. Sometimes, the patients or their families are simply against the use of prosthetic devices, possibly believing that stuttering can be overcome with the right amount of resolve and dedication to techniques. Others, for reasons sometimes unknown or the types of stuttering patterns they exhibit, simply do not benefit from altered feedback, even with continuous supplementation by endogenous techniques. That is, some are so severe that they have to "drone" at all times using altered feedback to derive any inhibitory effect over their stuttering. This is not how altered feedback was designed to work and the high effort and low quality of speech can contraindicate the use of altered feedback in these cases. What is unfortunate is that often times these patients will have already tried other means of intervention with little success and have found nothing that can provides the immediate help they are seeking to heighten their levels of fluency. Sometimes medications can help (see below). Other times, these patients may seek emotional help and means of coping with their stuttering, often from support groups such as the National Stuttering Association.

## The Use of Medications

Although we have yet to witness a person who stutters who does not become relatively fluent under auditory choral speech, there are some for whom creating functional combinations of second speech signals for potent stuttering inhibition is difficult. We have observed a few cases of very severe stuttering in which speech is disrupted by profound difficulty initiating, long silent blocks, or long prolongations of voiceless fricatives. The constant struggle to initiate and maintain strong vocalic signals can make the generation of endogenous-exogenous or endogenous second speech signals a very difficult task. Oftentimes, the patient that exhibits such stuttering patterns has tried every available recourse and has encountered little success in finding a source of inhibition. We have referred these patients to a psychiatrist nearby who is well-versed in the stuttering literature. The patients we referred claimed that the medications helped reduce some of the covert aspects of stuttering and allowed them to more easily implement some of the motoric techniques.

The idea of using medications to treat stuttering is not novel. Numerous medications have been tested with various results. Stuttering has been found to be associated with high dopamine levels and the use antipsychotic dopamine antagonists have been found to have some ameliorative effects for reducing stuttering frequency (Maguire, Riley, Franklin, Maguire, Nguyen, & Brojeni, 2004). In addition, stuttering has been found to be reduced in some cases by the use of selective serotonin reuptake inhibitors (Gordon, Cotelingam, Stager, Ludlow, Hamburger, & Rapoport, 1995), tricyclic antidepressants (Stager, Ludlow, Gordon, Cotelingam, & Rapoport, 1995), and anti-anxiety medications (Brady & Ali, 2000). While these medications appear to provide some relief from stuttering in some, their effects have not proven to be as powerful nor consistent as one might hope. There is always the issue of side effects and the potential risks that come with the use of specific medications. Another problem is that medications probably do not specifically attack the site of the problem as the site (if there is one) remains unknown. There is little doubt that these medications cause changes to brain physiology that somehow incur some inhibition of stuttering blocks, but it is not the relatively direct inhibition that we observe with the use of second speech signals. Currently evaluations of gamma amino butyric acid (GABA) receptor modulators are underway and perhaps this type of drug will offer new hope. Gerald Maguire, a psychiatrist, at the University of California, Irvine has spent years researching in this area and has suggested that in the future medications may be the key to efficiently managing the disorder.

# Motor Techniques Used with Altered Feedback

Everything that we have suggested so far, as well as the use of the motoric strategies as outlined below is an integration of therapies that could have been done in the past, even using the old DAF machine used by Perkins (Curlee & Perkins, 1973). However, we stress that our orientation is different. The goal is inhibition via the auditory system to the neural channel pipeline—not speech retraining. With this in mind, we suggest selectively tailoring the use of the motoric techniques outlined below to the needs and stuttering patterns of patients, whether they are implemented with or without the use of altered feedback.

## Intermittent Prolongation

The stretching or prolongation of the occasional vocalic gesture is one of the simplest means of inducing stuttering inhibition. For some patients, simply stretching the odd vowel is enough to induce high levels of fluency. For others, the synergistic combination of intermittent prolongation and altered feedback creates a powerful inhibitory force against the central block. Our notions of prolongation are considerably simpler than those held by behavioral regimes that dictate the duration of the prolonged sound based on a target speech rate. We suggest prolonging any word-initial continuant voiced sound, not just the classic vowels. Therefore, semivowels and even nasals can be prolonged as they are produced using voicing and then shaped in the vocal tract. With longer prolongations, come more inhibitory vocalic gestures. When using altered feedback, all these vocalic gestures resonate clearly through altered feedback and provide an enhanced synergistic second speech signal to keep the neural speech pipeline open. To people who stutter, the vocalic sounds are most important when used appropriately. Others can be relatively lightened (see light articultory contacts below) to reduce overall effort. As one can see, we clearly are quite obsessed with vocalic power. Behavioral regimes have always taken advantage of these inhibitory effects via prolongation or continuous phonation and the effects seem to be simply enhanced via the use of altered feedback. The inhibition often carries over, though the temporal window for this carryover seems to vary fairly considerably.

Instead of globally imposing droning across the entire speech production, the frequency and duration of intermittent prolongations during everyday speaking tasks is dictated by the needs of the user. Although we advocate droning at home for "inhibitory practice," we usually try to produce a speech pattern in which prolongations, whether used with or without the aid of altered feedback, are produced as needed to derive the desired inhibitory effects. However, in most people the extent they are needed is severely decreased in the presence of altered feedback.

The duration of the typical prolongation in our protocol is often proportional to the delay being used, as the amount of delay dictates when we will hear the target vocalic gesture. This is probably why in the past it was believed that droning was needed to induce fluency, as the delays used in the past were in excess of 200 ms, which caused most users to slow down their speech rate considerably (Costello-Ingham, 1993). Conversely, when using shorter delays (e.g., 60–100 ms), the duration of the prolongation can usually be much shorter, making the resultant speech pattern sound more natural than those induced via behavioral hierarchies (Stuart & Kalinowski, 2004).

The next question is where and when to insert the intermittent prolongations. Our inhibitory therapy operates on the notion that stuttering is more effectively and efficiently inhibited before a block occurs than during a block. Therefore, the idea of using intermittent prolongation can create added inhibition that provides the necessary carryover to overcome blocks before they occur (Dayalu et al., 2001; Saltuklaroglu, Kalinowski, Dayalu, Stuart, & Rastatter, 2004). Thus, any degree of added synergistic stuttering inhibition is like a deposit of "money in the bank" that can be spent at a later time but needs to be replenished before it runs out, for it is when the money in the bank is completely spent that we again become susceptible to stuttering.

Generally, the amount of vocalic prolongation that is added is derived weighing three factors: (1) levels of fluency under AAF, (2) comfort of the patient with his or her fluency level and the desire for added levels of inhibition, and (3) the type of stuttering pattern exhibited. The first two factors are obviously related. Some patients may only gain a 60% reduction in overt stuttering, but feel comfortable with that; others may improve by 80% but still want more. We must listen to our clients here and see how much additional effort they wish to expend to gain an added level of fluency. At the same time, we must recognize when adding too many prolonged gestures requires too much effort, is having little payoff, and is detracting too much from speech naturalness. The third factor is one where we have some general logical guidelines. Patients whose stuttering is generally characterized by syllabic repetitions or voiced prolongations often tend to require fewer intermittent prolongations as even their stuttered speech generally maintains enough continuous vocalic content to hold an endogenous-exogenous second speech signal. Some students have asked why people who exhibit involuntary prolongations may benefit from using controlled prolongations in any therapeutic modality. Recall that in chapter 6 we outlined the similarities of the involuntary behaviors and volitional compensations for stuttering, and the purpose is the same—the engagement of mirror neurons. Using AAF, the same holds true. Using a few short, volitionally produced and strategically placed voluntary prolongations, we can help derive additional sources of inhibition to combat the struggle-filled loss of control that comes with producing involuntary stuttered prolongations. In contrast, when we see stuttering patterns that are characterized by longer silences or prolonged voiceless fricatives, we usually expect the need for more endogenous vocalic prolongations to help generate enough carryover inhibition in the second speech signal to overcome the blocks responsible for generating these involuntary voiceless segments.

The next question is where to insert the prolonged sounds. We have used three strategies. The first is to systematically prolong the first syllable on "say" every fifth word. We select a passage, underline every fifth word, model the intermittent prolongation, and then ask the patient to try it. If the speech is fluent and stable, we may then ease off on the prolongation, perhaps only prolonging the first syllable in every sixth or seventh word. On the other hand if it is still unstable, and the person does not feel sufficiently fluent, we may ask him or her to try reading while prolonging the first syllable on every third or fourth word. We typically try not to use any more prolongation than on every third or fourth word for conversational speech as we may begin to see compromises to naturalness. Overall, this method works well for people who are less cognizant of their stuttering patterns and need some system to remember how to use prolongation. Oftentimes, we will recommend that children use some variation of this method as they may not be as tuned to their own stuttering patterns and may need some repeating source of supplementary inhibition across their speech productions. One variation of this method is using the function words as targets for prolongation. Small function words such as "in," "on," "and," "at," and so forth frequently appear, often produced fluently, and are short words with salient vocalic nuclei. These qualities make them prime candidates for selective targets or prolongation. Another advantage is that, being monosyllabic, they can often be prolonged with relatively little compromise to the natural prosody of speech.

Many adolescent and adults who stutter have an inventory of feared sounds. The presence of the sounds can provide another strategy for inserting a prolonged sound, especially if the difficult sounds include plosives (in which overt stuttering is often characterized by silent blocks) or voiceless fricatives. *We simply ask people to prolong the vocalic gesture immediately prior to the feared sound and build up sufficient inhibition of stuttering to carry over through the difficult sound.* One example can be found in introducing oneself. Often people who stutter have difficulty saying their own name. For the author (JK) an introduction such as "My name is Joe" may be typically characterized by overt stuttering on "Joe." However, with this knowledge and using altered feedback, he may produce "My name iiiiis Joe" using a prolongation on "is" and then fluently producing "Joe." We have seen many people who use altered feedback employ this prolongation strategy to help overcome sound and word fears. Providing a substantial inhibitory force before saying these words can help generate some invulnerability to the stuttering block. At first, this strategy may result in some unnaturalness, especially in severe stutterers who sometimes like to use an extended prolongation to generate the levels of inhibition necessary to overcome the difficult word. However, many find that the amount of prolongation required begins to diminish as the sound and word fears begin to abate and they are able to focus on the altered signal instead of waiting in fear for an upcoming stuttering block.

Often our patients use a combination of intermittent prolongation strategies as they begin to feel more comfortable with altered feedback. For example, they may begin by systematically exaggerating prolonged voiced segments, generating more inhibition than they need to overcome a potential block, yet allowing the temporal window of inhibition they created to safely take them further down the ensuing speech stream. Sometimes as they begin to realize this, they can switch to using prolongation only before feared sounds. As they continue to improve and feel more comfortable using the altered feedback, they may finally switch to using only a few prolonged vowels on function words to help maintain the signal and keep "money in the bank" for any potential block that may still be imminent.

## Gentle Onsets, Pseudostuttering, and Initiation Techniques

One of the flaws in typical behavioral protocols is that they emphasize global changes in speech production. Every syllable uttered is generally subject to motoric alterations. To us this is quite illogical. Speech sound mastery is learned early in life. People who stutter are not "brain-injured" and do not need to relearn the ability to speak. Also, most stuttering occurs at the beginning of phrases and sentences, so when inhibiting the neural block, it may be wise to focus on the initiation of the utterance. Therefore, one of our main therapeutic objectives is in allowing the person who stutters to initiate speech fluently. Mastery of this particular skill can often be a good prognosticator of fluency, as fluency can be self-perpetuating, especially in mild stutterers; providing an inhibitory technique that allows for fluent initiation can often result in entire utterances being fluently produced, especially when using altered feedback. We have used a number of methods to help with initiation.

Gentle onsets have been used in behavioral therapies for years as a means of fluently initiating without a laryngeal block (Webster, 1974, 1979). However, our gentle onsets differ from traditional gentle onsets. In a traditional gentle onset, the vocal folds are often brought together slowly and phonation begins at a low amplitude and increases gradually. In contrast, the main focus of our "gentle onset" is a rapid increase in vocal intensity to provide a strong dose of inhibitory vocalic gestures. Gentle onsets are most effective when the intended utterance begins with a vowel, semivowel or nasal gesture. When utterances begin with plosives or fricatives they can be more difficult to produce, as vocal tract constriction precedes phonation and there is ample opportunity for a block to occur. In fact, many people have reported abandoning the use of gentle onsets because of the difficulty in using them. In other words, they stutter when attempting to produce a gentle onset, perpetuating the notion that fluency-shaping techniques often fail when needed most. Nonetheless, for those who are able to master their use, gentle onsets can provide a means of efficiently inhibiting stuttering at the initiation of an utterance.

For those who favor a more Van Riperian approach, pseudo-stuttering can provide a powerful method of initiating speech fluently. It has been documented that producing voluntary syllabic repetitions prior to speaking can inhibit true stuttering by up to 80% on ensuing utterances (Fishman, 1937; Meisner 1946). The main problem with pseudostuttering is its conspicuous nature which detracts many users, especially the milder stutterers who have made a habit of hiding their stuttering. However, we suggest that for those who are not afraid to use it pseudostuttering can be effective. We have even had reports from patients who claim that silently or mentally pseudostuttering can help initiation. Though there is no documented evidence to support this, it seems a plausible notion considering that Ingham et al. (2000) found that simply thinking about stuttering could induce the same patterns of neural activation as true overt stuttering.

The last type of initiation method we have used is one that almost every fluent speaker also puts to use occasionally: the insertion of a short vocalic gesture prior to speaking such as an "um," "er," or "ah." It is not coincidental that fluent speakers use vocalic starters, most likely to prime their own speech mechanism for speech production. People who stutter can employ the same techniques. We proved that producing a vowel /a/ prior to speaking can inhibit stuttering by up to 30% prior to speaking (Dayalu, Saltuklaroglu, Kalinowski, Stuart, & Rastatter, 2001). Thus, combining this strategy with altered feedback can produce substantial levels of inhibition across utterances. The advantages of these starters is that they can sound as natural as normal speakers. However, they begin to sound conspicuous and unnatural when they are constantly employed or if they need to be exaggerated in order to produce the inhibition required.

Considering the proportion of stuttering that occurs on the initial syllable, choosing an initiation technique is an important clinical decision. Here again we are attempting to get the biggest "bang for the buck." That is, the method selected should have the most inhibitory power, sound as natural as possible, and, most importantly, should be a plausible target. If the starter cannot be produced without stuttering, then chances of stuttering on the remainder of the utterance also seem to increase as the system continues to seek a form of inhibition. For each patient, we recommend examining their stuttering pattern, experimenting with different types of initiation, and testing them in a variety of speech contexts and speaking situations.

## Light Articulatory Contacts

Typically we do not make the use of light articulatory contacts a strong focus in our therapy. It is doubtful that there is anything inherently inhibitory about hitting a point of vocal tract constriction lightly. However, for some severe stutterers who are prone to strong postural fixations, light contacts may be of some value. Though they cannot prevent the occurrence of a block, they may help prevent the system from cascading into the neural firestorm that it reaches during these postural fixations. In addition, hitting an articulatory configuration in the vocal tract lightly and quickly allows speakers to move more efficiently to the next vocalic segment where the sources of inhibition lie.

## Droning and Home Practice

Although we have made a point throughout this text about how unnatural droned speech can sound, there is no denying its inhibitory qualities. Given that the inhibited state seems to carry over or be maintained beyond its point of inception, droning can be used as a means of deriving an extended period of inhibition. As such, we advocate droning as an inhibitory technique, but we hope not one that is required for normal conversation.

Using AAF, the inhibitory powers of droning appear to be even stronger. Although extended droning may not be functional for conversational use, it makes an excellent warm-up or practice exercise and its inhibitory effects seem to be further enhanced when combined with altered feedback. We recommend users of altered feedback to warm up to the signal using long prolonged vocalic gestures. Spending up to 20 minutes in the morning or before an important speaking situation droning and using altered feedback can often provide high levels of stuttering inhibition that carry over, sometimes for a seemingly substantial amount of time beyond the time of the exercise. This can be similar to the warm-up exercises that behavioral therapies recommend, except that users are receiving an added source of inhibition when using altered feedback and are not "warming up" the speech periphery, but rather the central nervous system.

For severe stutterers who have difficulty initiating, or using prolongations, continuous phonation, or other additional sources of supplementary voiced gestures, we highly recommend some droning therapy with altered feedback. The derived inhibition is the "money in the bank" and can carry over, often facilitating speech with or without the use of an assistive device for an extended period of time. Again, thanks to the carryover inhibition that many experience, this droning often does not need to be done in front of anyone else, yet the benefits can carry forward into real-life speaking situations. The telephone device sold by Casa Futura™ and the computer software available on the Internet are highly conducive to this type of practice.

## A Note About Therapy for Children

Our therapy ideas are generally applicable to both children and adults. Both seem to receive the highest benefits and freedom from stuttering when they acquire multiple inhibitory sources. However, there is one slight difference in our orientation when treating children. We do not believe that we yet have the power to alter nature's intended recovery schedule. If we did, prevalence rates would have dropped, and that does not seem to be the case. When treating children who stutter, we also try to decrease their set point, thereby reducing their overt symptoms, and we hope, the attendant shame, embarrassment, and guilt. If the child in question is one of the lucky 80% who will recover, maybe we will accelerate the process. If not, we hope that we can provide the child with tools to continually inhibit stuttering and prevent the disorder from taking over his or her life. Even children as young as two or three years old can be tested with some form of altered feedback. If it is not with one of the devices listed above, it may be as simple as speaking into a hollow tube or a toy microphone. Even at this early age, providing this added inhibitory source may have substantial positive effects, even though altered feedback may not be extensively used. We often marvel at the ease with which fluency can be induced in many children, a phenomenon which is probably related to neural plasticity at that young age. When using any type of therapy in children, we try to achieve the highest level of inhibition in the simplest manner possible. If this includes using altered feedback, we simply encourage listening to the signal and using the odd prolongation. Fortunately for most incipient stutterers we have treated, that is generally enough to induce high levels of fluency.

Finally, we must stress again that when treating children, we remove any guilt or blame about stuttering from both parents and children. It is important to provide resources and support. We like to include information about the National Stuttering Association and show the videotape series on coping with childhood stuttering published by the Stuttering Foundation of America.

## Case Studies

The following are case studies of patients we have treated, providing examples of our therapeutic course.

### Patient P1

Patient P1 was 9 years old when we first met him. He was stuttering quite severely, with combinations of repetitions, prolongations, and even some silent blocking and postural fixations, although his silent blocks were generally short, rarely exceeding half a second in duration. He had been receiving speech therapy in the school system since he was 5 years old and reported some success when he remembered to use the skills he had been taught which consisted of prolonging vowels and repeating stuttered words. However, he also reported that using these endogenous methods by themselves was difficult to do in all situations and caused his friends to ask why he was speaking "funny."

P1 tested the SpeechEasy™ device and the effects were instantaneous. It is common to have this effect, especially for those who have had therapy before. The second speech signal often draws a person's attention to his own speech in the same manner that previous therapeutic techniques did. Nonetheless, this new altered form of speech passing through his neural pathways induced almost complete stuttering inhibition, to the amazement of himself, and his parents. Not only was P1 immediately fluent, but he also sounded natural and his new fluent speech was produced relatively effortlessly. His obvious elation showed that he had sensed the immediate transformation too. Not surprisingly, altered auditory feedback devices of this type, SpeechEasy™, Casa Futura™, and others tend to be successful in a number of people who are amenable to endogenous-exogenous second speech signals.

For this family it was a fairly easy decision to purchase an all-in-the-ear inconspicuous altered feedback device. P1 was monitored for over a year after acquiring his own device and with little wear for the test of time. Even after a year using the device, P1 was producing relatively fluent, natural, and effortless speech. Not surprisingly, after a brief period of carryover fluency, his stuttering returned when the device was removed, suggesting that the use of altered feedback is not curative in nature but the observed temporary plasticity may warrant further investigation. Considering P1's age and experience with the pathology, complete recovery from stuttering would be anomalous. However, in this case, the therapeutic protocol using altered feedback provided P1 with a simple, efficient means of effectively managing his stuttering over the long term. P1 reports continuing social and academic success. He also participates in team sports with a number of friends. His one complaint is that in some noisy environments, the amplified background noise makes it difficult to concentrate on the second speech signal coming through the device.

Patients such as P1 are examples who exhibit optimal effects from altered feedback. His stuttering was reduced instantly by more than 80% and he did not have to make any significant alterations to his manner of speaking. In other words, this was a case of the altered feedback providing almost all of the necessary gestural redundancy for stuttering inhibition. P1 had a number of factors working in his favor that contributed to such powerful effects. First, he had little difficulty self-generating strong vocalic sounds both at initiation and throughout his utterances. In other words, his overt stuttering patterns were not characterized by long silences and he was able to maintain the vowel-laden endogenous-exogenous second speech signal; nor did he have difficulty initiating speech. Second, as he was still relatively young, neural plasticity may have increased his susceptibility to the effects of altered feedback. Third, for a 9-year-old, P1 appeared to be acutely aware of the importance of listening to the second speech signal and how it affected his speech. Some people, especially children, seem to forget that they must continue to listen to the second speech signal in order to generate the benefit from the choral-like effects and must be reminded; this was not the case for this participant. Last, P1 had a supportive family that reminded him to use the device and to pay attention to the signal. They had a good understanding of how the device operated and did not hesitate to remind P1 of the benefits that he derived from using it.

## Patient P2

P2 is an example of an overtly mild stutterer to the point that the average listener may not be aware of her stuttering. However, the proverbial iceberg loomed beneath. She reported that she made constant use of covert avoidances and substitutions. She was able to read with little overt difficulty in the clinical setting, exhibiting only mild repetitions and short silent blocks. Overall, she demonstrated less than 2% stuttered syllables. However, she reported that she generally felt it was "difficult to speak," especially in traditionally problematic speaking situations such as using the telephone and speaking to an audience. There was an expression of constant concern and monitoring when speaking. This is quite typical behavior of those who are able to hide their stuttering behavior via the continued use of covert strategies. She also had received traditional behavioral therapy and reported that though it seemed to help her speech become more fluid, it had not provided her with the experiential sense of speech becoming easier. Thus, she continued to live with the fear of stuttering and reported only occasional use of fluency techniques.

When tested with an altered feedback device, it was difficult for us to tell the full impact. She seemed fluent, but her level of overt stuttering prior to using the device was so low that it was hard to tell how much of an impact the device was having. However, P2 took the device out on a "road test," where she tested her speech using the device in various real-life situations such as talking to strangers in the mall and calling strangers on the telephone to ask for information. When she returned she reported that her speech not only was fluent, but she felt considerably more confident when speaking. She reported that she did not have to switch words around (i.e., substitute), nor did she avoid any potentially difficult words. In other words, the use of this device not only smoothed over the relatively few overt stuttering behaviors, but also reduced the covert experiential aspects of stuttering, giving her the invulnerability that she had been seeking and had previously been unable to achieve elsewhere. This case highlights the need for obtaining feedback from patients regarding the experiential nature of stuttering. The relatively small decrease in overt measures did not tell the whole story and the full impact of the intervention could only be measured by the experiential sense of freedom from stuttering that the patient acquired.

These types of patients can be difficult to treat both behaviorally and with any assistive devices because they feel they are in a lose-lose situation. If they use techniques or conspicuous devices, they lose their ability to blend in with normally fluent speakers because of the conspicuous natures of therapeutic signature that mark the use of endogenous inhibitory techniques and devices that are visible to others. When prescribing measures for stuttering inhibition we need to acknowledge that people who stutter will generally only use a particular method if it is effective, efficient, and relatively inconspicuous. The idea is not to draw attention to oneself but to blend in with the fluent speakers.

## Patient P3

P3 was a 6-year-old child who was receiving therapy for stuttering in the school system. Due to parental concerns, he was referred to our clinic for additional therapy. P3 displayed typical incipient stuttering behaviors, namely, syllable repetitions at the beginning of words, especially when initiating an utterance. These behaviors were produced with little struggle and concern, although P3 was cognizant of his stuttering behaviors and was able to discuss them freely. He had a good sense of humor, and could be quite extroverted. Not surprisingly, his natural charm made him popular among the graduate student clinicians. His mother explained that P3 stuttered less frequently in the clinical setting than at home or school. Statements such as these are often typical of parents who bring their children for stuttering treatment and may have been what misled Wendell Johnson down the diagnosogenic path. Johnson may have observed children with little or no stuttering behaviors in the clinic, but the anxiety observed in the parents may have been enough to make the causal connection. Clinical environments simply provide a controlled and comfortable setting where stuttering behaviors are less likely to precipitate. Once a clinical environment becomes a "testing place," a Hawthorne effect can often be observed. Children and adults who stutter will stutter less simply by being in that environment and knowing what is expected. Therefore, we should listen to the parents when doing assessment. Mothers are often brilliant diagnosticians and we should listen to their assessments of their children's speech patterns, especially as many young children may still lack the necessary skills to articulate their own thoughts and feelings about their stuttering.

After a semester of therapy, P3 understood the rules of the therapy game. If he used his EasySpeech™ when the clinicians asked him to, he would receive stickers or another reward system being used that particular day. When he copied the clinicians' speech models or volitionally implemented the prolonged vowels, P3 was fluent. However, he was also fluent most of the time when he did not use any therapeutic controls. As he did not seem to feel any penalties from his mild form of stuttering, aside from the bribery with stickers and so forth, it was difficult to convince P3 to prolong vowels with any dependability in the clinic. His clinical fluency improved just by showing up to therapy, although his mother reported that use of the techniques did not carry over well to other environments, even though his family was supportive, continually provided "good speech models," and reminded him to use his easy speech.

Over two years of therapy at our clinic, P3's stuttering did not progress to more severe forms and he never started to show any adverse reactions to it. At the beginning of his therapy, we considered the possible use of altered feedback, as P3 responded well to it in the clinical setting. However, we did not take this route for a few reasons. First and foremost, his family was against the use of prosthetic devices for treating stuttering, which really stopped the issue being taken any further. Second, although we have successfully fit children as young as 8 years with all-in-the-ear devices, at 6, P3 may have been a little young and seemed to lack the maturity for using and handling these devices. Third, because of his mild, unchanging stuttering patterns, we suspected that he may be likely to recover. In the end, P3 received therapy under our supervision for two years. However, he did recover completely. Though spontaneous recovery usually does not take two years to go into effect, this seemed to be the case for P3. We doubt our therapy or the therapy he received in the school system had much to do with it. We also doubt that any other therapeutic intervention would have altered this natural course.

## Patient P4

P4 is 55-year-old gentleman who came to us seeking help after hearing about the effects of in-the-ear electronic fluency devices on "Good Morning America." At the time, he was unemployed, which he attributed at least in part to his severe stuttering. P4 had pronounced repetitions and long prolongations in excess of 2 to 3 seconds. In addition, P4 demonstrated a range of secondary behaviors including head jerking, nostril flaring, tongue protrusions, and strong facial grimacing that characterized his extreme struggle to produce speech. However, unlike many of the patients who come to us seeking help, P4 had no history of formal speech therapy, though it was obvious that stuttering had shaped his life dramatically. In fact, despite many attempts to contact him by telephone, all our initial contacts were via E-mail, due to P4's long-time aversion to using the telephone. It seemed clear to us from our interactions with P4 and his wife, that P4 felt a great deal of shame and embarrassment as a result of his severe stuttering.

On his initial visit to the ECU clinic, P4 tested an altered feedback device and was able to achieve about a 50% reduction in overt stuttering and a substantial decrease in overt struggle behaviors simply by placing the small device in his ear and listening to the resulting endogenous-exogenous second speech signal as he spoke. This was relatively impressive both to him and to us, but we saw the potential for further improvement. P4 knew his own patterns of stuttering very well. He had a clear inventory of feared sounds that were not going to be overcome simply by popping a device in his ear and listening to the robotic chipmunk speaking in near unison with him.

Even though P4 had no formal previous therapy training, he easily learned to use intermittent vocalic prolongations that were just long enough to highlight his own speech, creating short endogenous second speech signals and providing additional vocalic energy to the endogenous-exogenous second speech signals produced via the altered feedback. P4 learned to use these controlled prolongations on vocalic gestures produced prior to normally difficult sounds. With a little practice and a couple of visits to our clinic, he was able to use the added degree of stuttering inhibition to carry over into the difficult words and allow them to be produced fluently.

Like many people who stutter, P4 also had a tendency to stutter more frequently on content words than function words, especially on multisyllabic content words. We decided to take advantage of this and use short function words as the targets for intermittent prolongation. The advantage of words such as "and," "in," "on," "if," and so forth is that they are short, consisting of a single syllable, and like syllable repetitions, have a salient vocalic nucleus. Therefore, these function words are often produced fluently, and by prolonging their vocalic nucleus, we can often generate sufficient gestural redundancy so that the inhibition carries over for at least a few more words. Another advantage of choosing function words for intermittent prolongation is that they occur in almost every utterance so there is no shortage of prolongation targets that can be selectively chosen so as to maintain sufficient levels of speech naturalness.

After another visit to our clinic and a little more practice on his own, P4 became especially proficient at using intermittent prolongation on function words to help enhance the effects of the feedback device. Instead of waiting until a difficult word was imminent and prolonging a vowel immediately before the difficult word, P4 merely made a point of prolonging function words selectively throughout his utterances and allowing the synergistic inhibition to carry forward until it was time to prolong again. He learned to use the natural prosody of speech to select the function words that were going to be prolonged. Using this technique in conjunction with the altered feedback, relative to his prespeech levels, P4's levels of overt stuttering were decreased by about 80% in both reading and conversation. In addition, his speech was judged to be relatively natural sounding by naïve listeners, himself, and his wife. What is impressive to us is that this significant improvement was achieved in only three therapy sessions and two adjustments to his altered feedback settings.

The benefits that P4 had derived from this protocol were still strong after one year. On our last contact with P4, he had returned to college to further his education and had some interesting new vocational prospects in engineering. He also stated that he was now able to talk more freely and confidently, and did not feel the shame he had once felt about stuttering. He claimed that prior to using this protocol, all of this would have been impossible. We should also mention that perhaps with the exception of the author (JK), P4 reported wearing the altered feedback device probably more hours per day than anyone else we have treated, usually from the moment he awoke until immediately before sleeping—although he also mentioned occasionally falling asleep while wearing it.

## Patient P5

P5 is one of the most severe stutterers we have met. Before we met her, she had already received extensive behavioral therapy, both at the East Carolina Clinic and one of the popular intensive three-week clinics. Her stuttering was essentially characterized by silent blocking. It was not uncommon for her to have blocks in excess of 1 minute, during which she would assume an unnatural postural fixation. Neither was it uncommon for her to show 50% or greater overt stuttering frequency in both reading and conversational tasks. Needless to say, her overall speech output had been severely reduced and she was unable to complete even the most basic communication tasks without experiencing severe overt stuttering and the attendant shame and embarrassment. Stuttering had taken its toll on nearly every aspect of P5's life.

When we started working with her, all-in-the-ear fluency devices had not yet been released. P5 had simply been enrolled in our clinic every semester. Different graduate students had tried working with her using various combinations of gentle onsets and prolonged speech. The severity of her stuttering was such that P5 only reached the point of stringing together a few stutter-free utterances in the therapy room using extremely droned, unnatural speech patterns. To make matters more difficult, P5 never seemed to experience any carryover stuttering inhibition and her stuttering always regressed to its initial severity once the techniques were removed. It seemed as if we were all aware of this pattern, yet P5 continued to come to therapy, most likely because of the nurturing environment provided and her ability to develop a friendly rapport with her clinicians.

We suspected that altered feedback would help P5, as like almost everyone who stutters, she became completely fluent under choral speech. When ear level altered feedback devices were introduced, P5 was among the first to test one in our clinic. She achieved levels of fluency we had never before witnessed with her in any setting. She was able to read and maintain conversations with clinicians, friends, and family, while only experiencing minor disfluencies and speaking very naturally and effortlessly. For P5, this was a true breakthrough at the time. However, these levels of fluency were not to last.

The severity of her stuttering and the fact that she experienced long silent blocks soon surpassed the power of the altered feedback device for presenting second speech signals. When P5 could not initiate speech, which was very often in her case, no vocalic speech signal could be delivered to the device to create a second speech signal. Not surprisingly, the effects of the SpeechEasy™ when used in isolation soon lost a great deal of their potency and P5's frustration was obvious. However, we made it clear to her, that what was happening was not her fault and she should feel no shame about her stuttering. This was simply a case of the device alone not being sufficiently powerful to help her particular brand of stuttering. In conjunction to using the device, we began to focus on getting speech started with a strong, fluent vocalic signal and then using some intermittent vowel prolongations to assist the endogenous-exogenous second speech signal. The idea was to functionally combine second speech signals and provide the most potent forms of stuttering inhibition possible.

Thus, we continued to use the all-in-the-ear device as it continued to provide a source (though not an optimal one) of stuttering inhibition. We added the use of intermittent prolongations on easy words, especially when P5 could foresee a difficult word approaching. We also began to experiment with various methods of speech initiation. We tried gentle onsets and even the use of starter sounds such as "um" or "ah" to initiate a second speech signal and begin delivery of the altered feedback. P5 was able to use all the prescribed initiation techniques with varying amounts of success. The trouble was that her stuttering blocks would hit even when she was trying to initiate a simple motor plan to produce a fluent vocalic sound. In other words, her stuttering was so severe that it precluded the use of any initiation technique. She simply could not get started and generate enough of a speech signal to feed the inhibitory mechanism. We even tried using an electrolarynx as an additional endogenous-exogenous speech source, but the unnatural acoustic signal it delivered, combined with its conspicuous nature, did not make it an attractive option for P5.

Overall, our intervention with P5 did produce some long-term improvements in her speech, which we hope carried over into other areas of her life. When she was able to initiate fluently and use some intermittent prolongations to help maintain the acoustic vowel energy through the SpeechEasy™ device, her speech was considerably more fluent and relatively natural sounding. We recognize that, in this case, our therapeutic achievements regarding the speech end product were far from optimal. However, we believe from our interactions with P5 that our intervention had helped significantly more than others she had received. In addition, P5 was never made to feel any shame about her stuttering in our clinical environment. One of the reasons she kept returning to us for help, rather than the other venues she visited, was because we always made her aware that the resistance her stuttering showed to therapeutic intervention was not her fault. She simply had a severe case and could not be blamed for it.

Working with P5 also taught us a great deal about the advantages and limitations of altered feedback. These devices can help even the most severe stutterers when combined with appropriate motoric techniques. However, to stand alone as a means of delivering second speech signals for stuttering inhibition, improvements need to be made, which we hope will be incorporated in future generations of these devices. For someone like P5, devices that can provide exogenous second speech signals in addition to endogenous-exogenous signals may be of great benefit to help the process of fluent speech initiation. As P5 never failed to become fluent under auditory choral conditions, we are optimistic that in the future devices that better replicate this effect will provide her with relief from stuttering that she has most likely been seeking all her life.

## Patient JK

We must include the author (JK) as the final case study in this textbook. As co-inventor of the SpeechEasy™, he has used the FAF and DAF combination signals presented via an all-in-the-ear prosthetic device longer than anyone else who stutters. Private therapy began in elementary school because services were not provided at the parochial school he attended in Concord, Massachusetts. This therapy consisted of reading aloud, articulation type therapy, and some cognitive therapy. JK's stuttering could be rated as moderate at this time of his life. Public school system stuttering therapy began in junior high school and continued for six years. It generally focused on cognitive issues (e.g., looking at the positives rather than the negatives). However, focusing on the positives was no easy task in this new school system in which teasing JK about stuttering had become a class project for a few bullies. That was a dark period and ideas of a better tomorrow were too distant, abstract, and complex for an 11-year-old to grasp, especially when in seemingly unending turmoil. Nearly every utterance brought about struggle and facial grimacing for everyone to see, and soon sound and syllable fears grew unabated. Paradoxically, JK could be relatively fluent when using cognitive therapy (self-esteem therapy, more or less). After a year in his clinician's therapeutic environment, the severity of his stuttering diminished. JK was able to speak to his clinician for the 30-minute session without much of a problem. Because of her training, she often suggested a psychologic origin for the disorder.

High school came and the stuttering returned to its natural set point of moderate to severe. Sports and school took priority and the teasing decreased as most of the bullies found other projects. JK grew to 6' 4" and could see the light at the end of the tunnel in the classroom and in sports that his parents and speech pathologist assured him was there. Despite moderate-to-severe stuttering, high school was enjoyable as people had become more accepting of JK. But with the prospect of attending university and finding a career, more crises awaited.

Five years of stuttering therapy continued at university with 11 graduate clinicians. As stated before, the cycle of improvement and then relapse occurred every semester until JK wore out his welcome at the clinic in his last summer semester. JK's major at the time was business administration because it had no foreign language requirement (and for no other reason) he would not be required to speak in class. That is how people who stutter can think when picking areas of study and professions. JK was proud to say that in five years he never spoke in class. In one class a professor required students to introduce themselves and JK exited before the debacle. Strangely, he was fluent when he explained to his friends after class why he had left and stayed outside in the hallway. Other clients have also recounted traumatic experiences of this type in which the professor responded in a rude manner. With a marketing degree in hand, but no hopes of a job after graduation, JK enrolled in a fluency-shaping program in New York City. He felt like it was his last chance and began 17 days of droning, gentle onset, light articulator contacts, diaphragmatic breathing in the clinic and all over the city. Sure enough, after 17 days of droning JK was producing unnatural forward-flowing speech. By therapeutic standards he was more than a success, and displayed his skills on the Richard Simmons show and various other news segments. Sadly, JK's therapeutic gains were short-lived. Although he suffered the inevitable relapse, he was inspired.

With some struggle, he became a speech-language pathologist. Dealing with patients while stuttering, especially some of those with aphasia, was especially trying. That is why JK decided to become a professor and leave the patients alone, at least for a while. Although his stuttering was more accepted within the academic cocoon in which he lived his professional life, stuttering still permeated JK's life. Often lecturing was so exhausting that it took a nap after class to recover. The telephone was still avoided at all costs and his wife, children, or doctoral students usually made JK's phone calls. JK knew about the effects of altered feedback. His first experiences with it are described in the previous chapter and he became a staunch advocate for creating an all-in-the-ear altered feedback device. Although it took another 10 years for this idea to come to fruition, JK received the first all-in-the-ear device in April 2001. The change was immediate as JK's stuttering patterns, consisting primarily of voiced repetitions and audible prolongations, were highly amenable to the altered feedback effects. His speech did not become completely fluent, yet it was about 80% more fluent than previously. In addition, the severity of his remaining overt stuttering moments became a lot less severe. After the first couple of months JK experienced a "flush" of stuttering inhibition that was pure exhilaration for him. It was like coming out of darkness again. He started using the telephone and his first bill was in excess of $500.00. His students reported that they enjoyed his lectures more and JK reported feeling more at ease and speaking more freely while lecturing. In fact, everyone around him noted that JK became a much more fluent and confident speaker since beginning to use the altered feedback device.

By his own admission, he is now a mild stutterer most of the time, with fluctuating periods of moderate stuttering still creeping in on occasion. Over the last four and a half years, JK has actively participated in his improvements, making adjustments to the altered feedback settings and using a variety of endogenous techniques to supplement the altered feedback effects. JK has used intermittent prolongations and pseudostuttering, though he now favors the use of intermittent prolongations as he has developed the knack for inserting them relatively inconspicuously into his speech when he needs them, maintaining a relatively natural speech pattern. He also changes the settings on his altered feedback device every 6 months. Although the use of altered feedback is a well-known and powerful inhibitor of stuttering, it would not be surprising if there was some slight adaptation or degradation of the effects over time. Therefore, making occasional changes to the altered feedback setting is good practice, as it can help refocus one's attention to the signal and provide the brain with slightly different feedback to counteract any potential signal adaptation.

## Final Thoughts

The approach we have outlined may ruffle some feathers or raise some eyebrows, especially among the strict behaviorists in this field. However, we feel that this inhibitory approach was born of scientifically based theoretical knowledge and our past clinical experiences—both the successes and the failures. Though fluency remains the "Holy Grail" in stuttering, it seems to be achieved only temporarily via methods of inhibition. To continually focus upon being fluent is unrealistic and casts shadows of guilt, doubt, and shame over the therapeutic process. Although reports exist of stutterers who have been "cured" after the window for natural recovery closes, they are few and far between. In our years of experience, though we have seen people who cope with stuttering quite well, we have never met a person who is completely cured (and we suspect that sightings of such people may be similar to those of the Loch Ness Monster). Thus, the battle for continued long-term "fluency" may not be one that can be won. Perkins (2000) probably expressed this best in a National Stuttering Association newsletter. With his permission, we have reprinted his thoughts:

### Declaring War on Fluency

Who's to blame when your fluency therapy didn't free you from stuttering? I was the pioneer of the DAF rate control basis for fluency from 1964 to 1980; I labored under the illusion that if the slow, reasonably normal-sounding fluency we easily established could be maintained long enough, it should eventually become automatic. Learned skills, such as walking, start out being voluntarily controlled and gradually become automatic. Likewise, voluntarily controlled fluency should become automatic if practiced diligently enough and long enough. I thought it self-evident that fluency was the problem. That was the attraction of fluency therapy. This was the assumption that protected me from blame for almost two decades. It seemed obvious that if fluency were maintained long enough it would become natural, automatic speech and the problem would be solved. Meanwhile the objections mounted: I feel like a speech actor. I'm so busy being fluent. I can't think of what I'm talking about! Failure to maintain fluency was the clearest evidence of dissatisfaction as speakers gave up hope that this therapy would ever lead to natural speech free of stuttering.

### Therapy Failure and Blame

Not until I began listening seriously to what those who stutter were saying did I finally realize that they were not to blame for these failures of fluency therapy. I'm a slow learner. So it took nearly 20 years of fluency failures and escalating complaints for me to conclude, better late than never, that something was fundamentally wrong with the assumption that fluency is the problem. From the listener's experience, this assumption seems indisputable. But for the speaker, it misses the point completely; the speaker's experience is one of stuttered blockages that cannot be prevented.

Thus the blame lay in the professional failure to recognize that fluency is not the proper objective of therapy. Voluntarily controlled fluency could be helpful if it ever became automatic,

*BUT IT NEVER DID.* The reasons turned out to be why the speaker is helpless to prevent involuntary blockage. I discovered that the neural mechanisms of naturally fluent speech production couldn't be brought under voluntary control no matter how long you try. Expecting to speak naturally with voluntarily controlled fluency is like pasting feathers to your arms and expecting to fly. Fluency is simply a natural by-product of the speaking system functioning automatically. When I figured that out, the solution to stuttering fell into place. It explains why my colleagues and I have been to blame for fluency failures. For this reason I feel compelled to declare war on fluency. Voluntarily controlled fluency is the wrong scientific objective, to say nothing of the wrong treatment objective. Indeed, the very existence of self-help groups speaks to the failure of professional therapy to address the needs of those who stutter, which is not about making speech acceptable to listeners. It's about coping with the feelings that create stuttering and understanding how they offer a path to full recovery.

A great deal of help is available for those who stutter, but it is rarely in the form of completely fluent speech. As clinicians, let us provide those who stutter with a means to "inhibit" the pathology. At the same time, we must recognize that stuttering is an experiential disorder that is felt a great deal deeper beyond the struggle to produce speech (Guntupalli, Kalinowski, & Saltuklaroglu, in press). Aside from empowering people who stutter with inhibitory techniques, we can empower them with acceptance and coping skills to deal with the involuntary nature of the pathology. While we await the magic pill that permanently removes all traces of stuttering, we need to "chill out" in our expectations of fluent speech. Speech is a biological gift and we cannot expect to continually dissolve the neural hitches that present themselves in the speech pipelines of those who stutter. We can simply attempt to use biologically provided fluency mechanisms to the best extent possible and accept what we cannot control. By providing our patients with an understanding of the nature of the pathology and a realistic sense of what can be accomplished in terms of inhibiting stuttering without imparting upon them a sense of responsibility for failure, we are perhaps doing them the greatest service.

# References

Bloodstein, O. (1995). *A handbook on stuttering* (5th ed.). San Diego, CA: Singular Publishing Group.

Brady, J. P., & Ali, Z. (2000). Alprazolam, citalopram, and clomipramine for stuttering. *Journal of Clinical Psychopharmacology, 20,* 287.

Costello-Ingham, J. C. (1993). Current status of stuttering and behavior modification—I: Recent trends in the application of behavior modification in children and adults. *Journal of Fluency Disorders, 18,* 27–55.

Craig, A. R., & Calver, P. (1991). Following up on treated stutterers: Studies of perceptions of fluency and job status. *Journal of Speech and Hearing Research, 34,* 279–284.

Craig, A. R., & Hancock, K. (1995). Self-reported factors related to relapse following treatment for stuttering. *Australian Journal of Human Communication Disorders, 23,* 48–60.

Curlee, R. F., & Perkins, W. H. (1973). Effectiveness of a DAF conditioning program for adolescent and adult stutterers. *Behaviour Research and Therapy, 11,* 395–401.

Dayalu, V. N., & Kalinowski, J. (2002). Pseudofluency in adults who stutter: The illusory outcome of therapy. *Perceptual and Motor Skills, 94,* 87–96.

Dayalu, V. N., Saltuklaroglu, T., Kalinowski, J., Stuart, A., & Rastatter, M. P. (2001). Producing the vowel /a/ prior to speaking inhibits stuttering in adults in the English language. *Neuroscience Letters, 306,* 111–115.

Fishman, H. C. (1937). A study of the efficacy of negative practice as a corrective for stammering. *Journal of Speech Disorders, 2,* 67–72.

Fox, P. T., Ingham, R. J., Ingham, J. C., Hirsch, T. B., Downs, J. H., Martin, C., Jerabek, P., Glass, T., & Lancaster, J. L. (1996). A PET study of the neural systems of stuttering. *Nature, 382,* 158–161.

Gordon, C. T, Cotelingam, G. M., Stager, S., Ludlow, C. L., Hamburger, S. D., & Rapoport, J. L. (1995). A double-blind comparison of clomipramine and desipramine in the treatment of developmental stuttering. *The Journal of Clinical Psychiatry, 56,* 238–242.

Guntupalli, V. K., Kalinowski, J., & Saltuklaroglu, T. (in press). The need for self-report data in the assessment of stuttering therapy efficacy: Repetitions and prolongations of speech ≠ the stuttering syndrome. *International Journal of Language and Communication Disorders.*

Guntupalli, V. K., Kalinowski, J., Saltuklaroglu, T., & Nanjundeswaran, C. (2005). The effects of temporal modification of second speech signals on stuttering inhibition at two speech rates. *Neuroscience Letters, 385,* 7–12.

Ingham, R. J., Fox, P.T., Costello-Ingham, J., & Zamarripa, F. (2000). Is overt stuttered speech a prerequisite for the neural activations associated with chronic developmental stuttering? *Brain and Language, 75,* 163–194.

Kalinowski, J., & Dayalu, V. N. (2002). A common element in the immediate inducement of effortless, natural-sounding, fluent speech in people who stutter: "The second speech signal." *Medical Hypotheses, 58,* 61–66.

Kalinowski, J., Dayalu, V. N., Stuart, A., Rastatter, M. P., & Rami, M. K. (2000). Stutter-free and stutter-filled speech signals and their role in stuttering amelioration for English speaking adults. *Neuroscience Letters, 293*(2),115–118.

Kalinowski, J., Guntupalli, V. K., Stuart, A., & Saltuklaroglu, T. (2004). Self-reported efficacy of an ear-level prosthetic device that delivers altered auditory feedback for the management of stuttering. *International Journal of Rehabilitation Research, 27,* 167–170.

Kalinowski, J., Noble, S., Armson, J., & Stuart, A. (1994). Naturalness ratings of the pretreatment and post-treatment speech of adults with mild and severe stuttering. *American Journal of Speech Language Pathology, 3,* 61–66.

Kalinowski, J., & Saltuklaroglu, T. (2003a). Speaking with a mirror: Engagement of mirror neurons via choral speech and its derivatives induces stuttering inhibition. *Medical Hypotheses, 60,* 538–543.

Kalinowski, J., & Saltuklaroglu, T. (2003b). Choral speech: The amelioration of stuttering via imitation and the mirror neuronal system. *Neuroscience & Biobehavioral Reviews, 27,* 339–347.

Kalinowski, J., & Saltuklaroglu, T. (2004). The road to efficient and effective stuttering management: Information for physicians. *Current Medical Research and Opinion, 20,* 509–515.

Kalinowski, J., Saltuklaroglu, T., Guntupalli, V. K., & Stuart, A. (2004). Gestural recovery and the role of forward and reversed syllabic repetitions as stuttering inhibitors in adults. *Neuroscience Letters, 363,* 144–149.

Kalinowski, J., & Stuart, A. (1996). Stuttering amelioration at various auditory feedback delays and speech rates. *European Journal of Disorders of Communication, 31,* 259–269.

Kalinowski, J., Stuart, A., Saltuklaroglu, T., & Dayalu, V. (2003). *SpeechEasy™ hardware, software installation, and treatment protocol manual, Version 3.0.* Greenville, NC: East Carolina University.

Maguire, G. A., Riley, G. D., Franklin, D. L., Maguire, M. E., Nguyen, C. T., & Brojeni, P. H. (2004). Olanzapine in the treatment of developmental stuttering: A double-blind, placebo-controlled trial. *Annals of Clinical Psychiatry, 16,* 63–67.

Meisner, J. H. (1946). Relation between voluntary non-fluency and the frequency of stuttering in oral reading. *Journal of Speech Disorders, 11,* 13–18.

Perkins, W. (2000). Declaring war on fluency. *National Stuttering Association Newsletter.* New York: National Stuttering Association.

Ryan, B. P., & Van Kirk, B. (1974). The establishment, transfer, and maintenance of fluent speech in 50 stutterers using delayed auditory feedback and operant procedures. *Journal of Speech and Hearing Disorders, 39,* 3–10.

Saltuklaroglu, T., Dayalu, V. N., & Kalinowski, J. (2002). Reduction of stuttering: The dual inhibition hypothesis. *Medical Hypotheses, 58,* 67–71.

Saltuklaroglu, T., Kalinowski, J., Dayalu, V. N., Guntupalli, V. K., Stuart, A., & Rastatter, M. P. (2003). A temporal window for the central inhibition of stuttering via exogenous speech signals in adults. *Neuroscience Letters, 349,* 120–124.

Saltuklaroglu, T., Kalinowski, J., Dayalu, V. N., Stuart, A., & Rastatter, M. P. (2004). Voluntary stuttering suppresses true stuttering: A window on the speech perception-production link. *Perception and Psychophysics, 66,* 249–254.

Saltuklaroglu, T., Kalinowski, J., & Guntupalli, V. K. (2004). Towards a common neural substrate in the immediate and effective inhibition of stuttering. *International Journal of Neuroscience, 114,* 435–450.

Stager, S. V., Ludlow, C. L., Gordon, C. T., Costello-Ingham, M., & Rapoport, J. L. (1995). Fluency changes in persons who stutter following a double-blind trial of clomipramine and desipramine. *Journal of Speech and Hearing Research, 38,* 516–525.

Stuart, A., & Kalinowski, J. (2004). The perception of speech naturalness of post-therapeutic and altered auditory feedback speech of adults with mild and severe stuttering. *Folia Phoniatrica et Logopaedica, 56,* 347–357.

Stuart, A., Kalinowski, J., Rastatter, M. P., Saltuklaroglu, T., & Dayalu, V. N. (2004). Investigations of the impact of altered auditory feedback in-the-ear devices on the speech of people who stutter: Initial fitting and 4-month follow-up. *International Journal of Language and Communication Disorders, 39,* 93–113.

Stuart, A., Kalinowski, J., Saltuklaroglu, T., & Dayalu, V. (2003). *SpeechEasy™ training workshop, Version 3.0.* Greenville, NC: East Carolina University.

Van Borsel, J., Reunes, G., & Van Den Bergh, N. (2003). Delayed auditory feedback in the treatment of stuttering: clients as consumers. *International Journal of Language and Communication Disorders, 38,* 119–129.

Webster, R. L. (1974). A behavioral analysis of stuttering: Treatment and theory. In K.S. Calhoun, H.E. Adams, & K.M.Mitchell (Eds.), *Innovative treatment methods in psychopathology*. New York: Wiley.

Webster, R. L., (1979). Empirical considerations regarding stuttering therapy. In H. H. Gregory (Ed.), *Controversies about stuttering therapy*. Baltimore: University Park Press.

# Index